Mental Health Nursing

SIXTH EDITION

Linda M. Gorman, RN, MN, PMHCNS-BC, FPCN
Clinical Nurse Specialist/Nursing
Consultant
Private Practice
Oxnard, California

Robynn F. Anwar, MSN.Ed
Retired Nursing Professor of Camden
County College
Camden County College
Blackwood, New Jersey

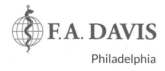

F.A. DAVIS

Philadelphia

F. A. Davis Company
1915 Arch Street
Philadelphia, PA 19103
www.fadavis.com

Copyright © 2022 by F. A. Davis Company

Printed in the United States of America

Last digit indicates print number: 10 9 8 7 6 5 4 3 2 1

Publisher, Nursing: Terri Wood Allen
Editor-in-Chief: Jean Rodenberger
Manager of Project and eProject Management: Catherine H. Carroll
Content Project Manager: Sean West
Illustration and Design Manager: Carolyn O'Brien

As new scientific information becomes available through basic and clinical research, recommended treatments and drug therapies undergo changes. The author(s) and publisher have done everything possible to make this book accurate, up to date, and in accord with accepted standards at the time of publication. The authors, editors, and publisher are not responsible for errors or omissions or for consequences from application of the book, and make no warranty, expressed or implied, in regard to the contents of the book. Any practice described in this book should be applied by the reader in accordance with professional standards of care used in regard to the unique circumstances that may apply in each situation. The reader is advised always to check product information (package inserts) for changes and new information regarding dose and contraindications before administering any drug. Caution is especially urged when using new or infrequently ordered drugs.

Library of Congress Cataloging-in-Publication Data

Names: Gorman, Linda M., author. | Anwar, Robynn F., author.
Title: Mental health nursing / Linda M. Gorman, Robin F. Anwar.
Other titles: Neeb's mental health nursing
Description: Sixth edition. | Philadelphia, PA : F. A. Davis, [2023] |
  Preceded by Neeb's mental health nursing / Linda M. Gorman, Robynn F.
  Anwar. Fifth edition. 2019. | Includes bibliographical references and
  index.
Identifiers: LCCN 2022016124 (print) | LCCN 2022016125 (ebook) | ISBN
  9781719645607 (paperback) | ISBN 9781719648325 (ebook)
Subjects: MESH: Mental Disorders—nursing | Psychiatric Nursing—methods |
  Licensed Practical Nurses | Nursing, Practical—methods
Classification: LCC RC440 (print) | LCC RC440 (ebook) | NLM WY 160 | DDC
  616.89/0231—dc23/eng/20220606
LC record available at https://lccn.loc.gov/2022016124
LC ebook record available at https://lccn.loc.gov/2022016125

To Corie, who saw me as an author many years ago.
~ *(LG)*

To my mother, Mayme Thomas, and Bessie Blount Griffin (Mom Bessie), I realize how much easier this journey would have been if you both were here. Wasim, my husband, and daughter, Andrea, I appreciate your belief in my abilities. To Aunt Shirley, Toni (sister), and Ted (brother), my family. Linda, thank you for being my mentor and friend. —Thank you.
~ *(RA)*

Ready for the Next Gen NCLEX®?

Davis Advantage can help!

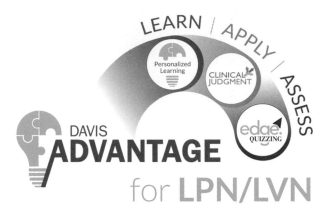

Davis Advantage for LPN/LVN

- Fundamentals
- Medical-Surgical
- Pharmacology
- Maternity & Pediatric
- Psychiatric Mental Health
- Leadership & Management
- Older Adults
- Life Span

Davis Advantage LPN/LVN combines student-friendly content in our ebooks with personalized learning, clinical judgment, and quizzing assignments that make it easy for you to...

- Make the connections to key topics.
- Improve your clinical judgment skills.
- Prepare for the Next Gen NCLEX®.

Davis Advantage Path to Success

LEARN	APPLY	ASSESS
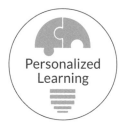	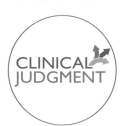	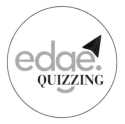
Personalized Learning	**Clinical Judgment**	**Edge Quizzing**
Dynamic activities & engaging videos help you learn the content and make the connections.	Case Studies that align with the new Next Gen NCLEX® & NCSBN Clinical Judgment Measurement Model let you apply your clinical skills.	Thousands of NCLEX-style questions, including brand-new Next Gen NCLEX® standalone questions, assess your understanding and reinforce key concepts.

Think like a nurse and succeed on the Next Gen NCLEX®

Visit **FADavis.com** to learn more or purchase access.

Acknowledgments

The staff of F.A. Davis including Terri Allen, Sean West, Gay Alcenius, and Marcia Kelley provided us with the support and of course attention to detail we needed to complete this project. They all worked closely with us to enhance the sixth edition.

—Linda Gorman
Robynn Anwar

Preface

The sixth edition of *Mental Health Nursing* is a psychiatric nursing text tailored specifically to the needs of the Licensed Practical Nurse/Licensed Vocational Nurse (LPN/LVN) student. We understand that many students at this level of preparation do not have the opportunity for clinical experience in a psychiatric setting, but they will encounter patients with mental health issues in their rotations and throughout their careers. Students will encounter patients and their families with psychiatric diagnoses as well as a variety of psychosocial issues and behaviors that challenge them. This text provides the basic knowledge and skills to address many of these challenges, with an emphasis on communication.

The impact of psychiatric disorders continues to be a major concern in the United States. Depression, anxiety, eating disorders, and substance abuse continue to be major health problems. The care of those with serious mental illnesses presents many challenges for the courts, law enforcement, and throughout health care, especially around the growing homeless populations. How society responds to debilitating mental illness has been the subject of much debate. Clearly, the need for nurses to have education in caring for people with mental health issues is essential.

Our goal with this text is to provide basic information about mental health theories, personality development, coping and communication styles, psychiatric diagnoses, psychosocial reactions, and nursing actions, all as they pertain to the practice of the LPN/LVN. The emphasis throughout is on enhancing skills that students can utilize in any setting to recognize and assist those with psychosocial and psychiatric issues. Communication approaches are emphasized.

The sixth edition of *Mental Health Nursing* includes updated information with an emphasis on new pharmacologic therapies, expanded information on common mental health disorders, and safety issues. Concept maps are included in many chapters as well as evidenced-based practice content. This edition incorporates mental health issues created by the COVID 19 pandemic as well as addressing the mental health impact on societal changes.

Chapters 1 to 9 provide the basics of mental health nursing concepts, with an emphasis on communication. Chapters 10 to 22 are "clinical" chapters in that they cover specific diagnoses and/or populations. Many of the chapters include the following new or enhanced key features which make the book easy to use to gain important knowledge:

- *Good to Know* gives a "clinical pearl" that succinctly describes a key take-away from the chapter.
- *Critical Thinking Questions* are expanded and interspersed in the chapters to emphasize a concept and challenge the student to apply the concept just covered. Many of these include case-based scenarios.
- *Toolbox* provides additional resources for students who want more information.
- *Differential Diagnosis* has been added to give the student more information on diagnoses that can be related or confused with the primary one.
- *Pharmacology* content in Chapters 8 and 10 to 22 covers important current information about medications used for the specific population that will pertain to the LPN/LVN scope of practice. All pharmacology content has been reviewed by our pharmacy consultant
- *Clinical Activities* are suggestions for the student to utilize when caring for patients with a particular disorder.
- *Classroom Activities* include suggestions for projects or actions that students and faculty can use in the classroom to enhance learning.
- *Case Studies* are in-depth, with questions to help the student apply knowledge learned in the chapter.
- *Patient/Family Education* reviews important areas to incorporate in teaching
- *Safe and Effective Nursing Care* highlights key activities for the student to focus on ways to promote safety and improved patient outcomes.
- *Evidenced-Based Practice* is new to the sixth edition. Many chapters contain a section summarizing a recent study that supports nursing actions.
- *Multiple Choice Questions*—At least 10 questions are provided at the end of each chapter, with the answers on the page for easy reference, and the answers and rationales in Appendix A.

- *Sample Care Plans* are provided in the clinical chapters along with concept map care plans
- *Appendix E* matches common behaviors with nursing diagnoses.

For the instructor, this sixth edition provides access to revised and updated PowerPoint presentations, test bank questions, and other expanded features.

As with the fifth edition, we utilize the terminology from the fifth edition of the *Diagnostic and Statistical Manual for Mental Disorders* by the American Psychiatric Association that was published in 2013 as well as the Text Revision in 2022 which reflects the most current thinking in psychiatry. Current terminology for diagnoses is used throughout the book. It is essential for the LPN/LVN student to be exposed to the most current information as they interface with other health-care professionals in the course of student rotations.

As authors of the sixth edition of this text, we have sought to promote ways to impart more knowledge to the LPN/LVN student. This text provides students with concise yet comprehensive information that will meet the needs of students who are facing an ever more intricate health-care system which became more complex as a result of the pandemic. We, as practitioners and educators in the field of mental health, have seen the impact of mental health issues on our patients and society. We hope that the students who utilize this book will gain a new perspective that includes up-to-date knowledge as well as empathy for the suffering these disorders can cause. We hope this book will contribute to knowledgeable and compassionate LPNs/LVNs.

Linda Gorman
Robynn Anwar

 ## LPN/LVN CONNECTIONS

F.A. Davis is pleased to offer **LPN/LVN Connections**, a consistent and recognizable approach to design and content that will make it easier for students and instructors to use multiple F.A. Davis textbooks throughout the LPN/LVN curriculum.

We have increased continuity whenever possible, without erasing the authors' autonomy or changing legacy content that has been popular in past editions. This makes it easier for instructors and students to move through the textbooks and ancillary products while recognizing shared themes and featured content.

Textbook Design, Style, and Pedagogy
- All textbook chapters include:
  - Numbered Learning Outcomes
  - Key Terms listed on the chapter opener and boldfaced where first defined in the chapter
  - Chapter Concepts
  - Bulleted Key Points
  - Chapter References, located online
- A Reading Level Evaluation is performed during the manuscript development, to ensure readability
- A uniform, space-saving internal design features special heads and colors that are shared across titles for features with similar content, to increase recognition

- Consistent and current terminology and laboratory values across titles; the authors followed *Davis's Comprehensive Handbook of Laboratory & Diagnostic Tests with Nursing Implications* by Van Leeuwen and Bladh for all values

Standardized Student and Faculty Resources
- For Students:
  - Advantage online student resources are available for purchase and include animations, personalized learning, clinical judgment case studies and quizzing
- For Instructors:
  - eBook
  - NCLEX-style test bank
  - PowerPoint presentations
  - Digital image collection
  - Advantage online instructor resources are available with adoption of *Davis Advantage LPN/LVN*. Resources include the **Davis Advantage LPN/LVN Curriculum Plan**, which includes implementation recommendations and engaging teaching strategies for programs of different lengths, whether you teach traditionally or in a concept-based nursing program.

F.A. DAVIS LPN/LVN ADVISORY BOARD

Amy Szoka, PhD, RN
Chair, School of Nursing
Daytona State College
Daytona Beach, Florida

Patricia Taylor, MSN-Ed, RN
Practical Nursing Coordinator
Kapi'olani Community College, University of
    Hawaii
Honolulu, Hawaii

Donna M. Theodore MSN, MA, RN, LMHC
Nurse Administrator/ Director
Diman Regional Technical Institute School of
    Practical Nursing
Fall River, Massachusetts

Loretta Vobr, MS, RN
LPN Instructor
Northwest Technical College
Bemidji, Minnesota

Dorothy L. Withers, MSN, RN
LPN Program Director and Director of Education
Prism Career Institute
Cherry Hill, New Jersey

Consultant

Gay Alcenius, Pharm D, BCCCP
Clinical Specialist Critical Care
Henry Ford Allegiance Health
Jackson, Michigan

Reviewers

Joshua Branham, MSN, RN
Practical Nursing Instructor
Indian Capital Technology Center
Sallisaw, Oklahoma

Lisa Brisk, BSN, RN, CLI, EMT
Instructor
Nassau County Vocational Education and
    Extension Board Practical Nursing Program
Hicksville, New York

Theresa K. Cebulski-Field, MSN, RN
Instructor of Nursing
Central Carolina Community College, Louise
    Tuller School of Nursing, Harnett Health
    Science Center
Lillington, North Carolina

Victoria Haynes, DNP, APRN, FNP-C
Tenured Professor/Coordinator of Diversity
    and Cultural Competency
MidAmerica Nazarene University
Olathe, Kansas

Robin Hill, RN, MSN
Practical Nursing Assistant Professor
Hagerstown Community College
Hagerstown, Maryland

Christa Jones, BSN, RN
Instructor
Pulaski Technical College – University of Arizona
North Little Rock, Arizona

Amber Nowlin, MSN Ed, RN
Program Coordinator: The Practical Nursing
    School at Buckeye Hills Career Center
Buckeye Hills Career Center
Rio Grande, Ohio

Table of Contents

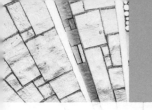

CHAPTER 1
History of Mental Health Nursing

KEY TERMS

American nurses association (ANA)
Asylum
Deinstitutionalization
Free-standing treatment centers
Mental health
National league for nursing (NLN)
Psychotropic

CHAPTER CONCEPTS

Evidence-based practice
Health promotion
Informatics
Professionalism

LEARNING OUTCOMES

1. Define *mental health*.
2. Identify the major trailblazers of mental health nursing.
3. Know the basic tenets or theories of the contributors to mental health nursing.
4. Define three types of treatment facilities.
5. Identify three breakthroughs that advanced mental health nursing.
6. Identify the major laws and the provisions of each that influenced mental health nursing.

 ## THE TRAILBLAZERS

Long before people knew what aerobic or anaerobic microorganisms were, nurses knew when to open or close the windows. Nurses helped women give birth and nursed the babies when mothers were unable to or when mothers died during or shortly after childbirth. The first flight attendants were nurses. For centuries, nurses have gone about the business of caring for people, but they have not always done so quietly. Who were the risk takers? Who advocated on behalf of the patient and the profession? In times when nursing was considered "women's work" and women were not politically active, the major trailblazers were female.

Florence Nightingale

Florence Nightingale (1820–1910) (FIG. 1.1) has been called the "founder" of nursing. Her story and her contributions are numerous enough to fill many

volumes. She was born of wealth and was highly educated. When she was very young, she realized she wanted to be a nurse, which did not please her parents. Conditions in hospitals were poor, and her parents wanted her to pursue a life as a wife, mother, and society woman.

Nightingale worked hard to educate herself in the art and science of nursing. Her mission to help the British soldiers in the Crimean War earned her respect around the world as a nurse and administrator. This was no easy task because many of the soldiers at the Barrack Hospital at Scutari resented her intelligence and did what they could to undermine her work.

The relationship between sanitary conditions and healing became known and accepted due to Nightingale's observations, record keeping, and diligence. Within 6 months of her arrival in Scutari, the mortality rate dropped from 42.7% to 2.2% (Donahue, 1985, p. 244). She insisted on proper lighting, diet,

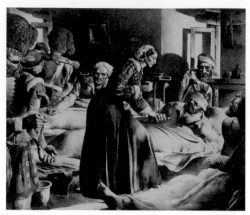

FIGURE 1.1 Florence Nightingale at work during the Crimean War.

cleanliness, and recreation. She understood that the mind and body work together and that cleanliness, the predecessor to today's sterile technique, is both a major barrier to infection and a gateway to healing. She carefully observed and documented changes in the conditions of the soldiers, which led to her adulation in popular culture and even poetry as "The Lady With the Lamp."

Nightingale was a crusader for the improvement of care and conditions in the military and civilian hospitals in Britain. Among her books are *Notes on Hospitals* (1859), which deals with sanitary techniques in medical facilities; *Notes on Nursing* (1859), which was the most respected nursing textbook of its day; and *Notes on Matters Affecting the Health, Efficiency and Hospital Administration of the British Army* (1857) (Donahue, 1985, p. 248).

The first formal nurses' training program, the Nightingale School for Nurses, opened in 1860. The goals of the school were to train nurses to work in hospitals, to work with people living in poverty, and to teach. Many of these nurses cared for people in their homes, an idea that is still gaining in popularity and professional opportunity for nurses.

Although Florence Nightingale's concerns were for all aspects of nursing, both physical and mental health, there were nurses whose focus was primarily on mental health. Mental health nurses provide care to patients who have emotional and mental health concerns, such as depression, anxiety, addiction, dementia, and personality disorders. The role of the nurse in mental health is to care for individuals, families, groups, and communities through counseling, patient/family education, and medication to promote mental and emotional health. Nightingale was so far

ahead of her time that many thought she was insane. One editorial even complained about Nightingale showing concern that nurses employed in asylums were not adequately trained. According to Smoyak (2001), Nightingale wrote that if medical treatments for men and women differed then so should training for nurses working with mentally ill patients and those working with physically ill patients.

Dorothea Dix

Dorothea Dix (1802–1887) (FIG. 1.2) was a schoolteacher, not a nurse. She believed that people did not need to live in suffering and that society had a responsibility to aid those less fortunate. Her primary focus was the care of prisoners and people with mental illnesses. She lobbied in the United States and Canada for the improvement of care standards for those with mental illness and even suggested that governments take an active role in providing persons with mental illness help with finances, food, shelter, and other areas of need. Dix learned that many criminals were also mentally ill, a theory that has been borne out in studies today. Because of the efforts of Dorothea Dix, 32 states developed **asylums** or "psychiatric hospitals." There is a monument to her on the Women's Heritage Trail in Boston that symbolizes her efforts.

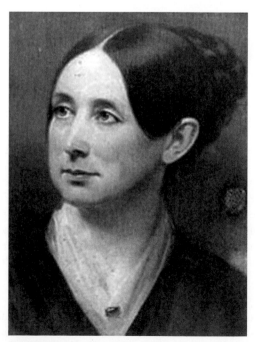

FIGURE 1.2 Dorothea Dix

Linda Richards

While Dorothea Dix sought political help for mental health care, a nurse named Linda Richards (1841–1930) (FIG. 1.3) worked to upgrade nursing education. She was one of the first five students enrolled in an American nursing program, and in 1882 she opened the Boston City Hospital Training School for Nurses to teach the specialty of caring for people with mental illness. By 1890, more than 30 asylums in the United States had developed schools for nurses. Linda Richards was among the first nurses to teach the planning of nursing care for patients. In cooperation with the **American Nurses Association** (ANA) and the **National League for Nursing** (NLN), she was instrumental in developing textbooks specifically for nurses that had stated objectives for outcomes of nursing education and patient care.

Harriet Bailey

The first textbook focusing on psychiatric nursing was written in 1920 by Harriet Bailey. It included guidelines for nurses who provided care for those with a mental illness. Bailey understood that nurses caring for these patients needed proper training. After she published her book, the NLN began requiring all student nurses to have a clinical rotation in a psychiatric setting (Videback, 2013).

Effie Jane Taylor

Euphemia (Effie) Jane Taylor (1874–1970) (FIG. 1.4) initiated the first psychiatric program of study for nurses in 1913. She is also well known for her development and implementation of patient-centered care, putting emphasis on the emotional and intellectual life of the patient. Effie Taylor received a diploma from Johns Hopkins School of Nursing and went on to become a nursing professor in psychiatry (American Association for the History of Nursing, 2017)

Mary Mahoney

Mary Mahoney (1845–1926) (FIG. 1.5) is considered to be America's first African American professional nurse. She contributed primarily to home health care and promoted the acceptance of African Americans in the field of nursing. During Mahoney's career, segregation made it impossible for black students to attend nursing school with white students. Instead, African American students attended separate schools such as Spelman Seminary (currently known as Spelman College) in Georgia and Tuskegee Institute in Alabama. An award in Mahoney's name is presented at the annual ANA convention to a person who has worked to promote equal opportunity for minorities in nursing.

Hildegard Peplau

Dr. Hildegard Peplau (1909–1999) (FIG. 1.6) was a nurse ahead of her time. She believed that nursing is multifaceted and that the nurse must educate

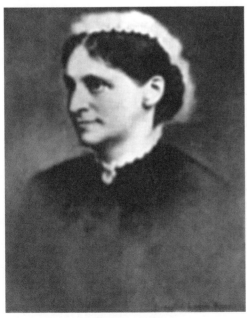

Linda Richards
America's First Trained Nurse
Born in Potsdam, 1841
FIGURE 1.3 Linda Richards

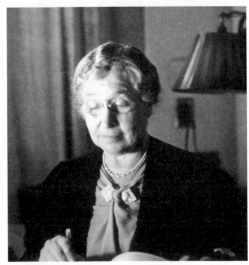

FIGURE 1.4 Effie Jane Taylor *(from Yale University, Harvey Cushing/John Hay Whitney Medical Library)*

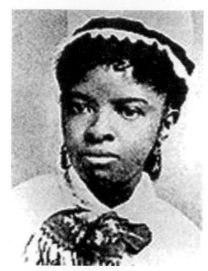

FIGURE 1.5 Mary Mahoney

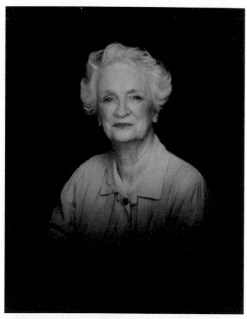

FIGURE 1.6 Hildegard Peplau

models in physical and mental health. Peplau saw the nurse as a:

1. *Resource person.* Provides information.
2. *Counselor.* Helps patients to explore their thoughts and feelings.
3. *Surrogate.* By role-playing or other means, helps the patient to explore and identify feelings from the past.
4. *Technical support.* Coordinates professional services (Peplau, 1952).

In addition to this, Peplau believed in building a collaborative therapeutic relationship between the nurse and the patient. In her book, she cites four stages of this relationship (Peplau, 1952):

1. *Orientation.* Patient feels a need and a will to seek out help.
2. *Identification.* Expectations and perceptions about the nurse–patient relationship are identified.
3. *Exploration.* Patient will begin to show motivation in the problem-solving process, but some testing behaviors may be seen; patient may have a need to "test" the nurse's commitment to their individual situation.
4. *Resolution.* Focus is on the patient developing self-responsibility and showing personal growth.

At Rutgers University in 1954, Peplau developed the first graduate-level nursing program to provide training for clinical nurse specialists in psychiatric nursing.

Hattie Bessent

In the early 1980s, the National Institute of Mental Health (NIMH) granted money to be used for the education and research of minority nurses who were choosing to upgrade to master's and doctorate levels of practice. Dr. Hattie Bessent (1908–2015) (FIG. 1.7) is credited with the development and directorship of that program. In 2008, the ANA presented Bessent with its Hall of Fame Award.

Bessie Blount Griffin

Bessie Blount Griffin (1914–2009) was a practical nurse, physical therapist, and forensic scientist specializing in handwriting. She also understood the mental stress of soldiers who lost their limbs during World War II. These soldiers wanted to write letters to their loved ones, but without their hands this

and promote wellness as well as deliver care to the ill. In her book *Interpersonal Relations in Nursing* (1952), Peplau brought together interpersonal theories from psychiatry and melded them with theories of nursing and communication. She believed that nurses work in society — not merely in a hospital or clinic — and that they need to use every opportunity to educate the public and act as role

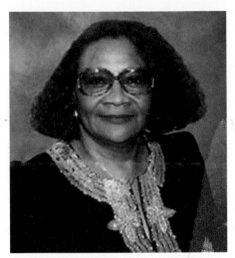

FIGURE 1.7 Hattie Bessent

was difficult. Griffin assisted these soldiers to learn how to write with their mouths and, in some cases, their feet (R.F. Anwar, personal communication, October 2007).

CRITICAL THINKING QUESTION

Nursing's trailblazers were risk-takers whose efforts expanded what it meant to be a nurse. One responsibility of a professional nurse is to give something back to the profession. How will you become a trailblazer? What steps should nursing as a whole take to strengthen the profession? What criteria should be important when deciding what level of preparation is required for a nurse specializing in mental health?

Classroom Activity

Research one trailblazer in nursing. On an assigned day, come to class with a prop and a brief explanation of the trailblazer and their contribution(s) to nursing.

 THE FACILITIES

Mental health refers to our emotional, psychological, and social well-being. It affects how we think, feel, and act. It also helps determine how we handle stress, relate to others, and make choices.

Mental health is important at every stage of life, from childhood and adolescence through adulthood.

People who have mental illnesses are found at all ages and in all walks of life; statistics say that about one in three Americans will experience some form of mental illness at some point in life. The trailblazers in nursing realized that mental illness is different from medical-surgical disorders. They understood that persons with moderate to severe mental disorders were often better served through care in special hospital units or special facilities.

Asylums

Early on, these special facilities were called **asylums,** which Webster Online defines as "an institution for the care of the needy or sick and especially of the insane." Patients in asylums were frequently treated less than humanely. Custodial care was provided, but patients were often heavily medicated.

Nutritional and physical care was minimal, and often these patients were volunteered for various forms of experimentation and research.

One of the largest asylums in the United States was Byberry, later renamed Philadelphia State Hospital (FIG. 1.8). This facility reportedly provided inhumane treatment to its patients. With the onset of deinstitutionalization and due to the poor conditions, this facility saw its last patient in 1990.

Hospitals

As treatment facilities evolved, the term asylum and the connotations associated with it became unpopular. In 1753, Pennsylvania Hospital established a facility to treat those with mental disorders. The hospital was established by Dr. Thomas Bond and Benjamin Franklin. Until the Community Mental Health Act of 1963 was passed, housing of this clientele was primarily handled by individual state hospital systems.

Today, hospitals treat patients with psychological needs according to the size of the hospital and its resources. To comply with regulations surrounding mental health issues, these patients may be seen in a hospital emergency department and then referred to other clinics or hospitals. Communities large enough to support such programs may provide in-house mental health treatment as well as outpatient treatment and after care. Metropolitan areas commonly provide treatment via several options, including hospitals and free-standing treatment centers.

Free-Standing Facilities

Free-standing treatment centers may be called *detoxification (detox) centers, crisis centers*, or similar names. Most people are familiar with the

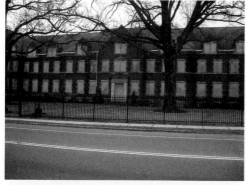

FIGURE 1.8 Byberry, later renamed Philadelphia State Hospital. (*Courtesy of Robynn Anwar.*)

Betty Ford Center. Many free-standing treatment centers provide care ranging from crisis-only to more traditional 21-day stays. As with the Betty Ford Center, a stay can last up to 120 days. This, too, depends largely on the size and needs of the individual community.

THE BREAKTHROUGHS

Nurse Training

It was not until 1937 that formal clinical rotations in mental health began for nursing students. Today, these rotations are required for students in all nursing programs. In 1955, theory relating to mental health nursing became a requirement for licensure for all nurses. Students in a practical or vocational nursing program are taught mental health theory and participate in observational clinical rotations. However, their clinical rotation differs from that of a BSN student nurse.

Throughout the 1800s and early 1900s, progress was made in developing humane, effective treatment of mental illnesses. With the best knowledge available to them as a profession, nurses were forward thinkers in providing specialized care to people unfortunate enough to have illnesses different from the tuberculosis, smallpox, and influenza that filled hospitals. Unlike physical illnesses, no medications existed to treat mental disorders. At that time, no one had been able to find pharmacological help for people with emotional, behavioral, or physical brain disorders. That would change in the 1950s.

Psychotropic Medications

In the early 1950s, chemists were experimenting with combinations of chemicals and their effects on people. In 1955, a group of **psychotropic** medications called *phenothiazines* (see Chapter 8) was discovered to have the effect of calming and tranquilizing people. One well-known phenothiazine is chlorpromazine HCl (Thorazine). What a world of possibility this medication opened for people living with mental disorders and for those caring for them! Suddenly, it was possible to control unwanted behaviors (to a degree), and patients were able to function more independently. Other forms of therapy became more effective because medicated patients were able to focus. Some patients improved so dramatically that it was no longer necessary for them to remain hospitalized and dependent on others. Between the mid-1950s and the mid-1970s, the number of patients hospitalized with mental illnesses in the United States was cut approximately in half, mainly because of the use of psychotropic drugs.

Deinstitutionalization

Phenothiazines were so effective that state hospitals and other facilities dedicated to the care and treatment of people with mental illness saw a large decline in population. It became costly to run these large buildings and continue to employ staff. The combination of these effects, as well as new laws pertaining to the care of this population, resulted in a movement called **deinstitutionalization**. People who had formerly required long hospital stays were now able to leave the institution and return to their communities. Once discharged, some went to group homes and some returned home. Unfortunately, others faced homelessness. Deinstitutionalization was and still is a controversial issue, but it was a huge step in returning a sense of worth, ability, and independence to those who had been dependent on others for their care for so long.

CRITICAL THINKING QUESTION

The law requires that people who have mental illnesses are treated using the "least restrictive alternative." Deinstitutionalization allows these people to live in the community. Consider the following scenario: Your city has just purchased the house next door to you, and the plan is to develop this into a halfway house for women who have abused their children. You are the parent of a 3-year-old, and you are also a mental health nurse. What would you do? What are your thoughts and feelings about this situation?

Organizations for Mental Health Nurses and Others

A natural progression from the breakthroughs that were happening in nursing was the development of organizations for nurses. The ANA is recognized as an organization for registered nurses (RNs). One of its goals is to promote standardization of nursing practice in the United States. The ANA also promotes the certification of nurses who meet specific criteria. The concepts of psychiatric nurse specialists, clinicians, and advanced practice nurses are a result of the work of the ANA. The American Psychiatric Nurses Association provides leadership in recommending standards of care for RNs who care for people with mental illness. In addition to other organizations, there is the National Alliance on Mental Illness (NAMI), whose commitment is to making life better for Americans with mental health disorders.

Classroom Activity

List the standards of psychiatric/mental health clinical nursing practice and give an example of a nursing behavior or action that correlates with each standard. Refer to the Web sites given here:

http://www.austincc.edu/adnlev3/rnsg2213 online/intro/standards

http://www.nursingworld.org/MainMenu Categories/ANAMarketplace/ANAPeriodicals/ OJIN/TableofContents/Vol-20-2015/No1-Jan-2015/2014-Scope-and-Standards-for-Psychiatric-Mental-Health.html

Specific to the Licensed Practical Nurse (LPN) and the Licensed Vocational Nurse (LVN) are two organizations: the National Association of Licensed Practical Nurses (NALPN) and the National Association for Practical Nurse Education and Service (NAPNES). NALPN welcomes LPNs and LVNs in the United States. The NALPN has a published set of nursing practice standards for the LPN (see Appendix D).

NAPNES was founded by practical nurse educators in 1941 and identifies itself as the world's oldest nursing organization dedicated exclusively to the promotion of quality nursing service through the practice of LPNs and LVNs. NAPNES is a multidisciplinary organization of individuals, facilities, and schools that advocates for professional practice of the practical and vocational nurse.

Tool Box

Organizations for Practical and Vocational Nurses

Learn more about NALPN and NAPNES at their Web sites:

National Association of Licensed Practical Nurse (NALPN) http://nalpn.org

National Association for Practical Nurse Education and Service (NAPNES) www.napnes.org

The National Coalition of Ethnic Minority Nurse Associations (NCEMNA) is made up of five associations: the Asian American/Pacific Islander Nurses Association (AAPINA), the National Alaska Native American Indian Nurses Association (NANAINA), the National Association of Hispanic Nurses (NAHN), the National Black Nurses Association (NBNA), and the Philippine Nurses Association of America (PNAA). Goals of the coalition include advocating for equity and justice in nursing and health care for ethnic minority populations and endorsement of best practice models for nursing practice, education, and research for minority populations.

> ## Tool Box
>
> ### Nursing Organizations
>
> AAMN: American Association for Men in Nursing: http://aamn.org/
>
> AAPINA: Asian American / Pacific Islander Nurses Association, Inc.: http://aapina.org/
>
> ANA: American Nurses Association: www.nursingworld.org/
>
> APNA: American Psychiatric Nurses Association: www.apna.org/
>
> HOSA: The Health Occupations Students Association: http://www.hosa.org/about
>
> MNA: Muslim Nurses Association: http://muslimnursesassociation.blogspot.com/
>
> NAHN: National Association of Hispanic Nurses: http://www.nahnnet.org/
>
> NALPN: National Association of Licensed Practical Nurse: http://nalpn.org
>
> NANAINA: National Alaska Native American Indian Nurses Association: http://www.nanainanurses.com/home.html
>
> NAPNES: National Association for Practical Nurse Education and Services: https://napnes.org
>
> NBNA: National Black Nurses Association: www.nbna.org/
>
> NCEMNA: National Coalition of Ethnic Minority Nurse Associations: http://ncemna.org/
>
> NLN: National League for Nursing: www.nln.org/
>
> PNAA: Philippine Nurses Association of America: http://www.mypnaa.org/
>
> Appendix C of this text provides more contact information for these and other organizations designed to promote and assist nurses, particularly at the LPN and LVN levels of preparation.

The American Association for Men in Nursing (AAMN) provides a forum for nurses who are men to meet as a group to discuss and influence factors that affect them as nurses. Among its objectives is to encourage men of all ages to become nurses and to support men who are nurses to grow professionally. Like other professional nursing organizations, AAMN advocates for continued research, education, and dissemination of information about men's health issues, men in nursing, and nursing knowledge at the local and national levels.

 ## THE LAW

Over the years, many advancements have been made in medicine and in the treatment of mental disorders. But mental health ethical practices have remained a challenge. Ethical considerations, especially, abound in the care of people with mental illness. Psychotropic (also known as *psychoactive*) medications benefit many patients, but their side effects are not always pleasant. As more drugs have been developed, more questions have arisen: How much medication is too much? Do we keep patients completely sedated? Which is worse — the illness or the medication? Other concerns have arisen, such as the relationship of some psychotropic drugs to diabetes mellitus.

As a result of these concerns, it was necessary for the federal government to more closely regulate mental health care. A series of laws governing various aspects of care for persons with mental illnesses were passed. The laws have changed somewhat and have been renamed in some cases, but the collective intention is to provide funding, treatment, and ethical care for this vulnerable segment of society.

CRITICAL THINKING QUESTION

Your employer has announced that your company is changing its medical insurance policy. The company will be providing employees with a set amount of money to spend on insurance benefits. The three insurance plans you have to choose from offer either family coverage or mental health services. You are a single parent with two preschoolers. You also have a diagnosis of bipolar disorder for which you need medication, therapy, and periodic hospitalization. What coverage will you choose, and why will you choose it?

Hill-Burton Act

In 1946, Senators Lister Hill and Harold Burton collaborated to create the Hill-Burton Act, a federal law. The first major law to address mental illness, this act provided money to build psychiatric units in hospitals. Today, people with mental illness who lack insurance coverage and who live below the poverty level cannot be turned away because of financial difficulties; they are protected by the Hill-Burton Act.

National Mental Health Act of 1946

The National Mental Health Act of 1946 was a result of the first congress held after World War II. It provided money for nursing and several other disciplines for training and research in areas pertaining to improving treatment for people with mental illness. The NIMH was established as part of this act. The NIMH continuously updates the public on mental health issues. Since 1999, NIMH has been researching autism spectrum disorder. In addition, the agency started the Army Study to Assess Risk and Resilience in Service Members (Army STARRS). The Army STARRS looks at the many challenges faced by those who encounter battle and the coping strategies used to address these challenges.

Community Mental Health Centers Act of 1963

The Community Mental Health Centers Act resulted from President John F. Kennedy's concern for the treatment of people with mental illness. The act's main purpose was to provide a full set of services to people within a community. These services were to include inpatient care, outpatient care, emergency care, and education. This was to be a national effort, funded federally at first. The goal was for the centers to generate enough services so that, eventually, the community could support it financially.

In 1981, the act was amended in congress. The Omnibus Budget Reconciliation Act (OBRA) was the amendment that allows money for mental health to be allocated differently. The bill did not do away with mental health services within communities, but it provided less funding. Currently, there is less money available in the federal budget for mental health, and that money can be withheld at any time. Unfortunately, with the turmoil in the insurance and health-care delivery systems today, mental health benefits are often among the first services to be cut back or eliminated.

Patient Bill of Rights

In 1980, the image of the patient was changing. The Civil Rights Movement of the 1960s began the provision of rights for all groups of people. Patients were beginning to be identified as "clients" who purchase services from health-care providers. Persons who are very young or very old and persons with certain physical, intellectual, or communication difficulties became politically recognized as "vulnerable." The outcome was the development of the Patient Bill of Rights, which is discussed in more detail in Chapter 3.

Affordable Care Act

In March 2010, President Barack Obama signed a bill allowing citizens and noncitizens to purchase health insurance (Siskin & Lunder, 2016) through the Patient Protection and Affordable Care Act, known as the Affordable Care Act (ACA). This bill recognized the needs of people with mental health challenges and established mental health care as an essential part of complete health coverage.

Tool Box

Community Mental Health Act of 1963

To read more about the Community Mental Health Act, explore these Web sites:

www.mass.gov/eohhs/gov/departments/dmh/about-the-department-of-mental-health.html

Omnibus Budget Reconciliation Act: www.gpo.gov/fdsys/pkg/BILLS-103hr2264enr/pdf/BILLS-103hr2264enr.pdf

---

Clinical Activity

In clinical postconference, discuss your answers to these questions:

1. Identify ways that (a) the delivery of psychiatric/mental health nursing and (b) roles, functions, activities, and settings have changed over time.
2. What issues or trends do you anticipate in psychiatric/mental health nursing in the future?

Safe and Effective Nursing Care

Study mental health nursing theories
Promote mental health care
Review the Nurse Practice Act and Scope of Practice of the state where practicing
Advocate for patients
Respect Patient's Bill of Rights
Join nursing organizations

Key Points

- Mental health nursing has a long and rich history. It has evolved from very rudimentary skills before the time of Florence Nightingale to the specialty area of nursing it is today.
- Patients with mental illness are treated in many different types of facilities, depending on the diagnosis and the availability of care in a particular community.
- The 1950s were important years in the mental health field. The first psychotropic medications were developed, making it possible for some people who had been in an institution to return to their homes and communities (deinstitutionalization). These medications also allowed other treatments to be more effective.

- Nurses at all levels of preparation are integral parts of the mental health treatment team. Our observations, documentation, and interpersonal skills make nurses effective tools in patient care.
- Since 1955, all nursing curricula are required to provide mental health theory.
- A series of laws over the past 70 years have provided money for education, research, and improvements in the care of people with mental illness. Financial difficulties in the insurance and health-care industries contribute to cutbacks in money and services for care and treatment of this population.
- The Affordable Care Act was signed in March 2010.

Review Questions

1. The main goal of deinstitutionalization was to
   a. Let all people with mental illness care for themselves
   b. Return as many people as possible to a "normal" life
   c. Keep all people with mental illness in locked wards
   d. Close all community hospitals

2. A major breakthrough of the 1950s that assisted in the deinstitutionalization movement was
   a. The Community Mental Health Centers Act
   b. The Nurse Practice Act
   c. The development of psychotropic medications
   d. Electroconvulsive therapy

3. The set of regulations that dictates the scope of a nurse's professional duties is called
   a. National League for Nursing
   b. American Nurses Association
   c. Patient Bill of Rights
   d. Nurse Practice Act   .

4. As a result of deinstitutionalization and changes in the health-care delivery system, nurses can expect to care for people with mental health issues in which of the following settings?
   a. Psychiatric hospitals
   b. Outpatient settings
   c. Medical-surgical hospital settings
   d. All of the above

5. Which of the following trailblazers in nursing was not a nurse?
   a. Hildegard Peplau
   b. Linda Richards
   c. Harriet Bailey
   d. Dorothea Dix

6. Which of the following nursing organizations specifically represent nurses who belong to racial or ethnic minorities? *(Select all that apply.)*
   a. NACE
   b. AAPINA
   c. NAPNES
   d. PNAA
   e. NANAINA

7. In the past, facilities that housed patients who were impoverished, sick, or insane were known as
   a. Detox centers
   b. Asylums
   c. Outpatient clinics
   d. Hospitals

8. What institute was established as a result of the National Mental Health Act of 1946?
   a. NLN
   b. NFLPN
   c. NAHN
   d. NIMH

9. Florence Nightingale's focus in the Crimean War was
   a. Improving mental health
   b. Upgrading education
   c. Providing a clean environment
   d. Writing care plans

10. The first psychotropic medications were introduced in the
   a. 1950s
   b. 1930s
   c. 1980s
   d. 1920s

REVIEW QUESTIONS ANSWER KEY 1.b, 2.c, 3.d, 4.d, 5.d, 6.b, d, e, 7.b, 8.d, 9.c, 10.a

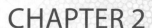

CHAPTER 2
Basics of Communication

KEY TERMS

Adaptive communication
Aggressive communication
Aphasia
Assertive communication
Broca's aphasia
Communication
Communication block
Dysphasia
Feedback
Global aphasia
Hearing impaired
Laryngectomy
Message
Neurolinguistic programming (NLP)
Nontherapeutic communication
Nonverbal communication
Receiver
Sender
Social communication
Therapeutic communication
Verbal communication
Visually impaired
Wernicke's aphasia

CHAPTER CONCEPTS

Communication
Health promotion
Safety
Sensory perception

LEARNING OUTCOMES

1. Identify three components needed to communicate.
2. Differentiate between effective and ineffective communication.
3. Identify six types of communication.
4. Identify five challenges to communication.
5. Identify common blocks to therapeutic communication.
6. Identify common techniques of therapeutic communication.
7. Demonstrate various communication styles.
8. Identify five adaptive communication techniques.

Humans communicate. Everything people do or say has meaning. Sometimes, a person's words and actions send different messages. It is essential for health-care providers to be able to communicate and connect with both their colleagues and their patients, whether they are a medical-surgical patient or have a mental health disorder. For example:

> Sally and Jim meet for shift report in the morning. Sally's eyes are red and swollen, and she is unusually quiet. Jim asks her if something is wrong, and she responds, "No, everything is just fine." Jim observed changes in Sally's behavior and appearance that indicate there is a problem. But Sally verbally communicated that nothing was wrong. What is the <u>real</u> message?

People from different cultures may communicate differently. Men and women may communicate differently. People who have hearing impairments communicate differently from people who do not. People in the medical profession communicate differently from people in the business profession by using medical terminology rather than business terminology. People communicate all the time in everything they do. **Communication** is the ongoing process of sending and receiving messages.

Are we connecting when we communicate? That is the question.

COMMUNICATION THEORY

In 1948, C. E. Shannon published an article in *The Bell System Technical Journal* for the sole purpose of explaining how to solve mathematical problems. In the article, Shannon identified the elements needed to communicate in mathematics. By 1951, Shannon had started to use his theory of mathematic communication to describe the process of language communication. Shannon's theory identified five elements necessary for communication: source, sender, channel, receiver, and destination.

Sender, Receiver, and Interpretation of Message

The process of communicating with others is challenging because it consists of the three parts shown in FIGURE 2.1. This model implies that the **sender** is only partially responsible for the communication.

Think about the scenario of Sally and Jim. Sally is the sender, sending a **message** to Jim, the **receiver.** As it turns out, Sally has severe allergies. She was visiting her friend who has cats. Sally is very allergic to cats, and the redness and swelling of her eyes were symptoms of her allergic response. She simply did not wish to burden Jim with her problem during shift report, so she opted to respond by telling him everything was "just fine." However, Sally cannot totally control Jim's interpretation of what Jim is seeing. Without **feedback** from Jim, Sally cannot confirm his understanding of her message. When feedback is not provided, it is difficult to determine what message was really received.

Classroom Activity

What was your initial interpretation of what Sally was communicating? On what did you base your interpretation? What "spoke" louder to you: Sally's words or her actions and appearance? What is the danger in making an assumption about Sally's message?

It is very important for the sender and receiver to double-check each other's understanding of the message with feedback. In nursing, this is crucial. When dealing with the health and safety of patients, nurses need to be very sure to avoid "mixed" or "missed" messages.

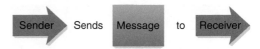
FIGURE 2.1 A basic flow of communication.

TYPES OF COMMUNICATION

Verbal and Written Communication
Verbal communication is the process of exchanging information by the spoken or written word. It is, therefore, the subjective part of the communication process. In the example given, Sally's reply that "everything is just fine" is an example of verbal communication. The expertise a nurse develops in the area of verbal communication is largely responsible for the credibility of that nurse. Critical thinking is essential to understanding Sally's reply.

GOOD TO KNOW
The meaning of a word or expression can change from one generation to the next or from one group of people to another. For example, in a class discussion on words and gestures and what they mean, one African American student spoke up. She shared with the class that "gals" in her country was considered a demeaning term for an African woman. However, in the 1950s and 1960s, being one of the "guys" or the "gals" was acceptable in the United States. It demonstrated acceptance and belonging to one's social group. Today it could be gender inappropriate.

Nonverbal Communication
Nonverbal communication involves a person's actions, tone of voice, the way they use their body, and their facial expressions. Nonverbal communication has a greater influence on communication than verbal communication does. In a sense, nonverbal communication is more objective than verbal communication because it is observable. However, it is also less precise because the receiver (FIG. 2.2) can interpret nonverbal communication in many different ways. In the example, Sally's body language communicated that she was not "fine." But it did not communicate whether she was not fine physically or emotionally.

The meaning of nonverbal communication varies by culture as well. Common hand gestures can

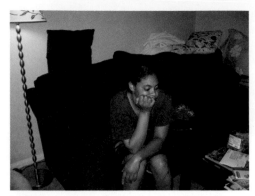

FIGURE 2.2 Nonverbal communication is estimated to be 70% of the message we send. The old saying is true: A picture is worth a thousand words *(courtesy of Robynn Anwar).*

Box 2.1

Examples of Communication With Cultural Implications

Words and actions that are seemingly harmless to some people can be very hurtful to others. People do not usually know that until they take the time to ask. These are examples of communication affected by cultural implications. How many more can your class identify?

• Eye contact with strangers or those in perceived positions of power or respect is not considered appropriate among some populations.
• Hand gestures may communicate different meanings to different groups of people.
• A slang term may be inappropriate or offensive or may exclude people who do not understand the meaning of the word.
• Gender-reference terms such as "you guys" may offend people when the group is mixed or not male.
• African American or Arab American women portrayed in subservient roles may offend members of these groups.

have wildly different meanings. For example, in the United States, the thumbs up sign is a sign of encouragement, agreement, or congratulations. This same gesture is a vulgarity in other cultures.

Cultural Considerations

Note the diverse cultures and ages in your community and identify a common gesture that you use that means something different to others.

People can learn from each other every day. Nurses, especially, need to be alert for terms or gestures that make their patients uncomfortable. They must make a conscious effort not to use words or gestures that are offensive to the persons in their care. Box 2.1 lists some examples of verbal and nonverbal communication to be cautious with.

Aggressive Communication Versus Assertive Communication

The terms *aggressive* and *assertive* are sometimes used interchangeably in American culture, but they have very different meanings.

Aggressive Communication

Aggressive communication is communication that is not self-responsible. Aggressive statements most often begin with the word "you." Aggressive communication, like aggressive behavior, is meant to harm another person. It is a form of the defense mechanism projection (see Chapter 7), or blaming, and it attempts to put responsibility for the aggressor's

feelings on the other person. Aggressive communication can be nonverbal. A person's tone, vocal pitch, or body language can be aggressive. An aggressive person may attempt to humiliate others for control. Frequently interrupting and creating fear are two of the behaviors an aggressive person may display.

Examples
"You make me so angry when you don't help with the housework!"
"It is because of you that I failed my math test!"

Assertive Communication
Assertive communication, on the other hand, is self-responsible. Assertive statements begin with the word "I." They express the speaker's thoughts and feelings honestly.

Example
"I feel angry when you don't help with the housework."

Assertive behavior and communication are techniques of personal empowerment. People choose to think or feel a certain way; others do not have the power to make people think or feel anything they do not choose to think or feel. Saying "I think" or "I feel" helps to keep people in control of their emotions, while allowing honest, open expression of the feelings they have as a result of someone else's behavior. The feelings and thoughts belong to the person choosing them, not to anyone else. People with assertive behavior convey respect for others.

Social Communication

Social communication is the day-to-day interaction people have with personal acquaintances. For example, teenagers usually communicate with their peer group in a different manner than they do with their parents. Today's teenagers usually communicate with their peers by means of texting using various apps. Physical, in-person communication has decreased. Nurses communicate differently with their patients than they do with their friends or family. In social interactions, nurses may use slang or "street language," and they may be less literal and purposeful than when they are talking to patients. Quite simply, social interaction has a different purpose than a nurse's professional communication.

Therapeutic Communication

Therapeutic communication is "communication between a health-care professional and a patient that is aimed at improving the patient's physical or psychological health and well-being" (Punyanunt-Carter, 2013). The nurse understands that in order to acquire certain pertinent information from the patient, unique techniques of communication will have to be instituted.

Therapeutic communication is purposeful: Nurses are trying to determine the patient's needs. If the patient is not comfortable sharing their needs and concerns, the nurse tries to uncover the problem by using techniques of therapeutic communication and "active" or "purposeful" listening (or "listening between the lines"). The techniques of therapeutic communication are individualized to the patient and their mental health disorder. Techniques of and blocks to communication will be reviewed later in the chapter.

Neurolinguistic Programming

Neurolinguistic programming (NLP) is a form of communication developed by John Grinder, a psychologist and linguistics professor, and Richard Bandler, a mathematician and editor (Grinder & Bandler, 1981). NLP is a way of framing statements and questions to communicate more effectively (see Chapter 9). The theory builds on the idea that humans tend to interact with the world in basically three ways: hearing, seeing, and touching. Choosing words that match a patient's primary way of interacting can make a difference in how communication is actually perceived by that patient. NLP can assist the health-care provider in communicating more effectively with the patient, which in turn may lead them to change behavior and choose a healthier lifestyle.

 CHALLENGES TO COMMUNICATION

Communicating is something that people often take for granted until they no longer can do it. Imagine answering the telephone while having laryngitis, trying to sign a legal document while your arm is in a cast, or attempting to read traffic signs after your eyes have been dilated. These are uncomfortable situations, but they are temporary. What about patients and coworkers for whom disabilities are permanent? One trailblazer, physical therapist Bessie Blount Griffin, understood the challenges faced by soldiers who had lost limbs in World War II. It was important that these veterans had an alternative method for communicating, which inspired Griffin to teach them to write using their mouths and feet.

People Who Have Hearing Impairments

The nurse must be patient when communicating with people who are **hearing impaired**. The person's frustration is likely even greater than that of

Clinical Activity

Community Resources Worksheet

Contact an agency that provides services for persons with disabilities in your community. Explain that you are a student nurse and that you are trying to determine the resources available in your community. Record the following information:

1. Name of person spoken with:
2. Name of agency:
3. Who are the target groups for this agency?
   a. Gender(s)
   b. Age(s)
   c. Specific disabilities, such as speech, hearing, and visual or other impairments
4. How do people access this agency?
5. What are the agency's fees for services?
6. What types of insurance does the agency accept?
7. What hours are the agency open?
8. Do people need appointments to come to this agency?
9. Where does the agency keep patient records? After your phone call, answer the following questions:
10. What is your impression of this agency?
11. Would you feel comfortable coming to this agency or referring a patient here? Why or why not?

Tool Box

Use this Web site to learn some American Sign Language vocabulary:

https://www.signingsavvy.com/

such as gestures, body position, and facial expressions, "speak" most strongly to patients. How does a sightless person or someone with low visual acuity interpret these nonverbal cues?

Nurses must learn to become detail-oriented storytellers. It is important to describe to the patient the location of the call signal and what the call signal sounds like, where their belongings have been placed, and who has just entered the room. Sightless people cannot see a wave of the hand or see when someone leaves or enters a room; these events must be verbalized.

Patient teaching for a person with a visual impairment may involve physically moving or touching them and verbally explaining in much more detail than usual. Learning to feed themself can be difficult for a newly sightless person. Usually, the teaching involves relating the food position on the plate to the numbers on a clock face. Sightless patients learn to rely on their other senses to compensate for the eyes they cannot use.

Sometimes individuals have more than one communication challenge. For example, some people have both hearing and visual impairments. When communicating with these individuals, a nurse needs to be creative. Investigate methods that have worked for this person in the past and explore methods such as a conversation board or printing the message on the person's palm.

As emphasized in any nursing fundamentals class, when entering the patient's room, the nurse needs to identify themself, explain what procedure is about to be performed, and make sure the patient is safe. The nurse should also indicate when they leave the room.

People Who Have Laryngectomies

Some people live with partial or total **laryngectomy**—the removal of their larynx ("voice box"). Imagine being able to speak one day and having no voice at all the next. The larynx is a body part that is very much taken for granted. How do these patients answer the phone, order a pizza, express their emotions, or call for help? When caring for patients with a laryngectomy, provide them with a notebook and a

the nurse. As with any other patient, try to establish a trusting, team-approach relationship. Let the person know you will try whatever it takes for you to be able to understand each other. Find out what has worked for that person in the past.

Not all people with hearing impairments use sign language; some use lipreading. However, lipreading may be inaccurate and could lead to miscommunication. Sometimes writing a note or providing the patient with a journal is an effective way to communicate with a person who is deaf or hard of hearing. Keep in mind the key factor is communication and not the patient's grammatical or spelling abilities.

People Who Have Visual Impairments

When a person is **visually impaired,** the nonverbal part of communication can be a challenge. Nursing is a highly affective art, so certain nonverbal cues, pen or pencil. A word or picture board can also facilitate communication. Having the patient type messages on a tablet, laptop computer, or a smartphone is another option.

Classroom Activity

Without using any verbal communication, ask a classmate to perform a simple task such as opening a door, going from a sitting position to a standing position, using eating utensils, or some other common activity of daily living. Then, trade places with your classmate.

People With Language Differences

Today's society is global. Even though English is the predominant language in the United States, it may not be the primary language for many of the people nurses work with and care for. As a nurse, you may find yourself in an area where you are the one who does not speak the patients' primary language. How will you communicate? How will you ensure safe care of your patients? If a physician with a thick accent gives a verbal order, how will you know you have heard it correctly? Although a patient's or physician's primary language may be different from yours, it is essential to develop a means of communicating. Techniques for ensuring understanding are provided at the end of this chapter and in Chapter 5.

Classroom Activity

Working with your classmates, select 10 English words and translate them into three other languages (e.g., Spanish, French, or Hindi) using an online translator app.

• Were you able to pronounce each translation correctly?

• Which language(s) did you find particularly difficult to pronounce?

People Who Have Aphasic/Dysphasic Disorders

A person with **aphasia** lacks the ability to speak, and a person with **dysphasia** has great difficulty with speech (partial loss of speech). The amount of speech a patient possesses is related to many things, including the person's age and the cause and severity of the difficulty. Both aphasia and dysphasia include damage to a portion of the brain. Aphasia and dysphasia are often used interchangeably when describing these disorders. There are several types of aphasia: **Wernicke's** (receptive), **Broca's** (expressive), and **global aphasia** (Table 2.1). It is important for the nurse to know which type of aphasia/dysphasia has been diagnosed by the health-care provider or speech therapist.

The health-care provider and the speech therapist will determine the cause of the brain injury and the extent of involvement, but the nurse will be part of the patient's plan of care. This requires a very individualized type of communication skill. An aphasic patient may try to read aloud a passage from a book, but what comes out of the patient's mouth may be unrecognizable. The patient would be very embarrassed if they knew what they were saying. The nurse must be very understanding and willing to try repeatedly to communicate with persons with various forms of aphasia. Nurses also must remember not to take any "nasty words" personally; chances are very good that the patient meant something entirely different (see the section Adaptive Communication Techniques).

Classroom Activity

Interview a representative from the Americans with Disabilities Act office, your state's Services for the Blind, or any local agencies that serve populations with special communication needs. Briefly share what you learned with the class.

Clinical Activity

During your clinical rotation, ask your instructor to assign you to care for a person with a communication challenge. Describe how you altered your usual communication patterns to work with this individual.

 ## THERAPEUTIC COMMUNICATION

It is possible to have a helping, therapeutic conversation with most people, but it takes some practice. These techniques need to be practiced in much the

Table 2.1
Types of Aphasia

Types of Aphasia	Description
Broca's aphasia (expressive)	Difficulty expressing themselves in written or verbal forms of communication. Sentences are incomplete.
Wernicke's (receptive)	Difficulty interpreting or understanding written or verbal forms of communication. Sometimes use the wrong word.
Global	Combination of receptive and expressive forms of aphasia

same way that one learns any other language: by hearing them, practicing them, and making them part of one's professional (and social) vocabulary.

Nontherapeutic Communication

Before reviewing therapeutic communication techniques, some examples of **nontherapeutic communication,** where there is a breakdown in a message, will be reviewed. The following are examples of communication blocks that impede helpful interaction with patients:

1. *False reassurance/social clichés.* These are phrases nurses may use to sound supportive. In social communication, these expressions sound friendly, but in a therapeutic relationship, they invalidate the patient's concerns. The patient is most likely seeking understanding of their diagnosis or a procedure.

Example	Effects on Patient
"Don't worry! Everything will be just fine."	• *Tells patient his or her concerns are not valid* • *May jeopardize patient's trust in nurse*

2. *Minimizing/belittling.* These, too, are used socially to try to relieve the tensions of others.

Saying that many people are experiencing the same thing as the individual is somehow supposed to make the problem seem lighter. In therapeutic use, the implications are different.

Example	Effect on Patient
"We have all felt that way sometimes."	• *Implies that the patient's feelings are not special*

3. *"Why?"* This simple word needs to be eliminated in therapeutic interactions. *Why* connotes disapproval or displeasure. The patient often does not know why they did or said something but may feel responsible for providing an answer anyway. The nurse needs to use less stress-producing methods to find out why. Asking "why" may sound as though you are accusing the patient of causing their problem.

Example	Effects on Patient
"Why did you refuse your breakfast?"	• *Patient feels obligated to answer something he or she may not wish to answer or may not be able to answer* • *Probes in an abrasive way*

4. *Advising.* Alcoholics Anonymous sometimes uses the statement, "Don't 'should' on yourself." Nurses also must not "should" on their patients. This sets the stage for expectations that the patient may not be able to meet. It also sets up, in the patient's mind, some sort of value system that identifies the nurse's value as the "right" one. In addition, giving advice can sound very judgmental.

Examples	Effects on Patient
"You should eat more." *"If I were you, I would take those pills so that I would feel better."*	• *Places a value on the action* • *Gives the idea that the nurse's values are the "right" ones* • *Sounds parental*

5. *Agreeing or disagreeing.* Socially, people agree or disagree for several reasons. Sometimes people are just expressing their opinion. Sometimes they are trying to make a favorable impression. Therapeutically, it is wise for

nurses to avoid statements that express their own opinions or values. The health-care provider does not want the patient to dismiss their own personal opinions and values.

Example	Effect on Patient
"You were wrong about that." *"I think you're right."*	• *Places a "right" or "wrong" on the action*

6. *Closed-ended questions.* These are forms of questions that make it possible for a one-word, "yes" or "no" answer. They discourage the patient from giving full answers to the questions. Closed-ended questions are those that start with such phrases as "Can you," "Will you," "Are they," and "May I." It does not help to add "please," as in "Please, may I ask you a question?" or "Will you please take out the trash?" This courtesy still leaves the possibility for the receiver to say "yes" or "no." To make the questions assertive and therapeutic, state or request what you want ("I need to ask you a question" or "Please take out the trash"). Closed-ended questions limit the patient's options for disclosure to the interviewer.

Adding words like *how* and *what* to the beginning of a close-ended question can turn it into an open-ended question.

Closed: "Can I help you?"

Open: "How can I help you?" or "What can I do to help you?"

Examples	Effects on Patient
"Can you tell me how you feel?" *"Do you smoke?"* *"Can I ask you a few questions?"*	• *Allows a "yes" or "no" answer* • *Discourages further exploration of the topic* • *Discourages patient from giving information*

7. *Providing the answer with the question.* This is a technique that television interviewers use frequently. For instance, an interviewer may ask, "Didn't you know that the committee would reject the proposal?" A better, more neutral way to ask this question is "What were your thoughts about how the committee might react?" Occasionally, the body language of the interviewer or the sender may influence the receiver's answer.

Examples	Effects on Patient
"Are you afraid?" *"Didn't the food taste good?"* *"Do you miss your mom today?"*	• *Combines a closed-ended question with a solution* • *Discourages patient from providing their own answers*

8. *Changing the subject.* Nurses sometimes do this inadvertently. When schedules are busy and several patients need a nurse's attention at the same time, it is very easy for a nurse to pass over a patient's question or concern and then proceed with the nurse's own agenda. Unfortunately, that may send the message to the patient that the nurse does not care or that this problem is not worthy of a nurse's time. This patient may be reluctant to offer more information to that nurse in the future.

Changing the subject may also reflect the nurse's discomfort with the subject. If the nurse just experienced the death of a loved one from a heart attack, for example, the nurse may be very uncomfortable answering a patient's questions about recovery and prognosis after bypass surgery. The nurse may answer quickly and move on to a more comfortable topic, such as, "Well, your physician has advanced your diet; that's good news!"

Example	Effects on Patient
The patient is asking a question about his/her prognosis, and the nurse responds, "Did the doctor say anything about discharging you today?"	• *Discounts the importance of the patient's need to explore personal thoughts and feelings* • *May be a reflection of the nurse's own discomfort with this topic*

9. *Approving or disapproving.* This is similar to minimizing or agreeing. Approving or disapproving puts the nurse in the position of the "expert," which, in many ways, the nurse is. The nurse's role, however, is to be supportive without being judgmental or imposing a personal idea of what is right or wrong, good or bad, on the patient. The patient may feel as though they are not meeting the nurse's expectation.

The nurse is in a partnership with the patient. The nurse collaborates with the patient to determine the best way to help the patient help. If the nurse can look at the relationship with that attitude, there is no right or wrong because each person is different. No two patients are the same, so what is helpful to each one is right for that patient.

Examples	Effects on Patient
"That's the way to think about it!" *"Good for you!"* *"That's not a good idea."*	• *Can sound judgmental* • *Can set the patient up for failure if the approval or disapproval does not help;* • *Can lower the nurse's credibility*

Techniques of Therapeutic/Helping Communication

Hildegard Peplau envisioned the nurse as a "tool" for ensuring positive interpersonal relationships with patients. Nurses are with the patient for approximately 8 to 12 hours daily. Compare that with the amount of time a health-care provider spends with the patient, and it is easy to see how the nurse becomes the therapeutic tool that helps the patient help themselves. This observation was noted by Florence Nightingale in her book *Notes on Nursing* (originally published in 1859).

Patients develop a different kind of rapport with nurses because they learn to trust them. Although nurses' technical skills are very important and must never be allowed to get rusty, it is the appropriate use of their verbal and nonverbal communication skills that cements the relationship with patients and ultimately promotes their healing.

The previous section pointed out some of the bad habits of communication. It is now time to learn new, effective methods of communication. These will feel awkward at first, but with practice, they will help improve the quality of interactions not only with patients but in most interpersonal communication as well.

GOOD TO KNOW

The communication methods covered in this chapter will not work for all people in all circumstances, but if you use them faithfully, you will see improvements in the way you relate to your patients and in the ways they respond to you

1. *Reflecting, repeating, parroting.* This technique seems to be the easiest to learn and therefore is used the most often. The nurse repeats a word or phrase that seems to be a key idea in what the patient is trying to communicate. It sometimes involves a degree of guessing on the part of the nurse to verify the perceived message. For instance, if the patient says, "I want to get out of here; everyone is against me," the nurse has several options for verifying the main concern of the patient. The nurse could say "Everyone?" or "Against you?" to try to encourage the patient to expand on these ideas. *Caution:* Because this technique might seem obvious to the patient, use parroting sparingly.

Example	Effects on Patient
Patient: "I'm so tired of all of this." *Nurse: "Tired?"*	• *Encourages exploring the meaning of the statement* • *Can be irritating if overused*

2. *Clarifying terms.* We live and work in a global society, with patients and coworkers from all over the world. But even native speakers of English may not always understand each other. Because of that, it is very important to clarify the meaning of terms. Nurses must be sure that the terms they choose are correct and mean the same thing to all parties involved in the interaction. This technique is easy to learn: Simply asking "When you say 'I can't do that,' what do you mean?" is one way of clarifying a statement. The patient may mean "I am not physically able to do that" or "I am not morally able to do that" or "I do not know how to do that" or any number of other things that the word *can't* may mean. If the nurse does not clarify that simple word, they could incorrectly infer the patient's level of ability or cooperation.

Example	Effects on Patient
"When you say 'tired,' do you mean it in a physical way or an emotional way?"	• *Encourages patient to restate the comment, occasionally providing more information* • *Improves chances that the message sent is the message received*

3. *Open-ended questions.* These are the essence of successful nurse-patient communication.

This technique is also among the hardest to learn. Open-ended communication allows the patient to become more involved in their plan of care.

One of the goals of helping communication is to get the patient to participate, so it is important that the nurse present questions in a way that will encourage the patient to provide information without the nurse sounding persistent or intrusive. Such a perception by the patient will interfere in future attempts at communication.

In some instances, "yes" or "no" may be all the nurse needs to know or all that the patient is capable of saying. In those instances, closed-ended questions may be used until the patient is able to provide more information. Otherwise, open-ended questions will get more productive outcome.

Example

"How are you feeling today?"
"What can I do to help, Ms. Green?"

Effects on Patient

- *Discourages "yes" or "no" answers*
- *Encourages patient to express needs in their own terms*

Using open-ended questions can be helpful in understanding the patient's pain level as well. Asking the patient "Are you in pain?" (closed-ended question) may not give an accurate picture. The closed-ended nature of this question does not provide useful, measurable information that allows the nurse to be helpful or therapeutic. A more helpful question would be "Ms. Green, on a scale of 0 to 10, how do you rate your pain?" or the request "Ms. Green, please tell me about your pain."

4. *Asking for what you need or want.* This relates to the discussion on assertive versus aggressive communication. Nurses can ask for what they need and want from patients and coworkers and still maintain a pleasant, professional tone of voice. This technique requires the user to start the sentence with the words "I want" or "I need." Taking the direct approach with people is usually the safest way to be sure that the receiver gets the message the sender intended to send.

These two examples show ways to be assertive, direct, and self-responsible while still maintaining politeness and allowing the patient to have some control over their care.

Examples

"Mrs. Smith, I need to ask you a few questions, please."
"I want to switch shifts with Mary next Tuesday, please."

Effects on Patient

- *States purpose for the interaction*
- *Keeps speaker assertive and self-responsible*

5. *Identifying feelings and thoughts.* This is another technique that can be difficult to master because people often do not use words carefully. A *feeling* is an emotion. A "feeling statement" must identify an emotion that one is experiencing or is trying to explore with a patient. For example, "I feel proud that I earned this promotion" or "I feel frightened to walk alone at night."

A *thought* is an opinion, idea, or fact that one wishes to express. "I think I deserve this promotion" and "I think security needs to be improved in the parking area" are examples of "thinking statements."

"I feel security needs to be improved in the parking area" and "I feel the patient needs a different pain medication" are incorrect uses of the word *feel*. There is no emotion identified in these statements. Feeling is certainly implied, but implied thoughts and feelings need to be stated directly to avoid mistaken conclusions. In both of these statements, *feel* should be replaced with *think* for correct usage.

Using words pertaining to thought and feeling correctly will minimize the amount of time the nurse must spend clarifying and will maximize the quality of the interaction. In the mental health specialty, it becomes even more important for the nurse to use such terms appropriately to help the patient identify and label their emotions and thoughts to facilitate therapy.

Examples

"I feel angry when you are not honest with me."
"I think honesty is important in all relationships."

Effects on Patient

- *Helps the patient to identify and label thoughts and emotions*
- *May give insight into underlying concerns or complications of healing*

6. *Using empathy.* Empathy is also related to feelings. There is a big difference between sympathy and empathy. Sympathy is a social emotion used when people wish to share emotional experiences. It is *not* a therapeutic technique because

it involves experiencing the emotion. Empathy involves identifying emotions without experiencing the emotion. Nurses use empathy with patients. They identify the emotion and relate to it while keeping the focus on the patient's needs. Being empathetic is accepting another person's reality. Nurses help patients deal with their feelings and still maintain professional control of the situation; the nurse needs to remain the helper.

Consider the following situation: A nurse notices a patient crying in the lounge. The nurse wants to help, so he approaches the patient, sits down, and offers his assistance. The patient tells the nurse that she just found out her pet died. The pet had been her "family" since her divorce. The nurse's response options are:

Sympathy: Remembering his own favorite pet who died, the nurse says, "I understand your feelings; my pet died suddenly, too."

OR

Empathy: The nurse identifies that the patient is mourning a significant loss and says, "I am so sorry. It must be very painful to lose something you feel so close to. I'd like to hear about your pet when you think you'd like to talk about it."

Patients need the nurse to be sensitive but still be the helper. Empathy is more appropriate in most therapeutic situations and validates the patient's emotions. The empathy displayed in this situation also keeps the attention on the patient not the nurse's experience with loss.

Examples	Effects on Patient
"It must feel very demeaning when others are dishonest." *"I can only imagine how difficult this has been."*	*• Acknowledges patient's feelings* *• Keeps nurse in position of control and helpfulness*

7. *Silence.* Silence serves many functions in communication, yet many people are very uncomfortable with it. Watch what happens at a social gathering or in the break room when a short silence occurs. Often, people fidget nervously or make "small talk" just to break the silence.

Silence, as a therapeutic technique of communication, serves two main purposes: First, it allows the nurse and the patient a short time to collect their thoughts; second, it shows patience and acceptance on the part of the nurse. Sitting quietly for a period of time, usually 2 to 3 minutes, and maintaining an open body posture sends the message that the nurse is willing to wait if the patient has more to say or that the nurse accepts the fact that the interaction may be over for the present. Silence can be just as powerful and effective as any verbal interaction.

Caution: Do not allow the silence to go on too long. If possible, allow the patient to end the silence. However, if nothing has been said by either party within 2 to 3 minutes, it is wise to suggest to the patient that it might be time for a rest. Then the nurse should take cues from the patient's response. Perhaps the conversation will begin again, or maybe the patient will be grateful for the suggestion to rest. Either way, the nurse can let the patient know that they are there if the patient wants to talk again at another time.

Example	Effects on Patient
Sit quietly near the patient	*• Shows that the nurse is comfortable with whatever the patient says and willing to hear more* *• Allows both to collect their thoughts*

8. *Giving information.* This is very different from the **communication block** of giving advice. Giving information relates to the helping relationship because it involves a form of patient teaching.

Nurses provide information in all phases of hospitalization, from preoperative teaching to discharge planning. Providing information may involve using pamphlets, videos, resource manuals, or other resource persons.

Example	Effects on Patient
"Mrs. Brown, I would be glad to explain this diagnosis to you. Tell me what the doctor has said, and I'll clarify it for you any way I can."	*• Increases rapport* *• Eases patient's anxiety* *• Honestly confirms that the health-care provider has given prior information* *• Suggests collaboration*

9. *Using general leads.* This is a method of encouraging the person to continue speaking. It lets the speaker know that the nurse is actively listening and interested in hearing more. The technique is fairly simple: It involves both verbal and nonverbal communication. Examples of general leads are saying "Yes?" while maybe raising the eyes, "Go on" while maintaining eye contact and possibly nodding the head in an affirmative motion, or just saying "And then?" if the person pauses in the middle of a statement or concern.

Example	**Effect on Patient**
Saying "Go on" while nodding head and maintaining eye contact	• *Feels valued and listened to*

10. *Stating implied thoughts and feelings.* This takes a combination of skills. It requires drawing an inference, using empathy, and making an observation about a behavior or condition the nurse sees in the patient.

    This technique is helpful in initiating a conversation that might be difficult to start with other techniques. Having a specific behavior or action pointed out makes it harder for the patient to deny or ignore the nurse's suggestion that something is different. Nurses are assessing their patient's physical and emotional states all the time.

    When a patient is reluctant to share in this situation, the nurse can preface the question with an observation and then follow with an educated guess at the emotion that is being experienced.

Example	**Effects on Patient**
"Ms. Johnson, you're not smiling today like you usually do. I sense something is bothering you. How can I help?"	• *Lets the patient know you are paying attention to him or her* • *Identifies a specific behavior or change in behavior, which lowers the chance of the patient denying it* • *Reinforces that the nurse cares and wishes to help*

ADAPTIVE COMMUNICATION TECHNIQUES

Certain populations require special consideration when nurses are communicating with them. **Adaptive communication** techniques are alternative ways of communicating with people who are affected by certain disabilities or who have varied amounts of ability.

People Who Have Hearing Impairments

When communicating with a patient who has a hearing impairment, it is important to know the extent of the impairment. Is the person deaf, or are they hard of hearing? Does the person speech-read (also called *lip-read*)? Do they use a hearing aid? How does the patient feel about their hearing impairment? Some patients are in denial about hearing loss or difficulties.

Communication can be very frustrating for patients with hearing impairments as well as for their nurses. These patients may use sign language, but most hearing people do not know sign language. Sometimes writing with pencil and paper or typing on a keyboard is effective, but it can be slow. Provide the patient with an amplifying device to enhance hearing. Install safety alarms in the home or provide when in a facility. Speech reading is helpful to some people with hearing impairments, but it is not always accurate.

People Who Have Visual Impairments

For patients who have visual impairments, adaptive resources such as audio books, Braille-prepared computers, magnifiers, corrective lenses, and guide dogs can be extremely helpful. The type of adaptive resource used depends on the type and severity of the visual impairment. For example, technology allows people with low visual acuity to increase the font size on a computer up to 500%. People with visual impairments may have heightened senses of hearing and touch.

GOOD TO KNOW
It is not necessary to talk slower or louder to a person with a hearing impairment. In fact, doing so may be considered offensive.

People Who Have Laryngectomies
Both external and internal aids now exist that amplify the vibrations of speech. For some patients with laryngectomies, placing an amplifier over the area of the larynx and talking produces a buzzing sound that replicates their voice. It is a monotone sound, but it greatly improves the ability of these patients to communicate in a more natural manner. Other methods for patients with laryngectomies to speak are esophageal speech and tracheoesophageal puncture. Not everyone can use these devices and methods, however. Some people need to rely on communication boards and pictures to communicate. Others make use of new computer-assisted devices.

People With Language Differences
We live in a diverse society and care for patients who speak and understand English with varying degrees of fluency. In health care, more than in any other area, it is crucial that providers and patients clearly understand each other. Serious mistakes can be made when the meaning of the message is lost in translation. Many facilities provide services for language translation. This practice is costly, but it can decrease the risk of medical errors due to misunderstanding. It is also important for the interpreter to have the proper credentials from the National Board of Certification for Medical Interpreters. Such certification ensures that they have an excellent command of English as well the patient's language. Although there may be a language barrier, communication should be effective.

The common practice of using the patient's friends or family members to assist in translation is not the best option. Typically, family members are unfamiliar with medical terminology and cannot explain it to the patient; moreover, patients may be uncomfortable sharing some information in front of friends or relatives. Finally, using a patient's family or friends to translate may violate patient confidentiality and privacy according to the Health Insurance Portability and Accountability Act (HIPAA) (see Chapter 3).

Evidence-Based Practice
Your 93-year-old patient who speaks English as a second language (ESL) is brought to the hospital for change in mental status.

Clinical Question
When would the patient need an interpreter for a positive outcome while in the hospital?

Evidence
In the past, when a patient whose second language was English was admitted to the hospital, the interpreter was usually a family member or friend. If the patient were alone, then interpretation was done with a telephone system or by one of the staff. This practice created gaps in the patient's care because information could be missed from admission until discharge. Many times, this situation produced a negative outcome. A study found that positive-outcome guidelines were needed to achieve a desired outcome when selecting the most effective communication strategy for a patient in need of an interpreter.

Implications for Nursing Practice
Use your facilities interpreter resources. Review and follow the guidelines of the Agency for Healthcare Research and Quality (AHRQ) when using staff as interpreters. Although the interpreter may speak the same language as the patient, all communication must be documented. Another effective communication strategy is timing. It is beneficial for an interpreter to be available for admission, patient teaching involving care and medication, and when the patient is being discharged.

Squires, A. (2017). Evidence-based approaches to breaking down language barriers. *Nursing, 47*(9), 34–40. https://doi.org/10.1097/01.nurse.0000522002.60278.ca

People Who Have Aphasic/Dysphasic Disorders

This is another area that offers many options for adaptive techniques. Nurses must be aware of the type and degree of aphasia/dysphasia for each patient. The health-care provider and speech pathologist or therapist are excellent resource people to help in deciding what type of adaptive technique will be the most effective. The nurse's documentation of the responses of a patient to the various techniques will also help in these decisions.

Adaptive communication techniques for aphasic/dysphasic patients range from changing the rate or pitch of speech to using objects, pictures, spelling boards, or computerized equipment if the patient has access to them (FIG. 2.3).

Keep in mind that nurses should not answer for the patient. Finishing sentences or playing guessing games with people who have these types of disorders is usually not in the best interest of the patient. It may take longer for these patients to process information and get the answer out. Be patient. When the patient is getting frustrated or is truly unable to respond properly, it may be because the words the nurse used were unfamiliar or because too much time has passed and the patient has forgotten the question. Gentle hints or rephrasing the question may be enough to help the patient. It may be just one word that makes the difference between the patient being successful or not.

Communication in all forms is essential to the work of a nurse. Taking the time to learn and use these techniques can make relationships with patients and coworkers more pleasant and rewarding.

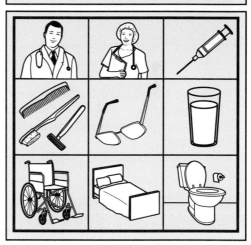

FIGURE 2.3 Picture board for patients with aphasia.

Safe and Effective Nursing Care

Provide clarity when instructing patients
Respect patients' cultural communication styles
Know the patient's learning style
Encourage patients to express themselves
Provide devices to assist in communication
Provide interpreter or interpreting devices when needed

Key Points

- Humans cannot *not* communicate. Interpersonal communication is a complex process.
- Therapeutic, or helping, communication is a language that is learned and shared by nurses. It is a purposeful skill that requires practice.
- People communicate verbally and nonverbally. Nonverbal communication sends a stronger message than verbal communication.
- Communication can be assertive or aggressive. Assertive statements are the more helpful of

the two; they start with the word "I." Aggressive statements are designed to place responsibility on another person. They start with the word "you."

- Nurses need to be aware of what blocks therapeutic communication.

- Nurses need to be aware what techniques to use to encourage effective, helping communication with patients.
- Special techniques are used when communicating with populations who have special communication needs.

Review Questions

1. Which of the following is an example of a therapeutic, open-ended question?
   a. "Why did you do that, Mrs. Jones?"
   b. "How can I help you, Mr. Thompson?"
   c. "Can I help you, Ms. Greene?"
   d. "Please, can I ask you a question, Mark?"

2. The purpose of therapeutic communication is to:
   a. Develop a friendly, social relationship with the patient.
   b. Develop a parental, authoritarian relationship with the patient.
   c. Develop a helping, purposeful relationship with the patient.
   d. Develop a cool, businesslike relationship with the patient.

3. You observe a patient in the family lounge. She appears to be talking to herself. You want to find out what is wrong. Your best approach to her might be:
   a. "Who are you talking to?"
   b. "Please stop talking. You are disturbing the other people."
   c. "I saw your lips moving. Can you tell me what you are talking about?"
   d. "Why are you talking to yourself?"

4. Your patient asks you the results of his blood tests. You respond:
   a. "They are all negative."
   b. "Why do you want to know?"
   c. "I think you should wait until your physician comes in."
   d. "I am not able to tell you right now, but I will call your physician and have her stop in to explain them to you."

5. Your patient is a single parent who has just been diagnosed with terminal cancer. She is concerned about returning to work and asks many questions. Finally, the patient says, "What do you think I should do?" You say:
   a. "I think you should just stay busy."
   b. "I wouldn't worry about it."
   c. "What are your thoughts about returning to work?"
   d. "Oh, you'll be just fine. There are lots of people worse off than you."

6. Your patient has refused all your attempts to care for him. You say:
   a. "I'd like to help you; what can I do?"
   b. "Why don't you like me?"
   c. "What is the matter with you?"
   d. "You must do this; it's physician's orders!"

7. Your patient is Jewish and refuses to eat nonkosher food. You say:
   a. "I will ask the dietitian to come and talk with you."
   b. "The dietitian will come to see you."
   c. "It's the best we can do. You need to eat."
   d. "You're right. The hospital food does leave much to be desired!"

8. Your patient is commenting that the physician has not been in to visit for 2 days. You say:
   a. "I hate it when that happens!"
   b. "What do you need to know?"
   c. "Well, he is very busy!"
   d. "You feel ignored by your physician?"

9. Your patient, who is usually very talkative, does not respond to you when you enter the room. You say:
   a. "What's wrong, Ms. Smith?"
   b. "Ms. Smith, is something bothering you?"
   c. "Can I help you?"
   d. "I'm wondering why you are so quiet this afternoon."

10. Ms. Smith responds to your question with "I feel like nobody cares." You respond:
    a. "Why do you say that?"
    b. "Like nobody cares? Please tell me more about what you are feeling."
    c. "Ms. Smith, you're wrong about that. Of course, we care."
    d. "Ms. Smith, maybe the doctor can change the dosage of your medication. You'll feel better."

REVIEW QUESTIONS ANSWER KEY 1.b, 2.c, 3.c, 4.d, 5.c, 6.a, 7.a, 8.d, 9.a, 10.b

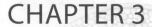

CHAPTER 3
Ethics, Evidence-Based Practice, and Regulations

KEY TERMS

Accountability
American nurses association (ANA)
American psychiatric nurses association (APNA)
Autonomy
Beneficence
Chronemics
Civil law
Commitment
Confidentiality
Culture
Culture of nurses
Doctrine of privileged information
Ethics
Evidence-based practice
Fidelity
Good samaritan laws
Health insurance portability and accountability act (HIPAA)
Intentional
Justice
Nonmaleficence
Nurse practice act
Ombudsman
Patient bill of rights
Patient self-determination act
Professional
Proxemics
Responsibility
Tort
Unintentional
Veracity

CHAPTER CONCEPTS

Culture
Ethics
Evidence-based practice
Informatics
Professionalism
Quality improvement

LEARNING OUTCOMES

1. Define professionalism.
2. Demonstrate understanding of the Nurse Practice Act.
3. Define five types of ethics.
4. Explain the difference between ethics for nurses and evidenced-based practice.
5. State the importance of accuracy in verbal reporting and written documentation.
6. State the importance of confidentiality.
7. Explain what HIPAA is and its role in health-care delivery.
8. Explain what the Joint Commission is and its role in healthcare delivery.
9. Explain the Good Samaritan Act.
10. Explain the difference between involuntary and voluntary commitment.
11. Define patient advocacy.

PROFESSIONALISM

Professional is a word with many different meanings. At its most basic, professional means "characterized by or conforming to the technical or ethical standards of a profession" (Merriam-Webster, 2017). *All* nurses and other health-care providers are expected to behave in a professional manner; they are to perform at the highest level of preparation they have achieved. Nurses are to abide by federal, state, and local guidelines. As professionals, nurses have a duty to stay informed in the nursing field. Participating in professional organizations and continuing education programs is important.

Employers, coworkers, and patients expect a nurse to maintain professional behavior, despite any personal problems the nurse is experiencing. A nurse's personal problems are to be handled outside of the work environment. Nurses are expected to be respectful of the beliefs of their patients and coworkers and not to force their personal beliefs on others at work. Nurses are expected to perform honestly. They are expected to report any infractions they notice in other nurses. In short, nurses are expected to behave and perform in a manner that promotes the pride and reputation of the nursing profession and not in a way that is a detriment to that profession.

 # ETHICS

Part of being a professional is to conduct yourself in an ethical manner. **Ethics** is conducting yourself in a manner that reflects fundamental moral principles that govern behavior. Ethics is knowing what is right and what is wrong. Nurses are faced with ethical issues daily, so it is important to know both your own values and the profession's code of ethics. The Codes of Ethics of the **American Nurses Association (ANA)** and the National Association of Licensed Practical Nurses (NALPN) Nursing Practice Standards – *Legal/Ethical Status* (Appendix D) have established guidelines for the nursing profession. These guidelines provide a framework for taking ethical action rather than simply giving answers to ethical questions. There are several ethical principles that nurses must deal with daily:

• Autonomy
• Beneficence
• Nonmaleficence
• Justice
• Veracity
• Fidelity

Autonomy refers to the nurse's ability to act independently at times and to self-direct, as well as to a patient's ability to make their own decisions. An autonomous patient is one who has the cognitive ability to make a conscious decision. For example, the patient has the right to choose or refuse medical interventions. It is necessary for the nurse to provide adequate information so that patients have sufficient understanding to make a decision that is appropriate for themselves.

In **beneficence,** the nurse acts for the good or welfare of the patient. For example, the nurse provides the patient with needed tools to make an informed decision.

A guiding principle of health-care professionals is **nonmaleficence;** that is, to "do no harm." Safety for both you and your patients must be in your thoughts at all times. Safety and effective nursing care (SENC) is the outcome desired for all patients.

Harm can be described as **intentional** or **unintentional** and falls under the category of a tort, which relates to civil law. **Civil laws** protect patients/persons and their property.

Justice refers to the principle that health-care providers should provide care fairly and justly. Treatment should be given equally, no matter if a patient's values, race, gender identity, sexuality, religious beliefs, primary language, or economic status differ from that of the health-care provider.

Veracity (honesty) is another quality of professionalism. No matter your level of nursing discipline, the professional choice is always to tell the truth. It may be painful, frightening, or embarrassing to admit personal conflicts, errors or omissions in patient care, but nurses will avoid further potential harm to their patient as well as to their professional reputation by admitting to mistakes and taking the appropriate corrective measures. Nurses are human. Despite their best efforts and multiple medication checks, nurses make mistakes. Recognizing them, admitting them, and taking corrective measures to ensure the patient's safety are the signs of sound judgment and professional nursing behavior. Honesty can also mean the difference between keeping and losing your nursing license. Veracity can allow a facility to research if the error made can be avoided in the future or if the traditional practice has led to other negative outcomes.

Fidelity refers to being faithful to the promise that you make as a nurse. One version of this promise is shown in Box 3.1. Examples of fidelity include being competent, attending nursing conferences, maintaining continuing education as mandated for licensure, and providing care based on the best available evidence.

Box 3.1

The Florence Nightingale Pledge

This nursing pledge was composed in 1893:

I solemnly pledge myself before God and in the presence of this assembly to pass my life in purity and to practice my profession faithfully. I will abstain from whatever is deleterious and mischievous and will not take or knowingly administer any harmful drug. I will do all in my power to maintain and elevate the standard of my profession and will hold in confidence all personal matters committed to my keeping and all family affairs coming to my knowledge in the practice of my calling. With loyalty will I endeavor to aid the physician in his work and devote myself to the welfare of those committed to my care.

https://nursing.vanderbilt.edu/news/florence-nightingale-pledge/

Tool Box

The Code of Ethics from the American Nurses Association can be found at www.nursingworld.org/codeofethics.

EVIDENCE-BASED PRACTICE

Florence Nightingale believed that caring for soldiers' wounds properly would decrease infections. When she tested this hypothesis in practice, the cleaning and caring for wounds resulted in fewer infections among the soldiers, creating a positive outcome. This provided evidence that Nightingale's hypothesis was correct. **Evidence-based practice** (EBP) refers to practices found through research that provide a positive outcome when applied to patient care. According to Muir-Gray, EBP "is about doing what works, and doing it the right way to achieve the best possible patient outcome" (1997, cited in Hopp & Rittenmeter, 2021, p. 4).

Currently, many nursing programs provide students with resources resembling the nursing boards. These resources monitor student-learning outcomes throughout their program and identify if there is a need for remediation in a specific topic. These outcome predictors allow the student to identify and fill gaps in classroom and laboratory/clinical skills, which may affect their success when they sit for the National Council Licensure Examination (NCLEX) examination for licensure.

Familiarity with both ethics and evidence-based practice will assist you in understanding the standards of care and the Nurse Practice Act.

Standards of Care

A variety of nursing organizations have created codes of conduct and standards of care to guide nurses in their practice. For example, the National Association of Licensed Practical Nurses (NALPN) has adopted Standards of Nursing Practice for LPNs/LVNs (Appendix D). These standards include a code of conduct. The **American Nurses Association (ANA)** has written about standards of care regarding topics important to the nursing profession, some of which are relevant to Licensed Practical Nurse (LPN) and Licensed Vocational Nurse (LVN). The purpose of the ANA is to foster high standards of nursing practice, to promote the rights of nurses in the workplace, to project a positive and realistic view of nursing, and to lobby congress and regulatory agencies on health-care issues affecting nurses and the public. According to the **American Psychiatric Nurse Association (APNA)**, evidence-based practice guided by research and applied to those treated for mental illness as well as other health issues is creating proven nursing interventions leading to positive outcomes.

Tool Box

ANA materials can be accessed at www.nursingworld.org.
Standards of Psychiatric–Mental Health Clinical Nursing Practice https://www.apna.org/?s=standards

Nurse Practice Act

Nurses must be aware of their state's Nurse Practice Act for practicing safely and within its parameters. The **Nurse Practice Act** dictates the acceptable scope of nursing practice for the different levels of nursing. When a nurse is questioning whether or not to perform a certain skill or perhaps is accused of wrongdoing, the Nurse Practice Act typically is consulted to find out if that nurse is performing at the accepted level of preparation. For example, if a state does not allow the LPN/LVN to take verbal orders and an LPN/LVN takes a verbal order, the Nurse Practice Act for that state may have been ignored. The nurse could be held liable for damages in a court of law. This can be an ethical dilemma as well. It may be the facility's policy to allow LPNs/LVNs to take verbal orders. When in doubt about the legality or ethics of an institutional policy, any nurse has the right *and* the responsibility to contact their State Board of Nursing as soon as possible to get an answer.

Classroom Activity

In Appendix D, review the NALPN Nursing Practice Standards Legal/Ethical Status. Identify how each of these standards relates to a practical/vocational nurse. Be specific.

Accurate Documentation

A nurse's best legal defense is the quality of their verbal and written communication. In her book, *Legal, Ethical, and Political Issues in Nursing,* Aiken (2004) indicates that spelling errors are crucial in liability cases, as they reflect on a nurse's general ability to care for patients. Legally, the assumption is "If it is not charted, it has not been done." Common situations can impede nurses' efforts at accuracy in charting. Nurses have demanding responsibilities, and they are frequently interrupted while caring for patients. Patient-centered care is the primary focus of a nurse's workday. Many times, it seems that the shift is over before it starts. Charting may be scaled down to a minimum, especially if the employer does not pay for overtime. However, accurate documentation is part of nursing care, and documentation enables facilities to be reimbursed. To ease the burden of charting on nurses and to improve reimbursement rates, facilities have turned to different types of charting.

Some facilities use a form of documenting called "charting by exception" in which only abnormal or unusual observations are documented in detail. This type of documentation is based on flow-sheet charting. The guidelines established at the facility are written on the flow sheet. You use a series of check marks and other symbols to indicate that assessments of all body systems have been made. You then initial the check marks and

place your full signature at the bottom of the page or wherever it is required. Only situations outside the established normal parameters are mentioned in some sort of nurse's written note. Although this type of charting saves time, it is sometimes challenged in court.

Currently, most health-care facilities use electronic medical records (EMRs) designed for patient charting to make patient information more standard, accessible, and efficient for documentation.

GOOD TO KNOW

You need to be proficient in reading, writing, and spelling. Most nursing programs require an entrance examination to determine whether nursing candidates are proficient in reading, writing, and math before being admitted into a program. Not only might gaps in reading, writing, and spelling be a source of embarrassment for you, but they are also unacceptable as professional, safe nursing practice. Deficient language skills are a much more common problem in the United States than you might think, and it is not just people from other countries who experience this difficulty. Basic computer skills are also a requirement for employment.

It is imperative to take as much time as necessary to record complete, accurate documentation on each patient. A nurse's competency to practice nursing can be questioned if for some reason the documentation is subpoenaed in a court case and spelling and grammar are of poor quality according to American standards. The Joint Commission (TJC) favors the use of the SBAR (situation, background, assessment, and recommendation) documentation style, deeming it concise and clear.

In addition to charting, all agencies and facilities have an established method for verbal reporting. It may be a recorded shift report; a grand or walking rounds report; or a one-on-one report with the incoming nurse. Again, it is important for you to spend as much time as needed to give crucial patient information gathered during your shift to the oncoming shift. Be thorough but as concise as possible. It is standard procedure to discuss each patient's vital signs, physical assessments, any visits from physicians or visitors, new orders, responses to medications and treatments, and any change in condition. An area that is sometimes forgotten is the mental, emotional, and behavioral status of the patient, especially on a medical-surgical unit. Usually, the patient's mental, emotional, and behavioral status is mentioned only if something seems inappropriate. Physical healing is affected by attitude and emotional condition; therefore, nurses should include the patient's psychological status in their verbal report. The outgoing nurse should always be sure that the incoming nurse has no further questions. In addition, the outgoing nurse should inform the incoming nurse of any task that was not completed on the prior shift.

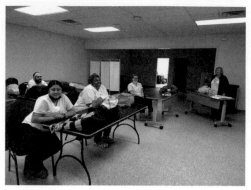

FIGURE 3.1 Through role modeling, professional values, rituals, and traditions, the culture of nursing is passed from one generation of nurses to the next. (Photo courtesy of Robynn Anwar)

CRITICAL THINKING QUESTION

You are supervising care during the 2100 to 0700 shift on a mental health unit. Another nurse who works this shift routinely has poor-quality charting. Nothing is hidden or omitted from the chart, but the nursing notes contain many misspelled words and many grammatical errors. You decide to "keep the peace" and say nothing because you get along well with this nurse and the patients like the individual.

Patient X demonstrates aggression toward Patient Y on your shift and shoves Patient Y, who then falls. Patient Y's family sues for negligence. The other nurse is found incompetent by virtue of written documentation that the court cannot decipher. To your dismay, you are also implicated as the supervising nurse on that shift because you did nothing to improve the quality of this nurse's documentation skills.

• What are your feelings?
• What might this mean for you?
• What will your defense be to the court?
• How will you handle similar situations differently in the future?

Culture of Nurses

A commonly accepted definition of **culture** includes the nonphysical traits, rituals, values, and traditions that are handed down from generation to generation. Nursing, too, passes its professional values, rituals, and traditions from generation to generation (FIG. 3.1). The affective, or attitudinal, components of nursing are behaviors that nurses typically learn by using other nurses as role models. This concept spawned the term *culture of nurses* (Neeb, 1994).

As mentioned earlier, nurses live and work in a global community. Nurses are born and raised in many different places. They have different ideas about religious, political, and social issues. However, when nurses come together as a profession, these personal ideas must give way to consistent behaviors that provide patients with the best possible evidence-based care. For example, spelling and grammar practices commonly used in personal text messages are not acceptable for documenting patient care in the United States. This is not an issue of labeling a nurse's personal or cultural belief system as right, wrong, good, or bad. Rather, it means that at work, nurses must conduct themselves like professionals and follow the basic tenets of professional communication.

A person's sense of personal space, the distance at which they are comfortable with others, is also cultural. **Proxemics** is the study of how different cultures relate to space. It is important for nurses to understand that the concept of personal space is highly dependent on culture. Why is understanding a patient's sense of personal space an important consideration for nurses?

Tool Box

Standards for cultural competency to understand the importance of a patient's culture can be found at https://www.cigna.com/assets/docs/about-cigna/thn-white-papers/cultural-competency-in-health-care-final.pdf.

Nurses must touch and observe patients in order to assess them. Registered and practical nurses make bodily assessments, even on a mental health unit, especially if the patient has a secondary diagnosis, such as chronic obstructive pulmonary disease (COPD) or heart failure. Nurses assist with noninvasive and invasive procedures. Male and female nurses care for male and female patients. In a way, nurses become desensitized to these functions, as it becomes a routine part of their jobs. However, some patients are very timid and modest. The patient may not permit a nurse of a different gender to provide care for them. And in some cultures, strangers may not touch others in certain ways. These individuals may prefer to have family members perform those tasks.

Another field of study is **chronemics**, how different cultures view time. If you have ever traveled between a big city and a small town in the United States, you may have noticed a cultural difference in time and waiting. People in the city tend to be much more rushed. They may watch the clock in restaurants, in classrooms, and while on hold on the telephone. In small towns, life is a bit slower paced. Again, this is not an issue of right or wrong, good or bad. It is an issue of differences in the way people are acculturated.

In cultures in which punctuality is not an issue, punching a time clock or serving a burger within the allotted time may not be a priority. However, in the culture of nursing, promptness is crucial. A patient who is in pain and asks for a pain medication expects the nurse to be prompt with it. If the nurse replies, "I'll be there in a minute," the patient will likely take the word *minute* literally. It may actually take the nurse 15 minutes to return with the medication. In that 15 minutes, the nurse may have had to answer another call light, assist someone to the bathroom, and prevent another patient from falling to the floor, all while bringing the medication that the first patient has requested. All that the patient in pain knows is that the nurse has not returned. Depending on the patient's culture, they may have used the call signal immediately after 1 minute had passed, or they may feel it is grossly disrespectful to ask again and thus wait while suffering silently.

In order for you to provide competent, holistic care, you need to be aware of the patient's health history as well as their cultural and spiritual beliefs. In addition to making you more effective professionally, understanding these differences enriches your personal appreciation of other cultures.

CONFIDENTIALITY

Confidentiality is so important that it is mentioned in both federal and state patient rights. Confidential means (1) marked by intimacy or willingness to confide; (2) private, secret (confidential information); (3) entrusted with confidences; and (4) containing information whose unauthorized disclosure could be prejudicial to the national interest (Merriam-Webster online).

Trusting a friend with a secret only to hear that secret was repeated to someone else is a break in confidentiality. Similarly, a patient's diagnosis and plan of care are to be discussed only with the patient and the health-care team; this information is very private and must be kept that way. But what happens when the patient shares something that *must* be passed on?

The **doctrine of privileged information** is a bond between patient and physician. Under this doctrine, the physician has the right to refuse to answer certain questions (e.g., in a court of law) and can cite "privileged physician-patient information." Nurses are usually not included in this relationship. If information is requested of nurses in a legal situation, they must answer as truthfully as they can. How does a nurse maintain honesty and confidentiality at the same time? First and foremost, you should communicate honestly to the patient that you cannot promise confidentiality in all situations. When you sense that the patient is revealing information that is potentially legally sensitive, it is a good idea to tell the patient right away that nurses are not protected by the doctrine of privileged information. Tell the patient that they can speak confidentially with the physician, but if the patient still chooses to share such information, a good technique is to tell the patient the information will have to be shared with a supervisor or others involved in the patient's treatment. The 1976 legal case of *Tarasoff v. Regents of the University of California* is the standard for the doctrine of privileged information. The doctrine also protects intended victims of patients who may be hospitalized or incarcerated. Inform the patient that only those parts of the conversation that are directly related to their care will be shared, but that if information is requested by a legal representative, you will be required to answer.

Temptations to break confidentiality are common, especially for the student nurse. It is fun and exciting to learn new information and to see your skills making a difference in someone's recovery. It is easy to start chatting about your experiences to another student or to a staff nurse, but be careful. The person nearby (e.g., in the elevator with you) may be a friend or a relative of the patient. Unless specifically authorized by the patient, these people do not ordinarily have rights to information about the patient. There are many horror stories about innocent conversations that were overheard by the "wrong" people that resulted in negative consequences to the patient and/or the nurse involved.

Whoever said hospitals were quiet places have probably never worked in one. Nurses and physicians talk often, and usually not quietly. "Dr. X is on the phone about Mrs. D's bowel surgery," calls the unit coordinator to the nurse across the hall. Such breaches of confidentiality happen not only in the hospital, but also in physicians' offices. For example, the nurse loudly announces to the provider that she just received Mrs. A's urine specimen results. "My goodness! Mrs. A has enough *E. Coli* in her urine specimen to kill a horse!"

How many patients or people in the surrounding area might have heard those exchanges? How would the patient feel if they knew that personal information had been handled so thoughtlessly? These breaches of confidentiality happen all the time, but that does not make them acceptable. Nurses must take the extra steps required to give or receive information quietly to the appropriate people (FIG. 3.2).

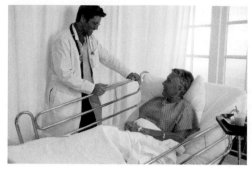

FIGURE 3.2 Maintaining privacy is a patient right and conveys caring to the patient *(photograph by Wendy Hope).*

Charts, too, can put confidentiality at risk, which is one reason facilities switched to electronic health records (EHR) systems. But even these systems are not perfect. How many eyes may have seen confidential patient information accidentally left visible on a computer screen when the nurse went to answer a call signal? What about the report sheet? Some nurses call these sheets their "cheat sheet." Nurses should be sure to keep their reports with them at all times. Here is an example of how a simple act of dropping a piece of paper led to a major event.

A nurse's cheat sheet fell from the nurse's pocket and was picked up by a patient's family member. This person could have brought the paper to the desk immediately, and the story would have ended there, but that was not the case. At the end of the shift, the family member, after reviewing the information, brought the cheat sheet to the charge nurse. None of the items on the list had been carried out, according to the family member who had been there the greater part of the day. Unfortunately, the nurse had charted these tasks as being completed. This display of unprofessional and irresponsible behavior was one thing; the family member maintained, however, that anyone could have picked up that piece of paper and learned many personal things about the patient. It contained information not only about that patient but information about other patients assigned to that nurse. The family member sued for breach of confidentiality and won the suit. Granted, this is a drastic example of what can happen, and laws regarding these situations vary from state to state. The story emphasizes that nurses must be careful with patient information of any kind and always maintain honesty in documentation. In these days of computerized and paperless documentation, nurses are still vulnerable to breeches of confidentiality.

CRITICAL THINKING QUESTION

You are an LPN/LVN on the surgical unit of the county hospital. In shift report, you are told that you will be getting a new postoperative patient within the hour. When the patient arrives, a police officer is in attendance. The officer tells you that this patient is a suspect in a homicide. The officer instructs you to report anything the patient says to you. When you begin your postoperative vital signs, the patient says, "Nurse, I shot the guy, and he deserved it. I would do it again if I had to. I can tell you because you can't tell anyone!" How will you handle this situation?

Health Insurance Portability and Accountability Act

The **Health Insurance Portability and Accountability Act of 1996 (HIPAA)** and the The Joint Commission (TJC) deal with documentation and privacy issues.

HIPAA was developed by the Department of Health and Human Services to provide national standards pertaining to the electronic transmission and communication of medical information between patients, providers, employers, and insurers. HIPAA allows more control on the part of the patient as to what part of their information is disclosed. It addresses the security and privacy involved with medical records and how that information is identified and passed between care providers. For example, Social Security numbers, which were in the past routinely used as a patient identifier, now are either not used or are used in some manner that is difficult to track, such as a partial number or a backward number. HIPAA was implemented in April of 2003. Some areas of health care, such as workers' compensation, are either exempt from HIPAA rules or are slightly less stringent in the sharing of information.

Clinical Activity

During your clinical rotation, observe the facility's HIPAA policy. Where is the policy located? Note if the HIPAA policy is violated, by whom, and how many times. What type of identifiers are used on a mental health unit?

In 2010, the U.S. Department of Health and Human Services published "Applying the Substance Abuse Confidentiality Regulations to Health Information Exchange (HIE)." This document contains frequently asked questions about confidentiality for patients being treated for drug and alcohol abuse. The document is located at https://www.samhsa.gov/sites/default/files/faqs-applying-confidentiality-regulations-to-hie.pdf. It carefully details what can and cannot be disclosed and strongly emphasizes patient rights (discussed later in this chapter) and the necessity for the patient's signed informed consent (discussed in the Crisis Intervention section in Chapter 8).

In addition to HIPAA for alcohol and drug abuse, the National Alliance On Mental Illness (NAMI) in 2014 stated that HIPAA protects the privacy of individuals living with mental illness. This law is important because it helps protect confidential mental health treatment records.

The Joint Commission

The Joint Commission (TJC) is the leading national accrediting body of health-care organizations. Earning accreditation by TJC indicates commitment to quality on a daily basis within the entire facility. Two other goals of accreditation are reducing the risk of undesirable patient outcomes and encouraging continuous improvement. Originally established to survey hospitals, the accreditation can now be achieved by long-term care facilities, mental health agencies, home health-care agencies, and hospices that provide quality care, including mental health and substance abuse treatment to children, adolescents, and adults. Accredited facilities and clinics have demonstrated compliance with the highest standards of clinical care and administrative quality.

In 2004, TJC established the National Patient Safety Goals (NPSG). These goals are revised annually. Among these goals are identifying sentinel events, identifying the sources of hospital acquired infections (HAIs), ensuring the use of two patient identifiers, and discontinuing the use of "dangerous abbreviations."

Tool Box

The Joint Commission Web site is at www.joint-commission.org
National Patient Safety Goals
https://www.jointcommission.org/standards/national-patient-safety-goals/

You have just started working on a medical unit. You have been assigned a patient called "Ms. X." You are curious about the fact that Ms. X is not using her real name. While reading her chart, you learn she is in an abusive relationship and has a history of substance abuse. You see the warning that "Ms. X's husband is not allowed in the unit at any time." When you go to meet the patient, you are shocked; Ms. X is your next-door neighbor. What do you do? What do you say to her husband? What do you say when your family asks you, "What happened at work today?"

RESPONSIBILITY

Responsibility is a key concept at all levels of nursing practice; however, responsibility does not necessarily mean independence. Responsibility for the professional registered nurse (RN) can mean different things than it does for the LPN/LVN. Nurses are expected to know their scope of practice for their state. *Responsibility* means performing to the best of one's ability within the boundaries of that scope of practice. Sometimes this means knowing when to say "No." Sometimes it means calling the state governing agency to ask specific questions.

Responsible behavior for a nurse also means keeping their personal life in a manageable state. Nurses need to be physically and emotionally prepared to be helpful to patients, and this cannot be done if their personal health is neglected. Nobody wants to be tended by a nurse who is not sleeping well or is preoccupied with personal problems. A good rule for nurses is to follow the recommendations in their personal lives that they would give to their patients.

It is a nurse's responsibility to communicate clearly with patients and with other health-care providers. Nurses must be alert to changes in patients' conditions, both physical and psychological. The actions nurses perform, the observations they make, and the documentation they complete are the most effective ways to be helpful and to ensure continuity of care for patients.

Agencies have different ways of organizing the way nurses perform their jobs. Some agencies practice team nursing; others assign primary-care patients for whom the nurse is responsible during the

entire hospitalization. Some facilities use a "buddy system" to ensure help for lifting and to cover the patient load during breaks or meetings. Regardless of the system used, each nurse is in some way interdependent with other staff members.

Being familiar with and using the techniques of communication discussed in Chapter 2 will ensure that you are able to share information and to assert yourself politely, effectively, and clearly. The responsibility nurses have for each other professionally is different from the kind of responsibility they have for their patients, but it is every bit as important, for it ultimately affects the quality of care nurses are able to give.

ACCOUNTABILITY

Accountability for nurses is part of working independently within their scope of practice. Nurses are accountable for their own actions. Being accountable is important in all settings—hospitals, long-term care facilities, private homes, physicians' offices, or psychiatric facilities. Accountability includes knowing when to ask for help, being familiar with your employer's policies and procedures, finding a reference to refresh your memory, and looking up an unfamiliar medication. It means doing everything you possibly can do to ensure that you are providing the safest, most accurate care to patients. It also means that when you agree to follow through with an order or a request, you do so.

You depend on other staff members to come to work. The patient acuity on the unit is high. What happens when you must work one or two people short? Who really suffers as a result? How do you feel when your "buddy" or helper overstays a break or mealtime? What is your response to that? How do staff absences affect patient care? How do they affect your ability to perform safely?

Impaired Nurses

Inappropriate use and misuse of mind-altering chemicals such as alcohol, prescription drugs, or nonprescription drugs can render a nurse legally unsafe. Continuing to practice nursing while using these chemicals displays unprofessional behavior and poor judgment. A nurse in this situation may be fearful of losing their license and also afraid or embarrassed to seek help. They may consider inaccurate charting, omission of certain charting, or blatant lying about a situation as a way to remain employed. The patient's safety is not the nurse's primary concern when this happens. Many states have developed programs to assist impaired nurses as a way to protect both the public and nurses. According to the Recovery and Monitoring Program (RAMP) in New Jersey, if a health professional is impaired and working with patients, an occupational hazard eventually will occur, possibly causing an injury or even a death. A resource for nurses with substance abuse issues is "Programs and Resources to Assist Nurses With Substance Use Disorders" (Eisenhut, 2016).

CLASSROOM ACTIVITY

Review and discuss the RAMP Web site for impaired nurses. Follow your state guidelines. Use https://www.nursingcenter.com/journalarticle?
Article_ID = 3386413&Journal_ID = 1444159 &Issue_ID = 3386006

CRITICAL THINKING QUESTION

You are working in an oncology unit, and a nurse whom you considered reliable and accountable in the past has had recent changes in behavior that lead you to suspect some type of impairment. This nurse frequently offers to give your patients pain medicine if you are busy. The nurse's other coworkers have noted that immediately before or after giving a narcotic, the nurse usually has to use the bathroom. How would you approach this situation?

 ## ABIDING BY THE CURRENT REGULATIONS

Good Samaritan Laws

Good Samaritan laws offer immunity from prosecution for citizens who stop to assist someone in need of medical help. Good Samaritan laws may not always protect nurses, physicians, and other medically trained personnel, especially if they are on duty. The Good Samaritan law came out of tort law. A **tort** is "a wrongful act other than a breach of contract for which relief may be obtained in the form of damages or an injunction" (Merriam-Webster Online). Good Samaritan laws vary from state to state, so it is important to understand the implication of this law in your state. The basis for all Good Samaritan laws, however, is that a third party cannot be charged with negligence unless help is given recklessly or that person makes the situation significantly worse, according to the guidelines for that particular state.

Tool Box

Link to Good Samaritan laws throughout the United States:
https://www.aafp.org/fpm/2008/0400/p37.html

Involuntary Commitment

Nurses need to be aware of their state laws and guidelines affecting **commitment**. Each state has its own regulations about people who need to be hospitalized against their will. This action is reserved for people exhibiting behavior that makes them potentially dangerous to themselves or to others. Involuntarily commitment should be used as a last resort. The average length of time for involuntary commitment is approximately 48 to 72 hours, but it can be more or less depending on state law. During this time, the person is observed and examined by the medical and nursing staff. The patient has full ability to exercise their rights under H.R. 10, the Civil Rights of Institutionalized Persons Act. At the end of the legal "hold," the patient chooses either to leave or to stay for further treatment. Most of the time, the patient realizes a need for help and stays.

Sometimes, it is the professional opinion of the treatment team that the patient remains a threat to self or to the community but that the patient cannot make the appropriate decision. This then becomes an issue of proving incompetence and becomes a matter for the legal system.

Voluntary Commitment

Most patients who are hospitalized for some type of mental illness are there voluntarily; that is, at some point they realized they needed help. This does not mean they are happy to be there, of course. There remains a stigma in the United States about being hospitalized for problems relating to a person's emotions or behavior. Many times, society assumes that these disorders are weaknesses in character rather than illnesses. It can be embarrassing to be labeled "mentally ill"; this diagnosis can follow a person for life and affect their personal and professional relationships. Being diagnosed with a mental illness could possibly prevent a person from obtaining life insurance. It is no wonder that sometimes people allow themselves to be hospitalized for a mental illness only as a last resort. Patients who agree to voluntary treatment are legally allowed to sign themselves out; however, this is often discouraged by the treatment staff except under certain situations. It is possible for the staff to institute an involuntary commitment for a patient who is voluntarily committed if they consider the person to be potentially dangerous to others and/or themselves. Voluntary and involuntary commitments are discussed in more detail in Chapter 8.

Restraint Usage

In both involuntary and voluntary admission to a facility, only a physician or a nurse practitioner may order the use of restraints except in an emergency. According to the American Medical Association (AMA) Medical Opinion 1.2.7, the physician will determine whether the restraint will be physical or chemical. Safety is an issue when the patient is in restraints. If not applied properly, a physical restraint can injure a patient, create a permanent disability, or result in a death. The patient should be monitored frequently, and monitoring should be documented. If possible, try alternatives before using restraints, perhaps sitting with patient or giving them something meaningful to hold. Review the restraint policy set by your facility or TJC. All oral orders for physical restraints must be signed by a health-care provider within 24 hours.

PATIENTS' RIGHTS

In the 1960s, the Civil Rights Movement was often in the news. The American Civil Liberties Union (ACLU) sought to gain rights for oppressed people of many different backgrounds. It was largely due to the efforts of this group that civil rights for people in prisons and for those warehoused in institutions for the mentally ill were addressed.

By the 1980s, the **Patient Bill of Rights** became a requirement for people receiving care in a mental health facility, as well as for the health-care workers providing that care. These rights vary from state to state but are based on federal guidelines and are supported in most states. Agencies in states subscribing to a Patient Bill of Rights must have the rights listed and displayed in a prominent place in the facility. Patients must be informed of the implications of their rights and must be given a copy of the Bill of Rights upon admission to the health-care facility. This also is mandated when care is provided in the home. Table 3.1 lists frequently adopted patient rights.

In addition to these frequently adopted patient rights, some states have adopted a set of patient rights for psychiatric patients. These rights may include the patient's right to

- Marry or divorce
- Sue or be sued
- Be actively involved in their care
- Be employed if possible
- Retain licenses (driver's license, license to practice one's profession)

In 1990, the U.S. Congress passed the **Patient Self-Determination Act (PSDA),** which all health-care agencies must follow. PSDA includes the following patient rights:

1. The right to facilitate their own health-care decisions
2. The right to accept or refuse medical treatment
3. The right to make an advance health-care directive

Clinical Activity

During your clinical rotation, ask a staff nurse to see the facility's Patient Bill of Rights. Is it written in languages other than English?

Clinical Activity

Compare nurse–patient interactions now and before the Patient Bill of Rights became effective. Interview a nurse who was working in the field before the bill's passage and a nurse working since the bill's passage. Determine how the Patient Bill of Rights has affected or changed nurses' interactions with patients.

Table 3.1

Most Frequently Adopted Patient Rights

Patient Right	Description	Nursing Considerations
1. Treatment in the least restrictive alternative	Patients are not to be held in any stricter conditions than their behavior or diagnosis warrants.	Patients are not to be hospitalized if they can be treated as outpatients and are not to be kept in lockup if not dangerous, and so on. Check the agency protocol and health-care provider's orders for the individual patient. You must still maintain safety for the patient and others. You also treat the patient with dignity.
2. Freedom from restraints and seclusion (except in emergencies)	Restraining can be with either physical or chemical restraints. Many areas require specific diagnosis-related restraint orders.	Be aware of the individual's diagnosis and correlating orders. • Make accurate observations and documentation about the patient's physical and behavioral response to restraint. • One guideline is to check circulatory function every half hour and to exercise and reposition the patient in restraint at least every 2 hours.
3. Give or refuse consent for medications/treatments (including electroconvulsive therapy [ECT] and psychosurgery)	All patients have the right to say yes or no to treatments that affect them. This must be *informed* consent, meaning the patient fully understands the treatment, potential outcomes, and potential effects of refusal.	Nurses can reinforce the health-care provider's explanation of treatment. Examine the patient's understanding; if there is little or no understanding of treatment, the nurse needs to have the provider return and explain again to the patient and significant others.
4. Possess and have access to personal belongings	Anything of a personal nature that the patient wishes to remain with him or her must be given to the patient. If any item poses a threat to the patient's safety or the safety of health-care providers, remove it and document.	Carefully document any teaching about safety of personal items. If your local laws allow, have the patient sign a waiver of responsibility for personal items.
5. Daily exercise	Patients need some form of physical activity at least once daily.	Exercise is according to patient's ability and activity order. Exercise can range from passive range of motion (PROM) to the most strenuous activity the patient can safely perform.
6. Visitors	Patient can visit with anyone they choose.	Determine at time of intake who will be visiting regularly. In cases of family concern over certain people the patient may wish to visit with, safety must be a key issue. At times, nurses may need to monitor visits and visitors. Carefully document the patient's emotional and physical outcome of visits.

Continued

Table 3.1

Most Frequently Adopted Patient Rights—cont'd

Patient Right	Description	Nursing Considerations
7. Writing materials	Paper, pencils, pens, and so forth must be available to patients.	Unless contraindicated for safety reasons, nurses can assist in ensuring that these items are available at all times. If safety is an issue (e.g., stabbing self or others with a sharp object), this condition needs to be noted in charting.
8. Uncensored mail	Mail must not be opened before the patient receives it.	If patient is unable to physically open the mail or if there is concern that the patient will lose a check, for example, the nurse or another agent of the facility may witness the opening of the mail. Arrangements can be made with a family member or guardian to sign checks or see to the patient's affairs if the patient is unable to do so.
9. Courts and attorneys	Legal access remains intact for anyone who is hospitalized, whether voluntarily or involuntarily.	Patients can call an attorney at any time. Nurses and agency representatives may be asked to help them. In cases when this seems inappropriate, patient, staff, and family can discuss alternatives in a family conference. Any outcomes need to be incorporated into the care plan and documented.
10. Employment compensation	Wages are not to be withheld during hospitalization.	Under certain legal conditions, compensation may be withheld for reasons other than a stay in a health-care facility. This would be confidential information but must be incorporated into the care plan and documentation.
11. Confidentiality (records, treatment, and so on)	Information about the patient is to be kept secure and private.	Discussion of the patient's condition must take place only in designated places and with designated persons. • Many states have cautioned nurses against giving *any* information regarding the patient over the telephone. In some states, a nurse can be in jeopardy of losing a license for releasing information over the phone. • Be careful of the wording in your charting. • Release information only to those people who are specifically required or legally entitled to have it.
12. Be informed of these rights	Patients must have full understanding of their civil rights while under facility care.	The nurse or the facility representative will explain in detail the meaning of these rights for the patient. Depending on your local law and agency policy, the patient may be asked to sign a document stating that these rights have been explained. Usually, a copy is then kept with the patient record and the patient keeps a personal copy.

PATIENT ADVOCACY

With the emergence of the Patient Bill of Rights, the role of a patient **ombudsman** was created to speak out for patients' needs. These individuals are either volunteers within the community or paid workers from an agency whose job is to ensure that patients, especially those considered vulnerable, are being treated in a safe, legal manner.

Part of a nurse's scope of practice is to be a voice, or an advocate, for the patients under their care. This is the meaning of patient advocacy as it applies to nurses. For example, your patient, who does not speak English, is asked to sign consent for surgery. The physician explaining the procedure and its risks sees the patient nodding his head and believes that the patient understands what is being said. The surgeon proceeds to give the patient a pen and the consent form to sign. Being aware the patient has a deficiency in communication, you have the responsibility to make the physician aware of the situation and to arrange for resources to enable the patient to understand what they are signing. To assist this patient, you must ensure that the patient is able to give *informed* consent for the surgery.

Nurses and other health-care workers also have a moral, legal, and ethical responsibility to report known or suspected abuse or neglect of people who cannot care for themselves.

COMMUNITY RESOURCES

According to the provisions of the Community Mental Health Centers Act, every community should offer some form of help to people with mental health disorders and those who abuse drugs. This help can be in the form of hospital emergency rooms, shelters, crisis centers, or social service offices. Most communities have a list available for the asking. Clinics and hospitals provide resources to people who are concerned that they or others are at risk for mental health or drug abuse issues. Depending on the facility's policies, the nurse may be able to help patients choose a community resource to access after discharge. Be sure to provide information on fees for the services provided by the individual agencies and accepted insurance. Some agencies are free, whereas some provide assistance on a "sliding scale" or according to ability to pay.

If the facility does not have or provide a list of community resources at the time of discharge, you can suggest that the patient find resources online or in a local public health office. Shelters for victims of abuse usually are *not* advertised; these are kept confidential to maintain safety for the people who need them.

Safe and Effective Nursing Care

Practice within the Nurse Practice Act established by your state
Advocate for your patients
Encourage patients to self-advocate
Provide patient with Bill of Rights document
Report suspected patient abuse or neglect
Maintain ethical standards of nursing
Obtain continuing education credits in evidence-based practice
Maintain patient confidentiality
Prevent HIPAA violations
Include patient in decisions about their own care, therapies, and medications

---

Key Points

- It is the nurse's responsibility to know the Code of Ethics and standards of nursing practice for the state in which they are practicing. These will vary from state to state.
- Caring for mental health patients means applying evidence-based methods to produce a positive outcome.
- *Collaborative practice* means working together with all levels of nursing and all ancillary disciplines to provide the best possible care for the patient.
- Honesty in nursing practice and excellence in verbal and written communication are crucial to the care of the patient and to the credibility of the nurse. A nurse's competency can be questioned if his or her English spelling and grammar are poor.

- Cultural considerations such as space, time, waiting, language, and touch (to name a few) are important parts of the nurse–patient relationship. They are also important in the culture of nursing. A nurse's personal beliefs may differ from the patients' and from the standards that are part of the culture of nurses.

- The patient's well-being and wishes, the state Nurse Practice Act, and agency policy dictate how nurses can care for the patient in a safe and respectful manner.

CASE STUDY

Nurse P, LPN, had worked for a long-term care facility in a small midwestern community for 10 years. Over the years, Nurse P gained the trust and respect of everyone she worked with or cared for on the job. Nurse P's reputation was very good in the community as well. One day, a resident asked Nurse P, "Go to my purse and get my glasses, would you please?" The resident had made this request many times before, so Nurse P had no reason for concern. Several hours later, a family member noticed that the resident was missing some cash and a wedding ring, which she kept in her purse "for safe-keeping." The resident recalled asking Nurse P to retrieve the glasses from the purse. Other residents and staff had also seen Nurse P looking in the resident's purse. The case went to small claims court. Nurse P was found guilty and was made to pay restitution. In addition, Nurse P's license to practice nursing in that state was revoked.

1. What could Nurse P have done to avoid this situation?
2. What are your thoughts about this situation? About the resident? About Nurse P? About the "fairness" of the situation?
3. What are your feelings about this situation?
4. What are Nurse P's chances of becoming licensed again? In her state? In another state? What would the results have been if this had happened in your state?

Review Questions

1. The code of behavior that reflects professional expectations based on fundamental moral principles is called:
   a. Commitment
   b. Ethics
   c. Nurse Practice Act
   d. Patient Bill of Rights

2. The document that defines the scope of nursing practice in each state is called:
   a. Commitment
   b. Ethics
   c. Nurse Practice Act
   d. Patient Bill of Rights

3. The set of rules designed to protect patients and others who are described as "vulnerable" is called:
   a. Doctrine of Privileged Information
   b. Collaborative practice
   c. Nurse Practice Act
   d. Patient Bill of Rights

4. Sandra, an RN from the local pool/registry, and you, the staff LPN/LVN, are working at a facility. You see Sandra charting her medications and treatments before she administers them. Choose the best therapeutic communication technique to use when approaching Sandra:
   a. "Why are you doing that?"
   b. "I am concerned about the legality and safety of charting before giving medications, Sandra."
   c. "You know it is wrong to chart before giving the medications."
   d. "You really shouldn't do that, Sandra."

5. A few hours later, Sandra gets sick and goes home. You know that she charted before giving her medications, and you saw her passing out some medications. You are not sure who got their medications and who did not. Mrs. G, a patient who is alert and oriented and a reliable historian for herself, sees you and says, "That new nurse forgot my medication this morning. It's my heart medication, and I need it. Would you get it for me?" You see the medication has been charted already. Your next action would be:
   a. Refuse the patient, telling her, "You're mistaken, Mrs. G. That medication is signed for, so you must have gotten it."
   b. Give Mrs. G her heart medication and assume she is right.
   c. Call the physician.
   d. Inform your supervisor of the entire situation.

6. The Health Insurance Portability and Accountability Act:
   a. Requires patients to be treated in designated regional treatment centers
   b. Approves of patient records being transported in personal vehicles by medical staff
   c. Allows patients to have some say in what medical information can be divulged and to whom
   d. Prohibits all transmission of medical records electronically

7. Mr. Richards has just had bilateral total knee replacement. He is in your transitional care unit. He repeatedly calls out in pain, disturbing the other residents, yet he refuses to take the prescribed pain medication, stating, "You're all just trying to knock me out." You:
   a. Shut his door, leaving him alone until he settles
   b. Offer another pain relief technique, realizing he has the right to refuse medication
   c. Have additional staff come to the room to assist while you administer a prescribed injection
   d. Inform him his behavior is not appropriate and is disruptive to others, and that he needs to stop calling out

8. The LPN/LVN knows that his or her scope of practice includes all of the following except:
   a. Administering nursing care under the direction of an RN
   b. Documenting the patient's data
   c. Independently ordering medications for the patient
   d. Assisting the physician or registered nurse with more complex care and procedures

9. The patient is semiconscious and is in need of emergency surgery to relieve a subdural hematoma. The nurse knows that:
   a. Emergency situations do not require prior consent.
   b. They must obtain written consent for invasive procedures.
   c. This is not a function of the LPN/LVN; the nurse should call his or her supervisor.
   d. The patient must be alert in order to give informed consent.

10. Mr. B is a 65-year-old attorney who has been admitted to your floor for blood work and neurological examinations. He is loud and verbally demanding of the staff. He says, "I know my rights. You nurses have to do whatever I ask. It's your job." The nurse responds:
    a. "That is not one of your rights, Mr. B."
    b. "You are taking time away from other patients, Mr. B."
    c. "The Patient Bill of Rights does make some provisions, Mr. B. Let me sit and talk with you about those rights."
    d. "Why are you so angry, Mr. B?"

REVIEW QUESTIONS ANSWER KEY 1.b, 2.c, 3.d, 4.b, 5.d, 6.c, 7.b, 8.c, 9.c, 10.c

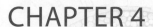

CHAPTER 4
Developmental Psychology Throughout the Life Span

KEY TERMS

Accommodation
Assimilation
Autonomy
Behavior
Behavioral theorist
Ego
Id
Lunar month
Maslow's hierarchy of needs
Negative reinforcers
Menarche
Operant conditioning
Positive reinforcers
Psychoanalytic
Psychosexual
Puberty
Self-esteem
Superego
Unconscious

CHAPTER CONCEPTS

Cognition
Culture
Evidence-based practice
Grief and loss
Growth and development
Health promotion

LEARNING OUTCOMES

1. Identify major theories of development from newborn through adult development.
2. Identify developmental tasks from prenatal development through death, according to the major theorists.
3. Identify possible outcomes of ineffective development, according to the major theorists.
4. Identify the five stages of grief/death according to Kübler-Ross.

 HUMAN DEVELOPMENT

The study of developmental psychology encompasses the study of human growth and development, a subdivision of psychology. This chapter covers only the very basics of human development. An introduction to the main theorists in the field of child development is presented, along with others whose theories are applied more in the areas of adult personality development. An overview of general physical and behavioral traits commonly seen in the different stages of human development will be addressed later in the chapter.

> **GOOD TO KNOW**
> Remember, the different views of psychological development presented in this chapter are theories. No single theory applies to *everyone* in *every* instance; these theories are based on a statistical sample of the average population. Each person is unique. Individuals are subject to different factors such as genetics and environment, which may affect development.

Each person develops at their own pace. While reading and learning about these theories, compare them with your personal experiences and observations. Some theorists' ideas may align with your experiences and beliefs better than other theorists' ideas do. Although you are not expected to adopt any of the theories discussed in this text, you do need to have a working knowledge of the main theories of human development.

You will also want to observe your patient's current behavior, how they act and react. Review the patient's mental health history, and compare their chronological age with some of the developmental theories.

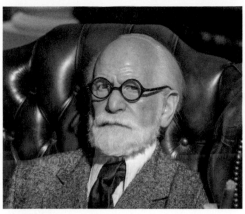

FIGURE 4.1 Sigmund Freud

CRITICAL THINKING QUESTION

Do other cultures use any of these developmental theories to understand human development? Do they use other, culture-specific theories of human development?

DEVELOPMENTAL THEORISTS: NEWBORN TO ADOLESCENCE

Sigmund Freud (1856–1939)

The theories of Sigmund Freud (FIG. 4.1) are considered controversial in today's world. Sigmund Freud was an Austrian neurologist. He asserted, after closely observing children, that the personality developed as early as age 5 and fully developed by age 12. He said that the personality must develop in a certain way at strictly defined ages and that failure to progress in this manner would certainly lead to dysfunction. Bear in mind that the life span of Western Europeans during Freud's lifetime was much shorter than it is today, so 12 years of age seemed much

older than it does by today's standards. According to Debra Kelly (2015), Freud's historical studies were of adults who were troubled during their lifetime. More or less, this is where Freud's assumptions about human **behavior** were based.

One of Freud's main tenets, or theoretical assumptions, was that behaviors resulting from ineffective personality development were **unconscious.** He theorized that ineffective personality development was in some way related to the relationship of the child to the parent and that it was related to what he called psychosexual development.

Freud's theories have validity for some people today, but others reject them. Freud is of particular interest because, in addition to his highly debated ideas, he was the first theorist to also offer a reasonably organized method of treatment. Because he was the first publicized theorist, all other theories have evolved as a result of his theories. Sigmund Freud's theories surface in almost every topic covered in this text. All other theorists compare their theories with Freud's, either in agreement or in opposition.

Table 4.1 shows Freud's psychosexual, or **psychoanalytic**, stages of development. Included in

Table 4.1
Freud's Stages of Development (Psychoanalytic or Psychosexual Stages)

Stage of Development	Approximate Ages	Tasks/Characteristics	Examples of Unsuccessful Task Completion
Oral	Birth–18 months	Use mouth and tongue to deal with anxiety (e.g., sucking, feeding)	Smoking, alcoholism, obesity, nail biting, drug addiction, difficulty trusting

Continued

Table 4.1

Freud's Stages of Development (Psychoanalytic or Psychosexual Stages)—cont'd

Stage of Development	Approximate Ages	Tasks/Characteristics	Examples of Unsuccessful Task Completion
Anal	18 months–3 years	Muscle control in bladder, rectum, anus provides sensual pleasure and parent pleasing; toilet training can be a crisis	Constipation, perfectionism, obsessive-compulsive disorder
Phallic	3–6 year	• Learn sexual identity and awareness of genital area as source of pleasure; conflict ends as child represses urge and identifies with same-sex parent. • Electra complex: "Penis envy"—daughter wants father for herself; discovers boys are different from her. • Oedipus complex: Son wants mother to himself; father is a rival.	Homosexuality, transgenderism, gender-identity problems in general, difficulty accepting authority Diagnostic and Statistical Manual (DSM-5) does not recognize homosexuality, transgenderism, or diverse gender identities as disorders in and of themselves.
Latency	6–12 years	Quiet stage in sexual development; learns to socialize	Inability to conceptualize; lack of motivation in school or job
Genital	12 years–adulthood	Sexual maturity and satisfactory relationships	Frigidity, impotence, premature ejaculation, serial marriages, unsatisfactory relationships

the table are some of the expected behaviors Freud thought one might witness as a child passes through these ages. The last column lists some behaviors Freud thought may reveal failure to progress through this stage of personality development. Discussion of Freud and his adolescence to adulthood theories continues later in this chapter.

Erik Erikson (1902–1994)

Erik Erikson (FIG. 4.2) was a German psychoanalyst who later moved to America and was a follower of Freud. Erikson took Freud's main concepts and expanded them to include nonphysical criteria. Erikson understood that people are individuals and that no matter how young the person, everyone is different. Erikson's theory began in a person's infancy and continued to late adulthood. Erikson's theory is classified as psychosocial theory. Erikson's observations indicated a variable different from the psychosexual and

age-specific theory offered by Freud. That variable is called an emotional component. Table 4.2 shows Erikson's eight stages of development. Frequently, his stages are identified by the words highlighted in the developmental tasks column. Note that the developmental tasks are always listed as opposites (e.g., trust versus mistrust) of each other. This is one way that Erikson projected his ideas about emotional fluctuation in people. Some publications call Erikson's last stage ego integrity versus despair rather than integrity versus despair. According to Kendra Cherry's (2020) explanation of integrity versus despair, "people reflect back on the life they have lived and have come away with either a sense of fulfilment from a life well lived or a sense of regret and despair over a life misspent" (Cherry, Section 1, para 2). In ego integrity versus despair, the person has resolved the issue that may have created some regrets and is now content and able to move on with their life.

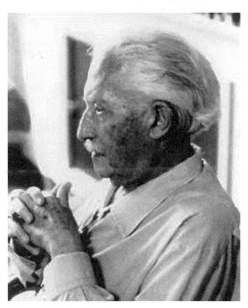

FIGURE 4.2 Erik Erikson

Classroom Activity

Describe which of Erik Erikson stages in his developmental theories you have experienced:

- Adolescence (identity versus role confusion)
- Young adult (intimacy versus isolation)
- Adulthood (generativity versus stagnation)
- Maturity (integrity versus despair)

Clinical Activity

Select an adult patient during your clinical experience and compare their biological age with Erikson's developmental stages. Do your patient's biological age and Erikson's developmental stage align?

Table 4.2
Erikson's Eight Stages of Development

Stage	Approximate Ages	Developmental Tasks	Examples	Examples of Unsuccessful Task Completion
Infancy	Birth–18 months	Trust vs mistrust	Nurturing caregivers build trust in the newborn.	Suspiciousness, trouble with personal relationships
Early childhood	2–3 years	Autonomy vs shame and doubt	"No!"—Toddler learns environment can be manipulated.	Low self-esteem, dependency (on substances or people)
Preschool	3–5 years	Initiative vs guilt	Child learns assertiveness can manipulate environment; disapproval leads to guilt in the toddler.	Passive personality, strong feelings of guilt
School age	6–11 years	Industry vs inferiority	Creativity or shyness develops.	Unmotivated, unreliable

Continued

Table 4.2

Erikson's Eight Stages of Development—cont'd

Stage	Approximate Ages	Developmental Tasks	Examples	Examples of Unsuccessful Task Completion
Adolescence	12–18 years	Identity vs role confusion	Individual integrates life experiences or becomes confused.	Rebellion, substance abuse, difficulty keeping personal relationships; may regress to child-play behaviors
Young adult	19–40 years	Intimacy vs isolation	Main concern is developing intimate relationship with another.	Emotional immaturity; may deny need for personal relationships
Adulthood	40–65 years	Generativity vs stagnation	Focus is on establishing family and guiding the next generation.	Inability to show concern for anyone but self
Maturity	65 years–death	Integrity vs despair *or* ego integrity vs despair (see section in text about Erikson)	Individual accepts own life as fulfilling; if not, he or she becomes fearful of death.	Has difficulty dealing with issues of aging and death; may have feelings of hopelessness

Jean Piaget (1896–1980)

Jean Piaget (FIG. 4.3) was a Swiss psychologist whose outlook on development was completely different from those of his colleagues Freud and Erikson. Piaget's theory is called cognitive development. *Cognitive* means "the ability to reason, make judgments, and learn." Piaget theorized that development was not as much a function of chronological age as of experiential age. Piaget was so sure of his ideas that he said they were applicable to any living organism; the catch is to make observations and comparisons about the cognitive process according to the expected ability for that organism. Piaget was the first to use children in his study. Piaget also asserted that intelligence consists of coping with the environment (Dennis and Hassol, 1983). He believed that a person must complete each stage of development before they can progress to the next stage. Table 4.3 shows the four stages of Piaget's theory of development.

CRITICAL THINKING QUESTION

Jamie is 2 years old. Jamie's parents are becoming frustrated because their child is "so naughty." They say that Jamie is always saying "No!" and "Mine!" and that Jamie is fascinated with playing with dirty diapers. The parents feel responsible for what they believe is "disgusting" behavior and wonder what they are doing wrong. They are quick to point out that Jamie's older sibling never did these things. They worry that something is wrong with Jamie or with them. What do you tell these parents?

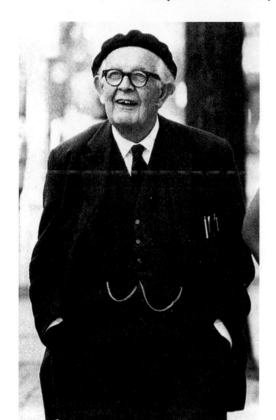

FIGURE 4.3 Jean Piaget

Lawrence Kohlberg (1927–1987)

Lawrence Kohlberg (FIG. 4.4) accepted Piaget's theories, but he perceived that very young people also have the ability to understand and judge right and wrong. Kohlberg's theory is therefore called the stages of moral development.

> **GOOD TO KNOW**
> Morality, the ideas that people have about what is right and what is wrong, is a function of the culture in which individuals grow up.

Kohlberg was a professor at Harvard University for many years. He developed and published his theory of moral development in 1958 as his doctoral thesis. It was based on some of the ideas of Jean Piaget. Kohlberg's true interest was in the mechanisms people use to justify their decisions. Although he was interested in the morality of his subjects, he was especially interested in how people support their decisions. He studied only male subjects ranging in age from 10 to 16 years. Kohlberg's theory is expressed in three levels. Each level has two sections. Table 4.4 shows these stages.

Table 4.3

Developmental Theory of Jean Piaget

Stage	*Approximate Age*	*Expected Ability*
Sensorimotor	Birth–2 years	• Uses senses to learn about self • Schemata develop which are plans or ways of learning to assimilate and accommodate. They include the behaviors of looking, hearing, and sucking.
Preoperational	2–7	• Thinks in mental images • Symbolic play • Develops own languages • Egocentric
Concrete operational	7-11 years	• Ability for logical thought increases. • Moral judgment begins to develop. • Numbers and spatial ability become more logical.
Formal operations	11 years–adult	• Develops adult logic • Able to reason things out • Able to form conclusions • Able to plan for future • Able to think in concepts or abstracts

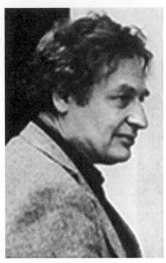

FIGURE 4.4 Lawrence Kohlberg

Kohlberg claimed that these stages build on the learning achieved from the stage before it. Therefore, the stages must be experienced in order, and one is not to backtrack, or revert, to a previous stage. Part of his theory was that moral development can be promoted via formal education. In fact, there is a mild resurgence of Kohlberg's theory emerging in some classroom environments today. But Kohlberg does have critics. His theory has been criticized on the grounds that it is sexist and culturally biased. According to Kohlberg, some cultures and peoples never progress to the highest level of morality, and certain behaviors that are acceptable in some cultures are objectively wrong. Kohlberg's theory also does not consider the emotional responses that daily problems and stressors can produce. In 1982, psychologist Carol Gilligan asserted that boys, girls,

Table 4.4
Lawrence Kohlberg's Theory of Development of Moral Reasoning

Stage	"Right" Behaviors	Why We Should Do "Right"	What If We Do Not Do "Right"
Level I: Preconventional			
1. Punishment and obedience orientation	*Do not do it* if it will result in punishment.	To avoid punishment and to see what one can "get away with"	I will be punished, and I do not like that.
2. Concerned with having own needs met	It is "right" if I (or if we) get something I want out of it.	To help me get my needs and wants fulfilled	I will not get what I want.
Level II: Conventional			
3. "Good boy, good girl" orientation	"Good" means living up to what is expected of us.	Self and others think we are "good."	Avoiding "blame" is more ethical than getting a "reward."
4. "Law and order"	"Right" means obeying the laws and rules.	It maintains social structure.	"Law" will have less importance than the will of "society."
Level III: Postconventional (Principled Level)			
5. Social contact	"Right" or "good" is behaving according to a general consensus.	We blend together for the greatest good and the welfare of all.	May become aware that "moral" and "legal" may not be the same
6. Universal "good"	Universal rules of justice and equality for all prevail. This is the "ideal" according to Kohlberg.	Live within the universal "good" according to own conscience.	Few people reach this according to Kohlberg. Therefore, in his own manual, the latest revisions do not measure this stage.

men, and women are all able to feel compassion and morality but that the genders process their morality from different perspectives, a variable that was not considered in Kohlberg's study.

Classroom Activity

As a class, develop a safety checklist for toddlers or preschool-age children. This checklist can be used as a tool for new parents, daycare providers, or others in your community.

DEVELOPMENTAL THEORISTS: ADOLESCENCE TO ADULTHOOD

Sigmund Freud (1856–1939)

In addition to his five psychosexual stages of development, Sigmund Freud had a model for the components of personality. He said that the personality consists of three parts: the id, the ego, and the superego. Remember that Freud theorized that all the components of human behavior are set in the unconscious. The behaviors may appear to be very purposeful and deliberate, but in Freud's theory, they are supposedly responses to situations of which people are not aware.

Id is the part of the personality that is concerned with the gratification of self. The id wants to fulfill our primal urges for food, sex, power, and entertainment. The term pleasure principle or the saying "If it feels good, do it!" arose from those who believe that all people have underdeveloped ids. These individuals promote the idea that people need to sometimes give in to the desires of the id.

Ego, in Freud's world, had a different connotation from the modern-day common use of the word. Ego, as Freud taught, is the balance to id and superego. Ego keeps id under control (in a mentally healthy individual). For example, perhaps you had an examination that was in a subject you felt fairly confident about, so you chose to study less than you would for other examinations. You went partying with friends for the weekend instead. Think about this as id behavior: it is more fun to party than to study. As you entered the testing area, a gnawing feeling started to enter your consciousness. You sensed "butterflies" in the pit of your stomach. You saw the first question on the examination, and your mind went temporarily blank. That is the ego response. In this scenario, the ego may be telling the

id, "Hmm. Maybe you aren't quite as confident as you thought you were!" And the id may respond, "This test was made just for me."

The third part of the personality theory of Sigmund Freud is the superego. The **superego** could be called the *conscience*. It is the part of the personality that allows people to determine what is right, wrong, good, and bad. The values exhibited by the superego are related to Kohlberg's moral levels; according to Freud, the superego is not chosen or learned.

A person who is well adjusted, or mentally healthy, has all three components of the personality, according to Freud. Freud would expect anyone who has any of the components missing or out of balance to display maladaptive behaviors. Defense mechanisms have been associated strongly with Freud's theories. Discussion of these defense mechanisms and maladaptive behaviors is found in Chapter 7.

Karen Horney (1885–1952)

Karen Horney (FIG. 4.5) was a psychoanalyst and one of the very few early female theorists. Her ideas were very close to those of Freud; however, she theorized that the causes of abnormal behaviors, or mental illness, were related to ineffective mother–child bonding. Unlike Freud, Horney was a feminist who asserted that psychological differences between men and women were not biological, but cultural. Horney developed the psychoanalytic social theory, which contends that a person's childhood contributes to and influences their personality

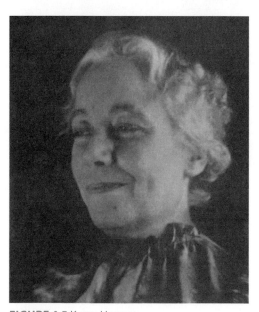

FIGURE 4.5 Karen Horney

in later life. Horney stated that safety and security are important factors in a child's life. Without both of these in a child's early years, difficult behaviors can be the result. Horney emphasized that it is the responsibility of the parents to provide that safe and secure environment (Dewey, 2007).

Ivan Pavlov (1849–1936) and B. F. Skinner (1904–1990)

Ivan Pavlov and B. F. Skinner worked on "conditioning," or manipulating, behavior. Both were called **behavioral theorists** because they showed that working with different behaviors and different stimuli could obtain different responses. Behavior modification is a direct result of their work.

Pavlov (FIG. 4.6) worked on involuntary responses. His well-known study was carried out with dogs, steaks, and a bell. When the dogs saw a choice piece of meat, they salivated in preparation for eating it. Pavlov incorporated the ringing of a bell when the meat was presented so that, in time, the researcher rang the bell and the dogs' association of meat with the sound of the bell stimulated the salivation response. This was a great breakthrough in the study of causes of behavior and ways in which behavior can be manipulated.

B. F. Skinner (FIG. 4.7) worked on **operant conditioning,** which is based on voluntary responses. Operant conditioning, very simply stated, means taking a behavior and operating on it by changing the variables or conditions surrounding the behavior. Skinner is known for the "Skinner boxes" in which he kept the animals he studied. These so-called boxes were cages big enough for the animal to move around in and contained an apparatus for the animal to operate voluntarily in response to different stimuli. There are three main parts to Skinner's theory: response, stimulus, and reinforcer. Table 4.5 defines these parts.

Skinner's theory led to the development of behavior modification. It is possible to "modify" or change any behavior by using appropriate stimuli and reinforcers to obtain the desired behavior. **Negative reinforcers** increase the probability that a behavior will recur by removal of an undesirable reinforcing stimulus. **Positive reinforcers** increase the probability that a behavior will recur by addition of a reinforcing stimulus. An example will help to clarify these concepts:

A supervisor wants to get employees to arrive to work on time. The supervisor has two possible paths to follow: negative reinforcement or positive reinforcement.

Negative reinforcement: "Several of you arrived late for work twice last week. If you arrive on time for every shift this week (the behavior), I won't have to write you up (removal of undesirable stimulus)."

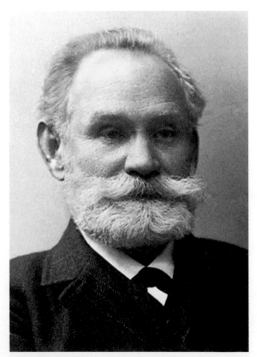

FIGURE 4.6 Ivan Pavlov

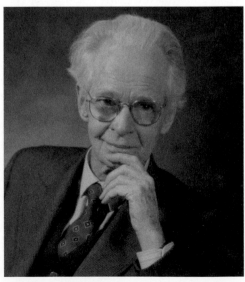

FIGURE 4.7 B. F. Skinner

Table 4.5
Operant Conditioning: B. F. Skinner

Skinner's Theory	Explanation
Response	Any movement or observable behavior that is to be studied. The response is measured for frequency, duration, and intensity (e.g., chicken rings bell in cage).
Stimulus	The event that immediately precedes or follows the operant behavior. The object is to find the stimulus that gets the chicken to ring the bell (e.g., food, noise, boredom).
Reinforcer	A variable that will cause the operant behavior to repeat predictably or increase in frequency. Sometimes this is called a *reward*. The reinforcer has to be meaningful to the person whose behavior is being "operated" on (e.g., chicken pecks bell and food drops into tray; when chicken wants food, it knows that pecking the bell will produce food).

Positive reinforcement: "Nurses who are on time for every shift this week (the behavior) will be entered in a drawing for a $50 gift card (the reinforcing stimulus)."

GOOD TO KNOW
One of the best ways to remember negative reinforcement is to think of it as something being *subtracted* from the situation. To remember positive reinforcement, think of it as something being *added*.

Abraham Maslow (1908–1970)

Abraham Maslow (FIG. 4.8) and several other theorists proposed the motivation theory, described as person centered or humanist. One tenet of humanistic psychology is self-esteem. In addition,

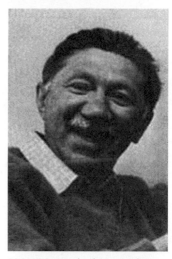

FIGURE 4.8 Abraham Maslow

person-centered theories involve observing and treating the whole person, so it is not surprising that nursing typically fits best with person-centered and behaviorist theories. One of the main developmental concepts embraced by the nursing profession is **Maslow's hierarchy of needs**. This hierarchy, or orderly progression of development, takes in the physical as well as the emotional components of personality development.

Maslow's hierarchy of needs has five levels. Maslow said that one must pass through these stages in order and that it is not possible for a person to move up to the next level until the previous level has been attained. These five levels set goals for a person to reach the level of self-actualization. This hierarchy is usually depicted as a large triangle or a staircase to help represent the progression from the "basic" needs to the "higher" needs of people (FIG. 4.9).

Physiological Needs
These are elements people need to survive: food, water, oxygen, clothing, absence of extremes in temperature, ability for body excretions, and sexual activity. These are considered necessary for life to continue. Without food, clothing, and shelter from extreme weather, an individual could die; without sexual activity, the species would die. The physiological needs are about survival. When preparing a plan of care for a patient, if the physiological needs are not prioritized, the patient will not survive. Can the patient proceed to the next level of the hierarchy without water or fluids? Can the patient survive without oxygen? Can the patient survive

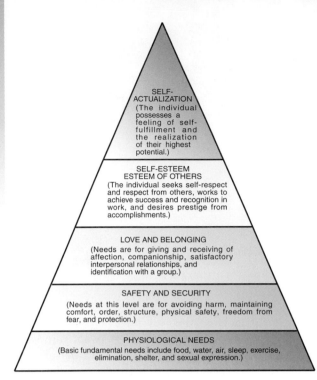

FIGURE 4.9 Maslow's hierarchy of needs *(from Townsend [2017]:* Essentials of Psychiatric Mental Health Nursing, *7th ed. Philadelphia: F.A. Davis Company, with permission)*

without elimination? These are the questions you must ask when doing a patient assessment. Being able to identify what takes priority can assist you in passing the National Council Licensure Examination (NCLEX) as well as in providing patient care. Maslow's hierarchy is an important component of the nursing discipline.

Safety and Security

It is important that people feel safe and free from fear. When individuals feel comfortable that their physical needs are being met, they begin to feel a sense of safety. Bear in mind that having basic needs met does not necessarily mean living in wealth or with steady employment. A number of people who are homeless learn to survive and are proud of their ability to survive in conditions that most people would consider deplorable. For these people, street life is a choice, and they are able to meet the safety and security step of Maslow's hierarchy.

Love and Belonging

It is a popular belief within psychology that loneliness is a major cause of depression. Sayings such as "Man does not live by bread alone" and "No man is an island" have implied this for many years, and that belief is now being borne out scientifically. People

need to feel loved, appreciated, and part of a group. Friendships that resemble families can even be seen in TV shows like *The Big Bang Theory* and *Grey's Anatomy.* A person's source of love and belonging may change over the life span. For babies and young children, love needs to come from parents or other caregivers; in adolescence and adulthood, the focus changes to a significant life partner, a peer group, or both. Regardless of the developmental stage of life, people need to feel loved.

Self-Esteem

Self-esteem is the ability to be confident that one is a person with good qualities and that others know and appreciate these qualities. This sounds easier to achieve than it often is. For example, when someone compliments you on a job well done, what is your usual response? Typically, we dismiss the compliment by saying something like "It was nothing, really." In addition to the negative effect such a dismissal has on effective communication, responding in this manner does not show positive self-esteem. One of the most difficult things is for people to learn to say "thank you" when given a compliment. "Thank you" not only acknowledges the other person's positive regard for a quality you possess, but it reinforces to yourself that you did a good job and deserve the recognition.

Unfortunately, people sometimes interpret this simple response as "false pride" and consider it to be in poor taste to acknowledge themselves in a positive manner. Women in particular have been socialized in this way for centuries. Although there has been some improvement in women's self-esteem over the years, there is still progress to be made.

Self-Actualization

The fifth and final rung on Maslow's hierarchy ladder is called self-actualization. This means achievement, taking risks, and working to one's potential. The self-actualized person is a problem-solver. Situations can be creatively dealt with when a person is confident enough to stretch the limits of ability. Taking the risk to stretch boundaries by joining the nursing profession is an example of seeking out self-actualization. Even though it may not feel comfortable yet, it is a process for self-improvement.

Carol Gilligan (1936–)

Gender differences have been a subject of discussion since the beginning of time. Men and women have always said that they just do not understand each other.

In her book *In a Different Voice: Psychological Theory and Women's Development* (1982), Carol Gilligan shared her research on the differences in how men and women think, communicate, and process life (Kincade, 2012). One of the fundamental gender differences Gilligan observed affects our understanding of Maslow's hierarchy. According to Gilligan, women tend to value relationships as a basic need, whereas men tend to value achievement as a basic need. This is not an issue of right or wrong; no value statement is being made. It is important, however, that nurses who are observing and collecting data on their patients understand that differences in patient attitudes and responses to treatment may be related to gender.

Carl Rogers (1902–1987)

Like Maslow, Carl Rogers (FIG. 4.10) was also a person-centered, or humanistic, psychologist. Although he believed that all people need to be valued, his theory is a bit different from Maslow's. The phrase associated with Carl Rogers is *unconditional positive regard.* Rogers believed that each individual has different ideas about life and the world they live in. Rogers did not think it was appropriate to put a value on another person's perception of the world.

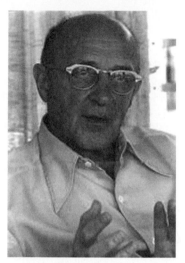

FIGURE 4.10 Carl Rogers *(courtesy of Bonnie Drumwright, PhD, Gold River, CA)*

Rather, he argued that every person deserves to be treated with respect and unconditional positive regard just by virtue of being a human being.

He also differed from Maslow in the area of self-actualization. Rogers claimed that self-actualization is the basic motivator for people and that all people have a built-in desire to achieve to their capabilities. Nursing practice has much in common with Rogers's theory.

Carl Jung (1875–1961)

Although he broke from some of Freud's ideas, Carl Jung (FIG. 4.11), a Swiss psychologist, also believed in the effects of the unconscious mind. He included

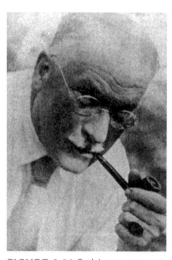

FIGURE 4.11 Carl Jung

in his definition of "unconscious" both repressed personal experiences and representations of universal human experiences, those experiences all people have. He used different terminology to describe the various parts of human personality, and he asserted that healthy personalities are a balance between the conscious and the unconscious. "Self" to Jung meant the deep, inner part of people. He believed that men and women are different, but that each contains part of the other. In fact, men's bodies do have traces of female hormones, and women's bodies have traces of male hormones. Jung used the term *anima* to describe the feminine tendencies in men and the term *animus* to describe the male characteristics in women.

Mask is a word Jung used to define the part of the personality that one presents socially. It hints at the idea that one's innermost self is usually different from their public self.

STAGES OF HUMAN DEVELOPMENT

Nurses care for people of all ages. Read the mission statement of your nursing program. It likely mentions that nursing addresses a continuum of health experiences throughout the life span. Nurses are responsible for having a working knowledge of the main physical and behavioral changes that can be expected within certain age groups. They must also have some idea of the complications that might occur if developmental tasks are not completed successfully. This is called the *study of developmental psychology*. Table 4.6 identifies the different life stages, some of the expected physical developments, expected behavioral developments, and possible outcomes of failure to meet certain developmental tasks. This chart incorporates traits from all the theorists identified in this text, but it is not a substitute for knowing the concepts of the individual theorists.

Classroom Activity

As a class, develop a teaching plan that could be used with children who are experiencing the divorce of their parents. The checklist should be detailed enough to accommodate age-appropriate communication and information. The class might prefer to do a separate checklist for each developmental group.

Death and Dying

Losing a loved one at any age or for any reason is a difficult experience. Separation, loss, and grief are human conditions that are unavoidable. Nowadays, people have a better quality of life and better health care than ever before. Because of this, the average life expectancy in the United States is 78.8 years, although it varies among ethnic and/or racial groups (Centers for Disease Control and Prevention [CDC]–National Vital Statistics Report). Johnson and Kanitsaki, in the Journal of Immigrant and Minority Health (2010), asserted that racism is a problem in health care, but not enough facts have been collected. It is suspected that issues related to racism can reduce life expectancy.

Modern people exist in a fast-paced and competitive society, which causes high levels of stress and encourages people to make unhealthy choices in their diets and lifestyles. This results in people dying of myocardial infarctions in their 30s and 40s. In addition, automobile accidents and recreational activities are taking the lives of children at higher numbers than ever before. According to the CDC, violence is a leading cause of death around the globe. Even though people know intellectually that they will die, they often struggle with death as if it is unexpected.

Elisabeth Kübler-Ross (1926–2004)

Psychiatrist Dr. Elisabeth Kübler-Ross (FIG. 4.12) was a leader in the study of the process of death and dying. She made her reputation by learning about the activities of the mind and body at and around the time of death. Her initial studies were based on only 200 subjects, all of whom had cancer; yet her theory, first published in 1969, has survived. According to Kübler-Ross, the result of experiencing the five stages of grief/dying is the ability to die in peace and with dignity. These stages apply not only to dying people and those they leave behind but also to other major losses in life. These stages are listed in Table 4.7.

Death is not only physiological; it is also deeply rooted in cultural and spiritual traditions. Just as every person is unique in life, so too are their rituals surrounding death.

Dr. Kübler-Ross emphasized the importance of communicating throughout the dying process. People who are in comas or in the end stage of death may not be able to respond to verbal cues or participate in conversation, but it is widely believed

Table 4.6

Overall View of Human Development

Life Stage	Age Range (Ages Vary Somewhat According to Theorist)	Expected Physical Development	Expected Behavioral Development	Potential Outcome of Ineffective Development
Prenatal	Conception	• Cells differentiate (specialize) by the end of the first trimester. • Intrauterine conditions of mother may affect prenatal development.	• Fetus kicks and may respond to stimuli such as familiar voices, music.	• Threats to mother's health of primary concern (e.g., smoking, drugs, malnutrition); mother's prenatal habits seem to have a strong influence on the developing baby. • Alcohol consumption during pregnancy is of special concern; can lead to a fetal alcohol spectrum disorder (FASD), which can cause physical anomalies as well as cognitive, emotional, and behavioral complications in a child. Neonatal abstinence syndrome (NAS), withdrawal symptoms in a newborn, related to opioids consumed by the mother during pregnancy.
Newborn	1st month of life	• May have flattened nose, unevenly shaped head, bruises from the passage through the birth canal; these physical characteristics will change over the first month of life.	• Bonding (e.g., touching, talking) of parents and baby is said to be crucial to development of trust. • Sucking reflex • Can see 7–10 inches • Likes bright colors • Likes to be talked to • Prefers female voices • Likes touch, cuddling, rocking, and the like • Will not be "spoiled" by this attention • Can hold head up for a few seconds • Follows light with eyes	• Angry crying • Mistrust • Withdrawal • Stress, which slows further development

Continued

Table 4.6

Overall View of Human Development—cont'd

Life Stage	Age Range (Ages Vary Somewhat According to Theorist)	Expected Physical Development	Expected Behavioral Development	Potential Outcome of Ineffective Development
Infant	2–18 months	Infants are all very much alike (physically and developmentally) until the age of 10 months.	2–4 months: • Begins to laugh • Follows people's movements with eyes 5–7 months: • Holds head erect • Turns head toward voices • Babbles/coos • Drinks from a cup 8–10 months: • Sits up alone • Says "mama," "dada"; understands "no" and "bye-bye"	• Poor parent-child relationship can lead to mistrust and poor self-concept. • Failure-to-thrive syndrome • Separation anxiety
Toddler	18 months to 3 years	• Long trunk • Short legs • Brain about ¾ of full size in order to be able to support future growth and development • Walking	• Toilet training • Learning gender roles • Self-centered • Does not share • Wants things now • Learns **autonomy** (independence) by using the word "no" • **Assimilation**, which is taking in and processing of information via the senses	• Anger • Regression • Reversion to infant-age behaviors

			• **Accommodation,** which is the ability to adjust to new information or situations	
Preschool (early childhood)	3–6 years	• Medical and dental examinations important • Nutrition can be challenging; children are starting to pick and choose their favorite foods; time to start teaching good nutrition. • Lead poisoning still a threat: lead tastes sweet and may still be found in some older plumbing or in old paint layers in housing units.	• Cognitive development is a primary activity; many questions; "why" is a frequently used word. • Socializes • Play important for self-expression and anxiety relief • Reading is the best parent-child activity. • Aggressive behavior (roughhousing) • Active imagination possibly leading to nightmares • Mixed feelings about going to school	• Enuresis—the involuntary bed-wetting in preschool and school-age children who have been toilet trained; often due to poor personal relationships • • Encopresis—involuntary bowel movements in the same population as enuresis
School age	6–12 years	• Body thinning out and growth slowing temporarily • Forming friendships with same-gender friends • Losing baby teeth and gaining permanent teeth • By age 6, brain almost full size; neurological system develops from head down. • By age 6 or 7, vision at its peak	• Learning to share • Peer group activities important • Beginning to show acceptance of moral issues by questions and discussions • Reversibility: the ability to put things in an order or sequence or to group things according to common traits	• Shyness and/or fear of school if trust and autonomy have not developed fully; may be a result of not being included in peer groups; has been defined as a "silent prison" • Gangs can be the result of negative types of peer groups. • Stuttering—repetitive or prolonged sounds or speech flow that is interrupted; seems to happen four times more often in boys; may be stress-related

Continued

Table 4.6

Overall View of Human Development—cont'd

Life Stage	Age Range (Ages Vary Somewhat According to Theorist)	Expected Physical Development	Expected Behavioral Development	Potential Outcome of Ineffective Development
		• Vision and hearing screening usually begins by the time the child enters school. • Agility increases • Scoliosis (lateral curvature of the spine) screening possibly encouraged. • Late childhood (10–11 years old)—beginning of sexual development, especially in girls, who now are maturing about 2 years ahead of boys. • Colds frequent, due to social habits		• Accidents are the leading cause of death in children; teaching safety to families and children is important. • Child abuse/neglect noted more frequently; all health-care personnel have the duty to report abuse or suspected abuse (discussed in more detail in Chapters 5 and 22).
Adolescent	12–18 years	• Growth spurt (musculoskeletal system) • Endocrine system maturing (hormones) • Secondary sex characteristics developing (facial and underarm hair, males' shoulders broaden, females' hips broaden and breasts develop)	• Learning independence • Learning self-sufficiency • Learning new social roles • Mood swings • Boredom • Introspection • Preoccupation with body image • Own "language" • Peer group very important—teens need intimacy	• Anorexia/bulimia frequent dangers for males as well as females; usually from white, middle-class families • Males who mature later seem to have the hardest time adjusting. • Suicide a major concern for this age group, usually because of feeling unimportant and not being taken seriously by adults

Stage	Age		
		• **Puberty**—individual is capable of reproducing • **Menarche**—female's first menstrual period, which happens around age 11–15 (it is important to know that nutrition and exercise affect this)	• Possible experimentation with alcohol, drugs, sex • Communication between parent and adolescent crucial • Talking on phone/texting for hours
Young adult	18–40 years	• Body usually in optimal physical condition	• Intimacy the main task to accomplish • Schooling and career planning important • Marriage and family decisions made	• Problems with developing intimacy • Difficulty leaving parent's home
Adult	40–60 years	• Gradual decline in hearing and visual acuity • Body beginning to shorten somewhat as musculature and bone structure change • Lung and cardiac capacity beginning to decrease somewhat	• Generativity, or passing down values and skills to the next generation (personally and professionally) is a major task of the adult.	• Disappointment with own achievements/next generation • Stress demands from different generations
Older adult	65 years–death	• Visual and hearing acuity continue to decline. • Becomes susceptible to an increasing number of physical and emotional illnesses	• Acceptance of limitations on independence and physical ability • Acceptance of the idea of death and beginning to prepare for it • Acceptance of retirement • Increases in stress throughout the life span	• Fear of death and dying • Difficulty with retirement—identity is often associated with career. • Depression relating to aging, loss of friends, and so on

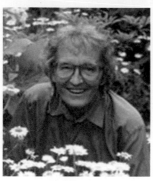

FIGURE 4.12 Elisabeth Kübler-Ross *(courtesy of Ken Ross, Scottsdale, AZ)*

conversation and continue to speak in terms of the reality of the situation.

> **GOOD TO KNOW**
> Dr. Kübler-Ross's theory also emphasizes the fact that hearing is the last sense to leave a person before death.

that they continue to hear what is going on in their environment. For this reason, nurses must be careful in talking to the patient and the family, even immediately after the patient's death. Again, people from some cultures and religions believe that the "spirit" or "soul" remains in the room for a period of time after death. Regardless of the belief system, it is a sign of respect to the patient and the significant others to include the patient in the

Children go through the same grief stages as adults, and as with adults, they may need special help to come to terms with losing a loved one. The help nurses give to younger patients must be age-appropriate. Infants and toddlers may not be able to understand what happened, but they do sense the change. Keep their routine as normal as possible and provide them with physical closeness and a safe environment.

Children from 2 to 6 years of age may have the sense that death is reversible. How often do they see cartoon characters "die" and then immediately return to animated life? When the reality that grandmother or grandfather is not coming back to life

Table 4.7
Five Stages of Grief/Death and Dying by Dr. Elisabeth Kübler-Ross

Stage	*Key Words*	*Expected Behaviors*
Denial	"Not me!"	Refuses to believe that death is coming; states "That doctor doesn't know what he or she is talking about!"
Anger	"Why me?"	Expresses envy, resentment, and frustration with younger people and/or those who are not dying
Bargaining	"If I could have one more chance . . ."	May become very religious or "good" in an effort to gain another chance at life or more time to live
Grief/depression	Realizes that "bargaining" is not working and that death is approaching	Becomes depressed, weepy; may "give up," quit taking medications, quit eating, and so forth
Acceptance	"OK . . . but I don't have to like it!"	Enters a state of expectation; may begin to call family members near; needs to complete "unfinished business"; prepares spiritually to die

is understood, it is important that the child understands that he or she did not cause the death of the loved one.

Children ages 6 to 12 have varying degrees of understanding. It is important to allow and encourage children to talk about their feelings. Recent incidents of school violence involving this age group have provided the opportunity for grief counselors to intervene with children who have survived these ordeals.

Teens are bridging the gap from childhood to adulthood and, therefore, may respond to grief and loss as adults at times and then as children. Provide structure, routine, and an environment in which they may freely express their thoughts and feelings.

When caring for dying patients, you need to be aware of the existence of and your state's recognition of an advance directive or "living will" (where the wishes of the dying person are placed on a legal document, signed by the person while competent, and witnessed) and the family's wishes. Advance directives also identify who the decision maker(s) will be if the person is unable to speak for themself.

Euthanasia (sometimes called *mercy killing*) is illegal in the United States, but physician-assisted death (also called *aid in dying*) is now legal in Washington, DC, and some states: California, Colorado, Hawaii, Maine, New Jersey, Oregon, Vermont, Montana, New Mexico, and Washington. These laws allow mentally competent adults who have a terminal illness and less than 6 months to live to request and receive prescription medication to hasten their death. In all states, competent adults have the right to decline any medical treatment even if such a refusal of treatment hastens death. All of these issues can bring out strong emotions for families and for the nurse who is caring for people at the end of their lives. These topics will continue to be debated for years to come.

The nurse's responsibilities at the time of death vary from state to state. For instance, in some states, nurses are allowed to pronounce the death of a patient; in other states, this can be done only by a physician. Death is also defined differently from state to state. Physical signs such as vital signs, skin color and temperature, presence or absence of activity on electroencephalogram (EEG) and electrocardiogram (ECG), and the ability to be viable—to live without mechanical assistance—are criteria used by states to define death. It is the nurse's responsibility to know the legal definition of death in the state in which they are working.

CRITICAL THINKING QUESTION

Your patient is in the final stage of life. Death is imminent, but the patient is still alert and oriented. The patient's family and spouse are in the room. The patient asks you to ask the physician to "put me to sleep." The patient's spouse weeps but supports the request; the other family members threaten to sue if the physician does "any such thing." What are your thoughts and feelings about this request? What will you do to help the patient? The family? The patient's spouse? As a nurse, what if this were your parent or child who was about to die? What might you think and feel then?

Safe and Effective Nursing Care

Prioritize care according to Maslow's hierarchy
Assist patient in meeting their needs, physically and emotionally
Understand patient's development according to the various developmental theorists
Provide patients with age-appropriate activities
Identify which stage a terminal patient is in according to Dr. Elisabeth Kübler-Ross

Key Points

- There are many theories about personality development in human beings. Although they are theories, there are strong indications of validity in all of them. The licensed practical nurse (LPN) and the licensed vocational nurse (LVN) must have a working knowledge of some of the more commonly accepted theories of human development throughout the life span.
- Dr. Elisabeth Kübler-Ross developed a theory of five stages that people go through when they

are grieving or dying. Although others have presented theories on this topic, hers remains the most commonly accepted theory in nursing.

- Each person is an individual and will go through stages of development or grief at their own pace. These theories are guidelines to help nurses understand what patients may experience as they go through certain stages in their lives.

CASE STUDY

Mr. Y, a 24-year-old construction worker, suffered a traumatic brain injury (TBI) after falling from scaffolding when his safety equipment failed. He was comatose for 8 days. During this time, family and friends kept a constant vigil. His wife was 6 months pregnant and fearful about the possibility of having to raise the baby alone. Many conversations were held in his room while he was in the coma. When Mr. Y awakened from the coma, he was able to recall most of what was said. He wondered why "nobody answered me when I talked to you." He

especially wanted to reassure his wife that "Nothing would keep me from seeing that baby!"

1. What suggestions would you have made to the family of this patient regarding patients who are comatose?
2. How can you help a patient who has concerns about "memories" they acquired while in a coma (e.g., what is real and what is not), and what things might have been said in confidence that otherwise if the patient was awake and alert would not be normally be spoken?

Review Questions

1. A 4-year-old patient comes into the clinic with her father. She is being checked for a recurring ear infection. As you prepare her to see the physician, she says to you, "I love my daddy. I'm going to marry him like mommy someday!" Which one of Freud's stages of development is she most likely demonstrating?
   a. Genital
   b. Oral
   c. Anal
   d. Phallic

2. Patient Y is 20 years old. Y is a perfectionist and very routine-oriented. Freudian theorists would say that Patient Y did not successfully complete which of the following stages of development?
   a. Genital
   b. Oral
   c. Anal
   d. Phallic

3. Patient Y (from question 2) is being treated by a behavioral psychologist. When Patient Y begins to miss meals and activities because of the need to complete routines perfectly, the staff is to intervene. Patient Y failed to come to dinner on your shift. You go to check on the patient and see Y carefully placing personal items in a special place in the bathroom. Your best response to Y from a behavioral and therapeutic background would be:
   a. "Y, where were you at dinner tonight?"
   b. "Y, you blew it. You didn't come to dinner and you know what that means: no pass for the weekend."
   c. "Y, I am just here to remind you it is dinnertime."
   d. "Y, it is not appropriate to miss dinner. What is the consequence of that, according to your care plan?"

4. In prenatal development, cell differentiation is normally completed by the end of the:
   a. First trimester
   b. Second trimester
   c. Third trimester
   d. First lunar month

5. The infant mortality rate is highest in mothers who are:
   a. Over 35 years old
   b. Over 30 years old
   c. Under 20 years old
   d. Under 15 years old

6. The term *anima* from Carl Jung's theory describes:
   a. Male characteristics in women
   b. Feminine characteristics in men
   c. Male characteristics in men
   d. Feminine characteristics in women

7. According to Erikson's theory, the developmental task a 3- to 6-year-old needs to accomplish is:
   a. Identity
   b. Industry
   c. Intimacy
   d. Initiative

8. Infants seem to be very much alike developmentally until the age of:
   a. 2 months
   b. 6 months
   c. 10 months
   d. 12 months

9. A toddler's ability to take in or acknowledge changes in the environment is called:
   a. Adjustment
   b. Assimilation
   c. Accommodation
   d. Autonomy

10. The parents of a 2-year-old arrive at the hospital to visit the child. The child is in the play room and ignores the parents during the visit. This 2-year-old's behavior indicates:
    a. The child is withdrawn
    b. The child is more interested in playing with other children
    c. The child has adjusted to the hospitalized setting
    d. A normal pattern

REVIEW QUESTIONS ANSWER KEY 1.d, 2.c, 3.d, 4.a, 5.d, 6.b, 7.d, 8.c, 9.b, 10.d

CHAPTER 5

Sociocultural Influences on Mental Health

KEY TERMS

Abuse
Culture
Ethnicity
Ethnocentrism
Homeless
Parenting
Prejudice
Religion
Scaffolding
Sociocultural
Stereotype
Zone of proximal development

CHAPTER CONCEPTS

Communications
Culture
Diversity
Family dynamics
Spirituality

LEARNING OUTCOMES

1. Define culture and cultural characteristics.
2. Define ethnicity.
3. Identify factors to consider when assessing culture and ethnicity.
4. Differentiate between religion and spirituality.
5. Identify three parenting styles.
6. Differentiate between abuse and neglect.
7. Define stereotype.
8. Define prejudice and bias.
9. Define homelessness.
10. Explain possible reasons for homelessness.
11. Identify nursing care for people who are homeless.

Many professionals in the field of psychology believe that social and cultural environments have a great influence on the way people develop and process life. These professionals believe that positive or negative social and cultural experiences early in life result in positive or negative behaviors and beliefs in adulthood.

> **GOOD TO KNOW**
> Part of the role of the licensed practical nurse (LPN)/licensed vocational nurse (LVN) is to learn about traits that are common among people and those that are different. It is important to understand people's customs and beliefs to avoid unrealistic expectations of patients.
> **Sociocultural** environments, culture, and ethnicity are among the factors that are said to have the greatest influence on people throughout their life span.

THE SOCIOCULTURAL THEORY OF DEVELOPMENT

Lev Vygotsky (1896–1934), a developmental theorist, studied the manner in which people responded to stimuli or their surroundings. He believed this was the key to how children developed. Vygotsky was certain that socializing played a vital part in the development of a person's cognitive ability, beginning in childhood. Based on his observations, Vygotsky developed the sociocultural developmental theory. The first part of the theory discusses the child's interaction with others in their environment; the second part describes the **zone of proximal development**, the time when the child's actions are at first dependent on others until the child becomes independent and performs without assistance, demonstrating cognitive growth. As the child becomes more independent, the parent or caregiver is still present to assist in advancing the child's positive behavior. This assistance is known as scaffolding. According to Saul McLeod, children's values, beliefs, and critical thinking strategies are made possible because of a relationship with other members of society (2020).

CULTURE

Culture is a shared way of life, the combination of traditions and beliefs that bond a group of people together (see Chapter 3). Culture is not based on one's skin color or country of origin. Culture is not a person's genetic makeup, but the surrounding environment a person is raised in or interacts with over a period of time. For example, in the 1960s, young people who were speaking out against the politics and morals of their parents began living in groups (FIG. 5.1). The area they chose to start this movement was the Haight-Ashbury district in San Francisco. They called themselves *hippies*, and they shared a way of life that consisted of experimenting with drugs, living together without being married (free love, as it was termed), dressing in ripped, dirty clothing, not cutting their hair, and doing just about everything else that was opposite to the values of the "older generation." This group believed in loving everyone, regardless of race, creed, or color—as long as the individual embraced the beliefs of the group. The group's symbols were the daisy and the peace sign, and slogans "flower power" and "power

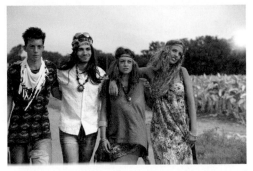

FIGURE 5.1 The hippies of the 1960s represented their own unique culture.

to the people" represented some of the ideals they followed. Much to the chagrin of the over-30 age group, these young people fit the definition of a culture. It was called a subculture or counterculture at the time. Today's generation X and millennials make their own cultural statements.

> ## GOOD TO KNOW
> You may discover that when it comes to other cultures, your knowledge is limited; it is as if you have been living in a glass jar. Nurses care for patients of other cultures, but they may not always be aware of how to interact appropriately with these patients. Understanding the beliefs and values of patients' cultures enhances patient trust in you, the health-care provider.

Nursing programs are a culture, using common terminology, performing the same sets of skills, and having similar curriculums. But nurses need to be aware of cultures beyond their own and that of the nursing profession. Bringing cultural competence to patient care is one of your primary responsibilities as a nurse. Cultural competence requires you to take into account the following areas: communication, personal space, social organization, time, environmental control, and biological variation. One model to improve your cultural competence as a nurse is the transcultural assessment model developed by Giger and Davidhizar (Giger, 2013). Culturally diverse care means that the nurse, no matter their own cultural background, adapts care in a manner congruent with the patient's culture.

Clinical Activity

You are assisting in preparing a care plan for your patient. Determine whether any of the patient's traditions or beliefs have been included in the plan of care.

Psychoanalyst Karen Horney (see Chapter 4) proposed the theory that some cultural traditions and beliefs cause disturbances in personal relationships and could lead to some forms of emotional disturbances. For example, in some cultures, it is customary for men and women to dine separately. If you are hosting a dinner party and include a couple from such a culture, they would likely experience a cultural shock with men and women dining together. This initially could create some tension between the couple and/or between the couple and the rest of the group. Madeleine Leininger, the nurse theorist who established the culture care theory, also realized the importance of transcultural nursing. While caring for children, she found that their behavior needs were related to their culture; without understanding each child's culture, functioning as a health-care provider was difficult (Leininger, 2006).

Clinical Activity

As a class, review and choose an online culture-assessment questionnaire to use in clinicals. After receiving your instructor's approval of the questionnaire, conduct a culture assessment of one patient during clinical rotation and share the results in postconference. Select a patient whose cultural characteristics are different from your own.

CRITICAL THINKING QUESTION

Your 65-year-old patient is from a different country and speaks only minimal English. Upon admission, a medical translator saw the patient and went over the hospital routines, rules, and patient's rights in the patient's native language. The patient's daughter refuses to let you assess or care for the patient. The patient appears to be in pain, but the daughter will not allow pain medication to be given. The patient refuses the hospital's food. Around suppertime, you smell food and enter the room to find the daughter cooking on a hot plate, which is a fire-code violation. What do you do next?

RELIGION

Religion is the organized and structured belief in a higher power. This belief system can be very strong—so strong that people fight wars over religion. Rituals or worship services are usually included in organized religions. Additionally, religion is often the subject of stereotype. A **stereotype** is a fixed, often incorrect or incomplete, notion or conviction about a group of people or a situation. For example, one stereotype of Muslims is that they marry only other Muslims. This idea is incorrect (Box 5.1).

Religious beliefs are often included in discussions of culture; however, it is important to note that religion is *not* the same thing as culture. For people who practice Judaism or Islam, for example, sometimes the relationship between their religious beliefs and their cultural beliefs is so entwined that it is hard to separate those traits.

Religions sometimes involve items considered sacred. Such items may include holy books, religious jewelry, the person's dress (headwear, loose-fitting clothing), or other types of personal effects. Patients should be allowed to keep these items whenever possible. In situations in which a patient may be in poor mental health and possession of these items is of actual or potential danger to the patient or others in the area, it may be necessary to remove the items. If that becomes necessary, enlisting the assistance of a representative from the patient's religion may be helpful.

Tool Box

Religious Diversity
https://www.americansurveycenter.org/research/religious-diversity-and-change-in-american-social-networks/
Global diversity in religion
https://www.pewforum.org/

Cultural Assessment—Questions to Ask

- Where was the patient born? If the patient is an immigrant, how long have they been in this country?
- What is the patient's ethnic affiliation? How strong is the ethnic identity?
- Who are the patient's major support people? Does the patient live in an ethnic neighborhood or community?
- Who in the family takes responsibility for health concerns and decisions?
- Are there any activities in which the patient declines to participate because of culture or religious taboos?
- Does the patient have any dietary considerations related to culture or religion?
- What are the patient's primary and secondary languages and their speaking and reading abilities?
- What is the patient's religion? What is its importance in the patient's daily life? What religious practices does the patient engage in?
- What is the patient's economic situation? Is income adequate for their needs?
- What are the patient's health beliefs and practices?
- What are the patient's perceptions of their health problems and expectations of health care?

Source: Gorman and Sultan (2008). *Psychosocial Nursing for General Patient Care,* 3rd ed. Philadelphia: F.A. Davis Company.

Classroom Activity

Interview a person whose religion is different from your own. You may use the interview format given in Chapter 6. Present the interview results orally or in writing to the class. Discuss what you thought you knew about the religion before the interview. Discuss what you learned after the interview. Review literature on that specific religion and compare it to the information from the interview.

SPIRITUALITY

Spirituality and/or religion are extremely important to some patients and unimportant to others. Unlike religion, spirituality is not organized. Although a person can be both spiritual and religious, an atheist can be spiritual. According to Luna Greenstein, a person confronted with a stressful event can reduce the effect of that event by turning to their religion or to their higher power (2016). As a nurse, you must learn to become comfortable listening and talking to patients about their religious and spiritual needs without pushing your personal values onto your patients. A patient's successful recuperation from an illness or a surgical procedure may be deeply tied to their spirituality. Nurses who are not comfortable in these situations should offer to call the chaplain in the facility or a spiritual leader of the patient's choice.

Classroom Activity

Have a "culture awareness day" for students to share information about their own cultures. When it is your turn, briefly describe the following traditions for your ethnicity or culture:

- Holiday foods
- Music
- Weddings
- Childbearing practices
- Health-care practices
- Death practices
- Myths and folktales

ETHNICITY

Ethnicity identifies a person with their shared cultural heritage. Language, country of origin, and skin color are parts of ethnicity. Different ethnic groups often exist within a larger culture. For example, a person born in America to Iranian parents is an American citizen, but the person's ethnicity is Iranian. However, these characteristics do not provide the complete picture of that person's ethnicity. For example, is an Iranian American person of the Christian, Jewish, Muslim, Baha'i, or Zoroastrian faith? The only way to find out is to ask them. People are generally very proud of their culture and ethnicity. Many communities have festivals that celebrate their unique traditions. These festivals do much to educate the community about the various people living together in it. You can learn a lot about a group of people from the kind of food they eat, the music they make, and the dances they do. In a similar way, you can learn how your patients communicate and how they view health care by asking thoughtful questions and listening carefully to the answers.

Evidence-Based Practice

Clinical Question: Does cultural competence education for health-care providers yield a positive outcome for patients?

Evidence: The tool, C.R.A.S.H. (mnemonic C – consider culture, R – show respect, A – access and affirm differences, S – show sensitivity and self-awareness, H – do it all with humanity) course is used in health-care facilities to educate health-care providers in bridging gaps in cultural understanding. Research shows that having cultural competence assists the health-care provider in providing high-quality health care, especially to patients belonging to underserved or underrepresented groups.

Implication for Nursing Practice: Health-care providers who acknowledge and understand patient diversity encourage patient compliance with taking medications and following treatment protocols. Culturally competent health care promotes patients' trust in their providers.

Mcgregor, B., Belton, A., Henry, T. L., Wrenn, G., & Holden, K. B. (2019). Improving behavioral health equity through cultural competence training of health care providers. *Ethnicity & Disease, 29*(Supp2), 359-364. doi:10.18865/ed.29.s2.359

GOOD TO KNOW

Education can help eliminate prejudice, which is judging a person or situation before knowing all the facts about them. Prejudice is a destructive behavior; it is hurtful, and it shuts the door on effective communication.

A number of laws in the United States are intended to minimize displays of **prejudice** relating to race, religion, gender identity, age, sexuality, and so on. However, it is impossible to legislate the private beliefs of individual people. When social or political leaders show bias toward specific ethnic groups, their followers will likely follow along. Nurses are in a perfect position to teach and model respectful interpersonal relationships. Through such modeling, it is hoped, we can make great strides in eliminating the prejudice of others.

Tool Box

Health Disparities

https://www.americanprogress.org/issues/race/
    reports/2020/05/07/484742/health-disparities-
    race-ethnicity/

It would be naïve to think that everyone who works in health care is free from prejudice. Kresslin and Groeneveld (2015) studied racial disparities in

health care. These researchers reviewed 59 cases of patients receiving procedures, diagnostic care, or therapeutic care. What they found was that 43% of the white patients received *more* care than was necessary. Previous health-care studies had shown that blacks often receive less care than whites. What was unique about this study was that it showed overuse of procedures for white people. In another study of health disparities, Carratala and Maxwell investigated systemic inequality in the United States. This study looked at health coverage, chronic conditions, mental health services, and the foremost causes of death (2020).

CRITICAL THINKING QUESTION

Should a patient's hospital-identification bracelet specify if the patient has insurance coverage? Will the patient without coverage be treated the same as the patient with coverage?

Prejudice has led to an emergence of **ethnocentrism**, which is the belief that one's own ethnic or religious group deserves rights and benefits more than others. Gangs, supremacist groups, and terrorist organizations may have all had their start in hate and prejudice.

Sadly, many cultural groups have a history of oppression. During World War II, 6 million Jews were rounded up and killed by the Nazis in concentration camps. The United States was built on the backs of African slaves, whose descendants have been fighting for their civil rights for over 200 years. Native Americans were forcibly removed from their ancestral homelands on the Trail of Tears. In recent times, some people have questioned if affirmative action is a form of discrimination against white people. As a nurse, you cannot know exactly what hurts your patients may have suffered or what prejudices they may have faced because of their religion, culture, or ethnicity. That is why it is important to keep the lines of communication open. People learn by sharing with each other. When in doubt, ask rather than make an assumption. Making assumptions about a person is stereotyping, which can end a helping relationship between nurse and patient.

Many mental health professionals believe that people raised in an atmosphere of prejudice and stereotyping tend to become angry, hateful, and aggressive adults. However, there is no proof that *all* people who are subjected to prejudice and stereotyped thinking develop into adults with such negative attitudes (Box 5.2).

Classroom Activity

Interview a person who is from a culture different from your own. You may use the interview format given in Chapter 6. Present the results to the class orally or in writing. This will reinforce the information presented in Chapter 6, as well as provide first-hand information pertinent to this chapter.

Box 5.2

Enhancing Cultural Sensitivity

- Know your own attitudes, values, and beliefs.
- Be aware of your own ethnocentrism.
- Be aware of your own prejudices that may influence your assessment.
- Maintain an open mind and seek out more information about your patient's culture, beliefs, and values.
- Communicate your interest about the patient's beliefs and values.
- Approach the patient as an individual. Avoid assuming that all people from one cultural background hold the same beliefs.

Source: Gorman and Sultan (2008). *Psychosocial Nursing for General Patient Care,* 3rd ed. Philadelphia: F.A. Davis Company.

THE CHANGING FAMILY

The definition of family is changing (FIG. 5.2). In June 2013, the U.S. Supreme Court paved the way for federal recognition of same-sex marriages. Today, same-sex marriages are legal in every state. Schools and clinics serve children who are lesbian, gay, bisexual, transgender, and queer (LGBTQ+) or who have family members who are. Many people who identify as LGBTQ+ are "out" in the open and living life with their spouses and children just as more traditional father-mother-children families do. However, despite signs of increased acceptance, LGBTQ+ individuals and their families may still struggle with bias and prejudice.

By the year 2030, according to the National Gay and Lesbian Task Force, there will be approximately 4 million gay elders requiring social services and living in long-term care facilities. How will that change the way nurses provide care? Probably very little; good nursing care will remain good nursing care. However, according to Lockhart and Davis (2016), nurses and their coworkers may need sensitivity training in order to interact seamlessly with the LGBTQ+ community. Clearly, nurses practicing in clinics and long-term care or assisted living facilities can expect some changes in the clientele.

Tool Box

LGBTQ+ Community
https://outrightinternational.org/content/
  acronyms-explained

Another issue facing schools, clinics, and other public facilities is "bathroom laws." In 2016, a controversial bill was passed in North Carolina (House Bill DRH40005-TC-1B) (03/22) to require single-sex occupancy in the use of the bathroom. This law would require transgender individuals to use the restrooms of the gender they were assigned at birth rather than the restroom that corresponds to their gender identity. Other states are currently reviewing bills related to single-sex bathrooms in public places, including schools.

There are numerous family structures. More individuals are choosing to start and raise families as single parents. Today it is not uncommon

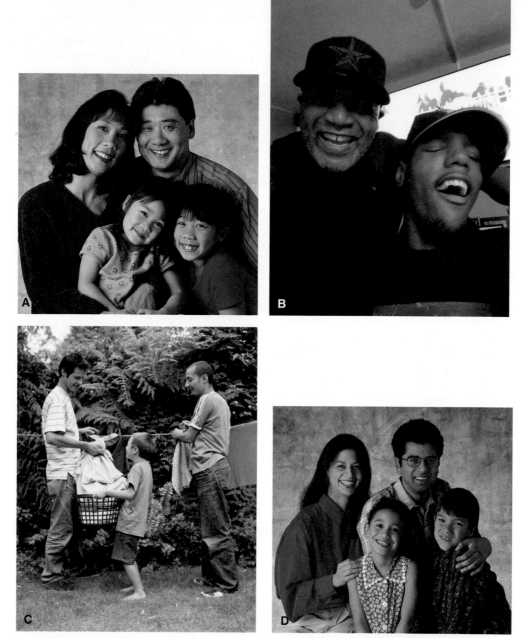

FIGURE 5.2 The definition of family is changing. (A) Traditional family, with a mother, father, and their biological children. (B) Single-parent family *(courtesy of Robynn Anwar)*. (C) Gay couple and child *(photograph by Creatas)*. (D) "Blended" family, in which each spouse has his or her own children, whom they bring into a new family.

for a child to be raised by a single father. Parents are adopting children from countries, ethnicities, and races different from their own. A family may include parents and siblings with assorted skin tones and languages. The global family is rapidly and constantly evolving. Many of these family changes are positive, but some can also be mentally challenging. One devastating example is the separation of parents and children because of their immigration status.

HOMELESSNESS

Homelessness is not a mental illness (FIG. 5.3). However, many people in the United States who are **homeless** also have some threat to their mental health.

The homeless population is as varied as the population of those who have homes. Some homeless people work full time but cannot afford housing. Economic downturns, foreclosures, domestic violence, lack of insurance, or other situations not related in any way to having a mental illness can result in homelessness. A small number of people choose to live on the streets. According to the National Coalition for the Homeless, tent cities have been appearing across America since 2000 (2009).

Many homeless individuals are also veterans of the armed forces. Services for these individuals are available through Veterans Affairs, but services can be difficult to access. The rise in homelessness is also linked to the rising cost of rental housing and the increasing rate of poverty (National Coalition for the Homeless, 2009). Funding to combat homelessness lessened after a new federal tax plan implemented in 2019.

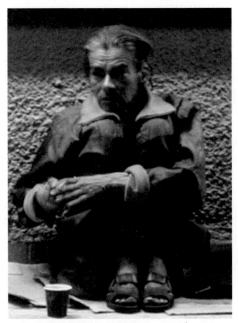

FIGURE 5.3 Homelessness is not a mental illness, but many homeless people face threats to their mental health *(courtesy of Telecom Pioneers, Nova 5 Chapter #5, Brooklyn, NY).*

Approximately one-third of the homeless population in the United States is mentally ill, with many more having substance abuse issues (National Coalition for the Homeless). People with certain mental illnesses, especially schizophrenia, have difficulty living independently, and they soon end up out of work, out of money, and out of a home. Once on the streets, they may be noncompliant with their medications, have no access to refills, lose the medication, or have it stolen (FIG. 5.4). Their only resources may be community-based mental health services (Barry, 2002). One community service is "street medicine" (Frye and McQuistion, 2016). This group of community psychiatrists visits homeless individuals where they live. There, psychiatrists assess and treat their homeless patients with needed psychotropics and any other therapies. According to MentalHealth.gov (2020), the Patient Protection and Affordable Care Act (ACA) made it possible for those with mental health disorders and substance abuse problems to be able to acquire health insurance coverage for treatment. In recent times, one of the biggest health crises for the homeless population has been coronavirus disease 2019 (COVID-19). Many people who are homeless lack facilities for hand washing and are unable to obtain masks. Their often-crowded living conditions allow for the rapid transmission of the severe acute respiratory syndrome (SARS) coronavirus 2, the cause of COVID-19.

CRITICAL THINKING QUESTION

You are the only source of income for your family. You are laid off because of a merger of two agencies. How long can you survive with no income? How will you pay for insurance? Jobs are not plentiful; the outlook for comparable employment in the near future is bleak. How close are you to living on the street? What will be the plan of action for you and your family?

In the 1950s, deinstitutionalization led to the discharging of people who were technically able to be "in the community" but who were not always able to cope with the stresses of caring for themselves, caring for their families, and maintaining employment. For some mentally ill individuals, this kind of pressure amplifies personal stress, leading to social confinement and increased mental illness.

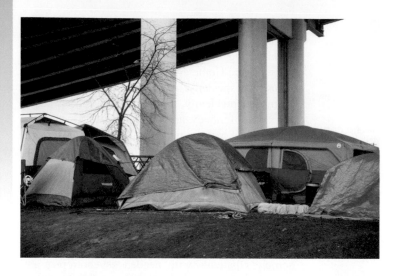

FIGURE 5.4 Tent city for the homeless in Camden, New Jersey *(courtesy of Joshua Rainey Photography/Shutterstock.com).*

In 1987, the Health Resources and Services Administration–Health Care for the Homeless (HRSA–HCH) was formed to provide information and help create plans to help people who are homeless. The problem is that funding of federal programs depends on statistics. The U.S. Department of Housing and Urban Development (HUD) collects data from the Housing Inventory Count (2012). One of HUD's goals is to find permanent housing for homeless individuals and families.

Patients may be brought to a facility through the emergency department or by a law enforcement agency. Sometimes medication is given to stabilize the patient, and they are returned to the community; other times the patient is admitted to a medical unit. Unfortunately, sometimes the patient's mental health issue is overlooked because of the health-care provider's focus on physical health.

Shelters of varying types exist in many cities. They are funded and staffed in different ways. For example, some are church funded and some rely on grants and underwriting by large businesses. Some are completely operated by volunteers, and some have paid staff. Depending on the resources available, shelters for homeless people provide anything from meals and overnight shelter to health care, dental care, and assistance with job placement.

Often, however, shelters require residents to follow certain rules. Clients in these shelters may be required to stay drug- and alcohol-free and to show proof that they are compliant with medications or some other criteria to help them return to an improved lifestyle. Those with pets may not be

allowed to have them at the shelter. Some people balk at these restrictions and leave the shelters.

What techniques do nurses need to help patients who may be homeless and physically or mentally compromised?

1. Treat the whole person, not the homelessness.
2. Treat the person as any other patient.
3. Maintain all patient rights.

 ## ECONOMIC CONSIDERATIONS

A study by Eron and Peterson in 1982 found that the lower the socioeconomic status, the higher the incidence of schizophrenia in U.S. society. The study found a similar, but weaker, correlation between socioeconomic status and mood disorders. The implication is that variables besides socioeconomic status influence mental health. For example, people who live in poverty or underprivileged circumstances will very likely have greater stressors than will people of higher socioeconomic status. So, is it the lack of money or the increased stress that leads to the disorder? Such questions make it very difficult, if not impossible, to make absolute statements about the correlation between disease and any variable.

 ## ABUSE

Abuse is misuse of a person, substance, or situation. Sometimes people say that they cannot be abusing because they have a rationale for their behavior. This is not true. Anyone who mistreats another person or who misuses or overuses a substance or a situation (such as gambling or power) is displaying abusive behavior. The fact is the person may be in denial about their behavior.

Some individual forms of abuse are discussed in Chapter 22. Abuse of all types is a growing phenomenon in society. People debate whether a higher incidence of abuse exists now or whether people are just talking about it more openly. Violence is a learned behavior. It is well documented that in the majority of physical abuse situations, the abuser was abused at some point.

When it comes to substance abuse, the findings are not conclusive. Some studies indicate that substance abuse may be genetic, learned, or possibly due to a chemical imbalance in the body. A phenomenon called the addictive personality groups abuse disorders together. It is important for nurses to understand that there may be more than one cause for a particular mental health problem. Good communication and data-collecting skills will help the nurse find potential causes for each patient's mental health problem. See Chapter 17 for more discussion of substance abuse.

 ## PARENTING

What is a "good" parent? Is it the parent who lets the child do anything the child wants? Is it the parent who buys all the newest fads for the child? Is it the parent who teaches strict values and ethics? Maybe it is the parent who is with the child at all times.

Parenting is the method of raising children that is used by parents or other primary caregivers. Parenting is a learned behavior; it is not an innate skill. So, how do parents *learn* to be parents? Typically, people tend to parent the way they were parented, for better or worse. That means all the cultural traditions and religious values in one parent's belief systems are brought out in the open and blended with those of the other parent. Then, it is up to the parents to take 1 day at a time and learn from their mistakes. Sometimes parenting is learned from friends and neighbors. Schools, health-care facilities, and communities may offer classes for parents.

CRITICAL THINKING QUESTION
You are home one evening, and you hear the 18-month-old child of your upstairs neighbors. The child has been crying for 3 hours. You have heard no footsteps in the apartment. Voicemail picks up each time you attempt to call. You become concerned and call the building supervisor to open the apartment. When you get in, you find the crying child and unsanitary conditions; the parents are not in the apartment. You look outside and see the parents several apartments down, partying with friends. What are your responsibilities? How will you respond to the parents? Whom will you notify? How long will you wait before you inquire? The parents tell you to mind your own business. What will you say to them? What will you do if it happens again?

Reactions to altered parenting styles are varied. Again, there is no "perfect" situation or guarantee of being "good" parents. Parenting is stressful. No matter what else patients are concerned about during their hospitalization, it is almost certain that their children will be a paramount focus of attention. Nurses can help parents through the stress of being hospitalized and apart from their children and also with the stresses of parenting in general by helping parents choose healthy lifestyles. Good nutrition, moderate exercise, and "adult time" apart from the children can be effective stress relievers.

In her classic work on parenting, Diana Baumrind (1971) classified three types of parents. They are described as follows:

1. Authoritarian parent: This parent sets up very strict rules. The child has little or no voice in family decisions. This style of parenting is evidenced by novelty clothing imprinted with the saying "Because I'm the Mommy/Daddy, that's why!" Authoritarian parents can lead to a rebellious, hostile child who may enter adulthood angry, violent, unwilling to obey laws, and unable to make consistent decisions.
2. Authoritative parent: This style of parenting has firm, consistent rules and limits, although the parent allows for discussion and occasional flexibility of those rules according to special circumstances. Children are allowed some freedom, within set limits, and some voice in decisions. Researchers think that this is the preferred style of parenting. It offers a balance between rules and responsibilities, which allows the child to learn to make appropriate choices and accept the outcomes of those choices.

3. Permissive parent: This is the type of parent many adolescents wish they had. This style of parenting provides little structure and few guidelines. The child is not sure of his or her boundaries. If one does not learn boundaries, it becomes difficult to learn how to control oneself and how to behave in certain situations. Permissive parents can be in danger of being accused of neglect. The parent acts as the child's friend rather than the parent of the child.

Later work by Maccoby and Martin expanded on Baumrind's theories, adding a fourth type of parent, the uninvolved parent (Tancred and Greef, 2015). According to Maccoby and Martin, this type of parent or guardian lacks responsiveness and demandingness, choosing not to be involved with the child. Maccoby and Martin called this parenting style *neglectful parenting*. The neglectful parent(s) did not demonstrate any involvement with the child, and interaction was minimal. The parent(s) demonstrated no interest in what the child felt was important. The effect on the child was having poor socializing abilities.

All of the parenting styles affect children emotionally, socially, and academically.

Clinical Activity

Select someone you know who is a parent. This can be a family member, friend, neighbor, or anyone you feel comfortable with. Using the parenting definitions of Diana Baumrind, identify what basic parenting style you think this parent is using and provide a rationale for your selection.

Safe and Effective Nursing Care

Assess and respect patients' cultural needs, values, and beliefs (dietary, modesty)
Identify patients' religious needs
Provide therapeutic communication
Provide a therapeutic environment
Direct patients with limited housing and other financial difficulties to a case manager
Identify dysfunctional families

Key Points

- Culture, ethnicity, gender identity, sexual orientation, and religion are deeply rooted human experiences. They are not "good" or "bad"; they are different for each individual who claims membership in that group.
- People have many more similarities than they have differences. It is important for nurses to concentrate on the similarities among people and to be comfortable asking questions about the background of their patients. Role modeling cooperative relationships can be very helpful in teaching others about cultural sensitivity.
- Homelessness can affect men, women, and children. The majority of homeless people are without employment, although those who are employed earn salaries that do not allow them to afford a place to live.
- Parenting is learned from experience and not something a person knows at birth.

CASE STUDY

Harold is a 76-year-old resident of a long-term care facility. He has type 1 diabetes and gives himself his own insulin. He has the diagnosis of paranoid schizophrenia but has been asymptomatic for 1 year. Harold is also a severe alcoholic, and he periodically leaves the nursing home against medical advice and is gone for 2 to 3 days. He has friends "on the street" because, before being institutionalized, that is where he lived. Harold goes to the local shelter for meals and knows he can go to the hospital to get his insulin. He has no family in the vicinity who can participate in his care.

CASE STUDY—cont'd

He no longer meets the criteria for skilled-care nursing. A decision must be made about his future, as he will no longer be eligible to remain in this facility. Harold wishes to be his own advocate and is found to be legally capable of making his own decisions. The outcome for this patient is that he chooses to "take my chances" and return to the streets. He has not been seen again by any of the facility staff. No further information is available about this patient.

1. Considering Maslow's hierarchy of needs (see Chapter 4), how would you classify Harold?
2. What are the arguments both for and against his decision to leave the long-term care facility?
3. Do you consider Harold to be mentally healthy and competent? Why or why not?

Review Questions

1. The concepts of space, time, and waiting are:
   a. Religious
   b. Cultural
   c. Economic
   d. Ethnic

2. The condition of judging a person or situation before knowing all the facts is called:
   a. Hatred
   b. Abuse
   c. Prejudice
   d. Stereotype

3. The phenomenon of homelessness in the United States can be blamed, in part, on:
   a. Deinstitutionalization
   b. Access to community services
   c. Mental illness
   d. All of the above

4. Nurses who care for patients who are homeless understand that in the United States:
   a. Homelessness is classified as a mental illness.
   b. Approximately one-third of homeless people are mentally ill.
   c. All people who are homeless have some form of mental illness.
   d. People must be mentally ill to choose to be homeless.

5. A patient is admitted with the diagnosis of paranoid behavior. The patient claims to be of a religion requiring the wearing of very heavy necklaces. You research the religion and determine this to be true, but the patient has been seen violently flinging the necklace at their roommate. Your best nursing action is:
   a. Call an assistance code.
   b. Remove all religious items.
   c. Do nothing: it is the patient's religious right.
   d. Enlist the assistance of a representative of the patient's religion to negotiate removal of the item(s) in question.

6. Parents accompany their ill 8-year-old child to the clinic. The child was diagnosed last month with type 1 diabetes and is insulin dependent. The parents admit they are not administering the insulin, as their religious beliefs do not allow the injection of foreign substances in any form for any reason. A check of the patient's chart clearly indicates that diabetes teaching had been done with this family at last month's visit. Your initial nursing action is:
   a. Report the parents for child endangerment, as nurses are mandatory reporters.
   b. Inform the parents that this child could die without the required insulin.
   c. Leave the room and call a doctor or registered nurse (RN) to the room stat.
   d. Collect information pertaining to what the religion would allow and facilitate discussion with the doctor.

7. When collecting data during an intake interview, the nurse understands (select all that apply):
   a. Most homeless people are unemployed.
   b. Culture is a shared belief system.
   c. Prejudice exists within the health-care delivery system.
   d. There is no correlation between mental illness and the condition of homelessness.

8. The most common reasons for homelessness include (select all that apply):
   a. Economic setbacks
   b. Lack of ambition and laziness
   c. Major health expenses
   d. Desire to live independently
   e. Mental health

9. Language, country of origin, and skin color define:
   a. Religion
   b. Culture
   c. Ethnocentrism
   d. Ethnicity

10. Diana Baumrind describes authoritative parenting as:
   a. The child has little or no voice in any of the family's decisions.
   b. The parents are always reminding the child that they are the parents.
   c. The child has a minimum number of guidelines.
   d. The child has rules to follow and has limits set.

REVIEW QUESTIONS ANSWER KEY 1.b, 2.c, 3.b, 4.b, 5.d, 6.d, 7.b, c, d, 8.a, c, e, 9.d, 10.d

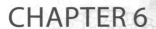

CHAPTER 6
Nursing Process in Mental Health

KEY TERMS

Affect
Assessment
Awareness
Data collection
Evaluation
Formal teaching
Implementation
Informal teaching
Judgment
Memory
Mood
North american nursing diagnosis
  association-independence (NANDA-I)
Nursing diagnosis
Nursing interventions classification (NIC)
Nursing outcomes classification (NOC)
Nursing process
Objective
Orientation
Patient interview
Patient teaching
Plan of care
Planning
Scope of practice
Subjective
Thinking/cognition

CHAPTER CONCEPTS

Collaboration
Communication
Health promotion
Professionalism

LEARNING OUTCOMES

1. Define the role of the licensed practical nurse (LPN)/
   licensed vocational nurse (LVN) in the five steps of
   the nursing process.
2. Identify the components of a mental health status
   assessment.
3. State the need for the nursing process in mental
   health issues.
4. State the concepts of patient interviewing.
5. Prepare a patient interview.
6. Collaborate in creating a nursing process for a given,
   hypothetical patient.
7. State the concepts of patient teaching.
8. Prepare and implement a teaching exercise.

NURSING PROCESS

The **nursing process** is a tool used throughout all areas
and levels of nursing (FIG. 6.1). Although some parts of
the nursing process apply only to the registered nurse
(RN), the LPN/LVN will still participate in the process.
The nursing process is a formula nurses use to provide
individual patient care and to organize and implement
care in a systematic, universal way. The nursing process
also allows you to determine whether the plan and interventions produce a favorable outcome for the patient.
In preparing to use the nursing process for patient care,
you need to incorporate critical thinking to arrive at the
desired outcome. It is part of the culture of nurses to be
part of a positive outcome. An overview of the nursing
process is given in Table 6.1.

  Scope of practice describes the services that a health
professional who is educated or trained is deemed competent to perform. It specifies under what conditions the
services may be delivered, and it regulates the roles of

| Assessment | Nursing diagnosis | Planning | Intervention | Evaluation |

FIGURE 6.1 Steps in the nursing process

Table 6.1
The Nursing Process—ADPIE

Assessment	Nursing Diagnosis (NANDA-I)	Planning	Implementation/ Intervention	Evaluation
Subjective/ objective: Collects patient data to assist the nurse in providing care and providing for the patient needs	Relates to the assessment data to determine how the nurse will plan for the care needed; use the problem, etiology, signs and symptoms (PES) model	Plans the patient's outcome: short- and long-term goals; must be measurable, realistic, and achievable, with target dates	Defines what actions the nurse/ health-care provider will provide; the nurse/ health-care provider should be able to provide a rationale for each action/treatment provided.	Determines whether the plan and the interventions provided the expected outcome; determine which interventions can be continued, changed, or terminated.

the RN and the LPN/LVN in the nursing process. In the early 1950s, Hildegard Peplau (see Chapter 1) hypothesized that nurses are a tool best utilized in relationship to the patient and the environment and in collaboration with other nurses and health-care professionals. She stressed the phases of a working relationship that included a termination phase where nurses prepare both themselves and their patients for termination of the relationship. Peplau's model is still widely used in nursing practice today.

GOOD TO KNOW
LPNs/LVNs should know and understand their scope of practice in order to provide safe and effective health care.

In the early 1970s, the American Nurses Association (ANA) developed standards of practice for RN- and LPN/LVN-prepared nurses. The association differentiated between the RN role and the LPN/LVN role in the nursing process; however, the LPN/LVN plays a part in all decisions made. Individual state Nurse Practice Acts and Boards of Nursing may

also offer their own interpretation of the ANA guidelines relating to the role and scope of practice for the LPN/LVN in the nursing process. The following section of the chapter provides a step-by-step explanation of the nursing process.

Tool Box
The nursing process is a systematic approach to providing care.

https://www.nursingworld.org/practice-policy/ workforce/what-is-nursing/the-nursing-process/

STEP 1: ASSESSING THE PATIENT'S MENTAL HEALTH

Assessment is the first step in the nursing process. The role of the LPN/LVN in step 1 is to assist with the assessment—the collection of data. The RN is responsible for the initial assessment when the patient is admitted to or transferred into a facility. The LPN/LVN is not responsible for the initial assessment, although the LPN/LVN does learn the importance of **subjective** and **objective** assessment data. In some states, the term *observation* is preferred instead of *assessment* for the LPN/LVN. **Data collection** is made during every contact a nurse has with a patient. It is essential to the well-being of the patient and in assisting the medical team in making the best choices concerning that person. In most cases, data collection is accomplished by filling out a document that is used by the facility. Nurses assess the patient's attitude, tone of voice, facial expression, and other physical objectives—the nonverbal communication—as well. Unfortunately, many of these generic forms are written in closed-ended format. They are very impersonal and may not reflect the specific information needed about that patient.

It is during the data collection/assessment part of the nursing process that the mental status examination is performed. The mental health assessment gives a picture of the patient at the time of admission as well as other medical health information. The mental status examination is a series of questions and activities that check eight areas: the patient's (1) level of **awareness** and **orientation**, (2) appearance and behavior, (3) speech and communication, (4) **mood** and **affect**, (5) **memory**, (6) **thinking/cognition**, (7) perception, and (8) **judgment**. These examinations are of varying lengths and formats, but they all assess the patient's mental capabilities.

Table 6.2 lists areas to be included in a mental status examination. It also suggests the type of assessment that should be made and provides ideas for questions or requests that can be used by members of the health-care team to make the assessments. Finally, it gives some parameters for normal and abnormal responses.

Nurses have many ways to improve the quality of data collection. One of these is to conduct interviews. For the purposes of this text, the word interview pertains to any nurse-patient interaction that requires a nurse to obtain specific information from a patient. The **patient interview** is usually the primary method of data gathering. It is important to collect data about the whole person. Data related to thoughts and feelings are as important to any nurse-patient interview as the physical data collected. Two types of interview are discussed in more detail.

1. **Intake/Admission Interview**

   Most facilities have standard admission interview forms that suit their particular needs. The forms are written in a very matter-of-fact way and are usually in a closed-ended format (see Chapter 2). Patients who are frightened, angry, or just too ill at the moment may easily refuse to answer those closed-ended questions. The patient may have answered the same questions when initially entering the facility and may feel frustrated by what they perceive to be inefficiency or poor communication among the staff when the same questions are repeated. This can set up both the nurse and the patient for a difficult time. It is up to the nurse to rephrase the questions in an open-ended format that will seem more individualized to the patient.

Example
Standard form: "Do you smoke or use alcohol? _____ YES _____ NO."

Nurse interviewer: "I am required to provide you with information about the hospital's policies on the use of tobacco and alcohol." This statement might then be followed by the standard closed-ended question, "Do you use any tobacco or alcohol?"

Questions can be changed from the closed-ended type to open-ended in most cases. Practice and patience on the part of the nurse interviewer will make this a more caring experience for both the nurse and the patient.

Table 6.2
Mental Status Examination

Area of Assessment	Type of Assessment	Suggested Methods of Assessment and Normal Parameters	Alterations to Normal Assessment
Appearance	Observation of patient's dress, hygiene, posture, actions, and reactions to health-care personnel. Observe for wounds and scars.	Clean, hair combed; clothing intact and appropriate to weather or situation; teeth in good repair; posture erect; cooperates with health-care personnel	Displays either unusual apathy or concern about appearance
Behavior	Objective	Cooperates with health-care personnel Makes direct eye contact (The appropriateness of eye contact depends on the patient's culture.)	Displays uncooperative, hostile, or suspicious-type behaviors toward health-care personnel. Restless
Level of consciousness (LOC)	Subjective and objective assessment of the patient's degree of alertness (wakefulness)	Awareness is measured on a continuum that ranges from unconsciousness to mania. "Normal alertness" is the desired behavior. There is usually a standard guideline for helping with this assessment, but subjective observations can be documented as well, such as if the patient cannot stay awake for even short intervals or is overly active and has difficulty staying in one place for any period of time.	Outcome is not within normal limits if the patient is difficult to arouse and keep awake or finds it difficult to feel calm.
Orientation	The degree of patient's knowledge of self	Orientation measures the person's ability to know who they are, where they are, and the day and time, usually within 1 or 2 days of the actual day and time. Measurement techniques are accomplished by asking the patient, "What is your name?" "Where are you right now?" and "Tell me what the day and date are." Asking "Who is the president of the United States?" is used in the United States as well. Nurses frequently document this as "oriented X 3," but it is best to also write down the objective data on which this routine answer is based.	Abnormal results of orientation are the patient's inability to correctly answer questions pertaining to themselves or to commonly known social information.

Table 6.2
Mental Status Examination—cont'd

Area of Assessment	Type of Assessment	Suggested Methods of Assessment and Normal Parameters	Alterations to Normal Assessment
Content of thought	Subjective assessment of what the patient is thinking and the process the patient uses in thinking	Formal testing may be undertaken by the psychologist or psychiatrist to determine the patient's general thought content and pattern. Nurses may contribute to the assessment of thought by documenting statements the patient makes regarding daily care and routines.	Behaviors including flight of ideas, loose associations, phobias, delusions, and obsessions may become apparent. These alterations in "normal" thought processes are defined and discussed in future chapters that relate to specific illnesses.
Memory	Subjective assessment of the patient's ability to recall recent (short-term) and remote (long-term) information and/or events	**Recent memory:** Recall of events that are immediately past or up to within 2 weeks before the assessment. One measurement technique is to verbally list five items. After 1 minute, patient should be able to recall four to five of those items. Continue with assessment and at 5 minutes, patient should be able to recall three to four of the items. **Remote memory:** Recall of events of the past beyond 2 weeks before assessment. Patients are often asked questions pertaining to where they were born, where they went to grade school, and so on.	Inability to accurately perform recent or remote recall exercises within parameters may indicate symptoms of delirium or dementia.
Speech and ability to communicate	Objective and subjective assessment of aspects of patient's use of verbal and nonverbal communication	Patient can coherently produce words appropriate to age and education. Rate of speech reflects other psychomotor activity (e.g., faster if patient is agitated). Volume is not too soft or too loud. Stuttering, repetition of words, and words that the patient "makes up" (neologisms) are also assessed.	Limited speech production; rate of speech is inconsistent with other psychomotor activity. Volume is not appropriate to situation (speaks at a very loud volume even when asked to speak more quietly). Stuttering, word repetition, or neologisms may indicate physical or psychological illness; hypertalkative; mumbled or slurred speech

Continued

Table 6.2

Mental Status Examination—cont'd

Area of Assessment	Type of Assessment	Suggested Methods of Assessment and Normal Parameters	Alterations to Normal Assessment
Mood and affect	Subjective (mood) and objective (objective) assessment of the patient's stated feelings and emotions Affect measures the outward expression of those feelings.	Mood is the stated emotional condition of the patient and should fluctuate to reflect situations as they occur. Facial expression and body language (affect) should match (be congruent with) stated mood. Affect should change to fluctuate with the changes in mood.	Mood and affect do not match (e.g., facial expression does not change when stating opposite feelings).
Abstract thinking/ judgment	Subjective assessment of a patient's ability to make appropriate decisions about their situation or to understand concepts	Give patient a proverb to interpret, such as "You can't teach an old dog new tricks." Patient should be able to give some sort of acceptable interpretation such as "Old habits are hard to break" or "It is hard to learn something new." *Or* give the patient a situation to solve (judgment). For example, ask the patient what they would do if a small child were lost in a store. An appropriate response might be "to call the manager" or "to try to calm the child."	Patient cannot interpret the proverb in an acceptable manner. Patient cannot complete problem-solving questions appropriately. The patient might answer very literally, "Dogs can't learn anything when they get old" or "I would go through the child's pockets to see if there were any phone numbers in them."
Perception	Assesses the way a person experiences reality. Assessment is based on the patient's statements about their environment and the behaviors associated with those statements. Nurses and health-team members must document this often-subjective information in objective terms.	All five senses are monitored for interaction with the patient's reality. Patient's insight into their condition is also assessed.	Presence of hallucinations and illusions. These are discussed further in Chapter 15. Individuals who are not within normal boundaries of judgment or insight will not be able to state understanding of the origin of the illness and the behaviors associated with it.

2. Helping Interview

The helping interview is used to determine or isolate a particular concern of the patient and to help the patient learn to help themself (FIG. 6.2). Patients may trust nurses more than other health-care providers because nurses have built a rapport with them and are usually more easily accessible than others. It is important to remember, though, not to help to the point of interfering with the patient's ability to help themselves.

Consider a situation in which the patient is not progressing according to a "normal" postoperative course. The nurse notices the patient weeping and senses that a need is not being met. The nurse can use this opportunity and observation to begin obtaining information from the patient that may help explain the delayed postoperative progress.

Guidelines for Nurse-Patient Helping Interview

1. *Be honest:* Tell the patient the purpose of the interview.
2. *Be assertive:* If the interview is mandatory (e.g., intake, preoperative), let the patient know that it is needed to provide the patient with the proper care. If possible, agree upon a mutually acceptable time to conduct the interview.
3. *Be sensitive:* Sometimes the questions are very difficult or embarrassing for the patient to answer. Assure the patient that you understand their concerns and that the information they share is part of their medical record. Only the patient, the patient's designee, and people who are involved in their caregiving will have access to this information. Periodically observe your patient while conducting the interview. Be aware of your body language and tone during the interview. Do not impose your beliefs on the patient.
4. *Use empathy:* Let the patient know that you are interested in what is being said and that you are there to be helpful. Acknowledge the patient's feelings but do not judge the patient.
5. *Use open-ended questions:* Personalize the questions as much as possible. Use this time to discuss and clarify as much information as you can to avoid having to repeat parts of the interview later.

STEP 2: NURSING DIAGNOSIS: DEFINING PATIENT PROBLEMS

Processing the collected data is a function of the RN, according to the ANA. Once data are collected, the RN identifies **nursing diagnoses**. Nursing diagnoses are a universal language on which interventions are based. There are different models or theories of nursing diagnosis that may be used and recommended by your work setting. These include nursing diagnoses published by the **North American Nursing Diagnosis Association-Independence (NANDA-I)**, formerly known as *North American Nursing Diagnosis Association (NANDA)*. The NANDA-I list is updated frequently.

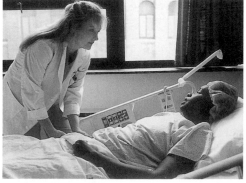

FIGURE 6.2 The helping interview allows the nurse to determine a patient's special needs and concerns *(from Williams and Hopper [2011]*. Understanding Medical-Surgical Nursing, *4th ed. Philadelphia: F.A. Davis Company, with permission).*

Tool Box

Nursing Diagnoses
Review the NANDA-I list for universal nursing diagnosis language.

http://www.nanda.org

It is the RN's responsibility to assimilate the data that have been collected and choose one or more potential nursing diagnoses for the patient. The LPN/LVN needs to understand the function of the nursing diagnosis. In collaborative nursing practice, LPN/LVNs can make suggestions and offer rationales to the RN that may be incorporated into the patient's **plan of care**.

An emerging format for writing a diagnostic statement for a patient's plan of care is the **PES** model. The components of this model are: **P**, the problem or need; **E**, the etiology or cause; and **S**, the signs, symptoms, or risk factors. The nurse blends these components into a "neutral" statement that avoids value-laden or judgmental language. The nursing diagnosis is *not* a medical diagnosis. Rather, it is a universal language used among nurses to help clarify the patient's needs (see Appendix E, Assigning Nursing Diagnoses to Client Behaviors). The nursing diagnosis also identifies whether the assessment problem is an actual problem or a potential one. The "actual problem" diagnosis will include P, E, and S, whereas the "potential problem" diagnosis will include only P and E.

STEP 3: PLANNING (SHORT- AND LONG-TERM GOALS)

The LPN/LVN role is again as a partner in care planning. The ANA believes that the RN has responsibility for this step of the nursing process. **Planning** care involves setting short- and long-term goals from the patient's perspective, not from the nurse's perspective. It is for this reason that the patient and their significant others must be involved in the plan of care. Recovery will happen much more quickly if the patient plays an active role in decision making and does not have the impression that treatment is being done *to* or *for* them but rather collaboratively *with* them.

Prioritizing the goals is the next step in planning care. This is one area in which the patient and the nurse might not see things the same way. Sometimes, the patient's priorities are different from those of the nurse. Whenever possible, the patient's priority should be considered. However, when there is a threat to life or health related to the patient's priority, the nurse must intervene and explain the reason why the patient's wishes will have to wait a while.

The aim of selecting goals that will improve mental health status is to keep the mind–body connection intact. It will be of great help to the patient if the nurse is able to detect alterations in the mental attitude and set goals with the patient

to maintain the best outlook and strongest possible effective coping skills. Both short- and long-term goals should be set for the patient. Goals should be realistic, measurable, and achievable. A target date for the plan should be included so that the patient is aware that by specific dates certain outcomes are expected.

> **GOOD TO KNOW**
> To write effective patient goals, use the acronym **SMART**. Goals should be
>
> **S** = specific
> **M** = measurable
> **A** = achievable
> **R** = realistic
> **T** = time-based

STEP 4: IMPLEMENTATIONS/ INTERVENTIONS

The LPN/LVN's role is to assist with identifying and carrying out the specific steps that will help the patient reach the goals. Nurses are able to provide input about new evidence-based practice interventions that may be helpful, and the LPN/LVN is often the person who begins to help adapt certain procedures to assist the patient. You may use this opportunity to conduct some new patient teaching or to reinforce prior teaching. Relaying information about **implementation** (putting the care plan into action) and patient progress to the RN will provide the information the team needs to offer the best possible care for the patient. You also need to understand and specify the rationale (reason) for the interventions that are selected and be prepared to explain them to the patient and their family, provided the patient consents to their involvement.

Depending on the state they live in, the LPN/LVN may play a different role when it comes to formulating outcome statements or performing an **evaluation** of interventions. In much the same way NANDA-I developed problem and nursing diagnostic standards, work is being done to standardize outcome statements. **Nursing Interventions Classification (NIC)** is a comprehensive standardized language. It provides a number of direct and indirect intervention labels with definitions and possible nursing actions. The interventions address general practice as well as specialty areas (Doenges & Moorhouse, 2013).

Clinical Activity

If your clinical affiliates will allow, arrange to shadow a nurse from the mental health unit. Write a summary of the following:

• Observations of the nurse–patient relationship
• Communication style
• Understanding
• Patient responses

CRITICAL THINKING QUESTION

Your state Nurse Practice Act allows you, the LPN/LVN, to oversee care and to function as a charge nurse when the RN is on call. Your patient has gone out on a 3-hour pass with relatives and returns to your agency refusing to follow the guidelines as stated in the care plan and behavioral contract for reentering the facility after a visit. Your patient is argumentative but answers questions appropriately. Your data collection includes fruity odor on breath, mood swings, and hunger. You need to reevaluate and revise the care plan but are unable to make contact with the RN on call. What would you consider to be appropriate nursing diagnoses? What interventions can you perform and still remain within your state's scope of nursing practice?

Patient Teaching

Many interventions that are helpful to the patient involve **patient teaching**. Frequently, facilities have special teams or departments to carry out certain teaching, but teaching is becoming a bigger part of a nurse's responsibility. This is true at all levels of nursing preparation. The health-care provider is still responsible for providing the patient and/or family with initial information, but the nurse does the "fine-tuning" required to send patients home safely. Nurses teach patients about medications, coping strategies, adaptive equipment, and anything else the patient requires, not only for the period of hospitalization, but also for the time when the patient leaves the facility. Individual states and facilities set

the guidelines regarding teaching responsibilities for health-care providers and nurses.

Everyone needs a little help when they first start teaching, regardless of what sort of teaching will be done. Like the forms used for the patient interviews, the facility may use standardized classes or teaching sheets. This practice helps ensure that continuity exists in teaching and that critical information has been given to the patient. There are some legal ramifications to teaching as well. Despite the use of standardized teaching tools, nurses still need to be aware of some principles of teaching and learning. Fortunately, most of the steps of the nursing process can be used for setting up a teaching plan.

Teaching in any form is most effective when it is started as soon as possible after admission. Nurses teach patients in different ways. Teaching can be divided into two categories: **formal teaching** and **informal teaching.**

Formal teaching is any situation in which a class or a group is scheduled or a specific objective must be met. The facilitator is often a staff nurse who has worked in the specific area being taught. Formal teaching involves a nurse and one or more patients. Usually, a pre-set curriculum is used in these one-on-one or group sessions. The time to teach in the formal setting will most likely be limited by the facility according to staffing needs, because the nurse instructor probably also has a patient assignment. Examples of formal teaching include diabetic teaching and back-care classes or teaching about defense mechanisms.

Classroom Activity

Review the main learning styles that people can have. Then, organize the class into three groups, each of which will focus on a different learning style. Working with your group, prepare a presentation on the steps of the nursing process. Use teaching methods to appeal specifically to your assigned learning style—auditory, visual, or physical (tactile), see below.

Informal teaching, or adjunctive teaching, happens anytime, anywhere, whenever the patient needs information. The patient may see the nurse in the hall, or the nurse may notice that the patient is working with a colostomy bag in his or her room or reading an exercise pamphlet. These are excellent times to reinforce what the patient has learned or to make gentle suggestions for improving their technique.

GOOD TO KNOW

Active listening enables the nurse to focus on the patient's strengths and weaknesses.

Clinical Activity

Review the medication record of your assigned patient and provide an informal teaching about one of the medications. Write the outcome of the informal teaching.

Principles of Learning

Nurse-educators need a basic understanding of the principles of learning and teaching. Some of these principles are listed here:

- Each person learns differently. Some people process information visually, others by hearing, and still others by hands-on (tactile) learning.
- Each person learns at their own pace. The larger the group, the more levels of ability the nurse will have to work with. Some patients catch on more quickly than others. Learning to teach a person with a mental health disorder may be difficult. For example, some patients may not feel comfortable learning in a group where others may become aware of their disorder.
- People learn best when the information is *meaningful* to them. Think of your own education—the things you are interested in are the things you work harder at to attain. However, subjects that you may find hard or boring are still required for licensing. In a similar way, patients may not see the importance of the class/group that they may be required to attend as a criterion for discharge.
- Learning is most effective when the information is presented in small segments, or "chunks." The size of these chunks may be dictated by the facility. But when you can be flexible, it is best to present only as much as the patient can absorb at one time.
- Positive reinforcement will help the patient succeed at learning the required task. The stronger the positive reinforcement, the greater the learning. Once patients have been successful, they will want to continue to learn. *Success breeds success.*

Principles of Teaching

1. *Know the patients:* What are their abilities? What is their prior level of knowledge about the subject? What, if any, are the cultural or language differences of the patients in the class?
2. *Know the material:* It is not as important to give a "perfect" talk or demonstration as it is to be able to correctly interpret and respond to questions patients may have. Sometimes the nurse-educator will need to adapt the teaching plan to meet a particular patient's need. An educator who is not comfortable with the material will be less helpful to the patient than one who can individualize the curriculum to the various needs of the class.
3. *Have a teaching plan:* A good teaching plan will improve your confidence and delivery of the material. A very simple format, such as ADPIE for the nursing process, may be easily transformed into a teaching format by omitting the "diagnosis." Thus, the teaching format would be APIE.

GOOD TO KNOW

You can easily remember the steps of the nursing process with the acronym **ADPIE**, which stands for **A**ssessment, **D**iagnosis, **P**lanning, **I**ntervention/ **I**mplementation, **E**valuation.

- **A** = assessment. What is the need for the teaching? Is the patient aware of their diagnosis? What does the patient know about their diagnosis? Ask the patient about their education preference. Assess patients' learning limitations. Assess if the patient would like family members or friends to be involved. Is this the appropriate time for patient education? Will this be informal or formal teaching? For example, "Good afternoon, Mr. Smith. My name is Sandy, I am your nurse. I would like to know if you are aware of your diagnosis." Assessment can also be enhanced by the use of a pretest or questions to the patient to determine their past knowledge in this area.

- **P** = plan. The plan is often called the *goal*. Nurse-educators need to ask themselves a few questions, such as: What do I plan to accomplish in this initial educational meeting? What teaching strategies will I use? During the first meeting you will define a short-term goal and review the desired long-term goal. For example, "Our goal for today is to learn about the medications you will be taking." It is important that the patient understand that goals must be specific, realistic, measurable, achievable, and time-based.

- **I** = implementation. This is the step-by-step method that will be used to accomplish the plan, for both short and long term. The nurse will have as many or as few steps as needed. The steps are written out and a rationale is included with each step, but it may or may not be necessary to perform each step every time. This will depend on the individual or patient group. Chances are good that an individual or a group will never be taught exactly the same way twice. However, there will be critical items you need to cover with all patients to meet legal and safety requirements.

- **E** = evaluation. In a teaching plan, nurses evaluate the patient's learning as well as the teaching performance. Some questions that you need to reflect on for this part of the teaching plan are the following: How do you know the patient has grasped the teaching? What do you look for? Do you need to ask for feedback or a return demonstration? Does the feedback or return demonstration need to be perfect? How did you do as a teacher? Did you achieve the plan? Was the patient able to reach all the goals? Did you have enough time? What will you do differently next time? Does the patient show evidence that their behavior may change as a result of the teaching plan? Evaluation criteria may change from time to time as well.

4. *Be flexible:* To the extent that the facility's program allows, be familiar enough with the material to be able to build in extra practice time for the tactile learners, extra videos for the visual learners, or time to review verbally for the auditory learners. Be able to teach in several different styles.

5. *Be able to evaluate the learning:* In health teaching in a facility, evaluation can be in the form of a question-answer session, a short quiz, or a return demonstration.

6. *Plan to allow a few minutes after the session for questions:* Even though you may ask for and welcome questions during the session, there are always people who are not comfortable asking questions in a group. These people will want your time in private, so allow some time to clarify their concerns after class or set up a time to help them later in the day.

Once the teaching plan has been developed, you need to think about how and when to implement the teaching. This requires familiarity with some commonly used methods of teaching, especially the patient's learning style.

Educators tend to teach according to the style of learning they prefer. For instance, if nursing students prefer lecture classes, they probably feel most comfortable teaching in a lecture format. If a specific nursing instructor was particularly helpful to a nurse as a student, the nurse may prefer to use that teacher's methods when teaching patients. No teaching method is better or worse than any other method. What makes the difference is the learning style of the patients and the rapport that you build with them. Because classes in facilities generally have more than one pupil, you will need to be able to use different methods of presenting information. Because people's personalities are different, each group will have a different dynamic, and each class will be different.

The typical methods used in health teaching are lecture and demonstration.

1. *Lecture:* This is a teaching method designed for information giving. It is unilateral; you talk, and the patients listen. It is interactive only when there is some form of question-answer period or brainstorming. Lecturing is an excellent method of introducing a topic to patients and giving them some theory. It is a way to explain the significance of the topic so that the material becomes meaningful to them.

   In preset programs, the lectures are usually prepared in either text or outline form so that the nurse educator needs to invest only minimal time in researching, writing, or setting up for the class. Learning sessions may include videos, slides, or charts. Learning from the lecture method is traditionally evaluated through quizzes or question-and-answer sessions.

Because not all patient participants are comfortable answering in a group, it may be difficult to assess how much learning each individual achieves.

> ### GOOD TO KNOW
> Not everyone has the same learning style. Finding the style that is best for a particular patient may help to change behavior.

2. *Demonstration:* Demonstration is an excellent technique to follow in an introductory lecture. For visual and tactile learners, it is the preferred method of learning.

   In prepared programs, the demonstration outline will be provided. You are responsible for having the instructions needed for each patient. For a patient who is being discharged from a facility on psychotropic medications to reduce their mental health symptoms, you need to have ready information about each medication, its dosage, the time to take it, and possible side effects to report. If the patient is a diabetic, diabetic teaching is essential as well as learning about finger-stick tests, oral medications, or insulin injections.

   Demonstrations are effective because, after the initial demonstration, you can have the individual, their partner, or a family member perform a return demonstration. One-on-one help can be provided if needed. This allows you to make more objective assessments of the patient's learning and therefore predict the patient's ability to safely perform the technique after discharge. It also allows you to individualize the technique or provide options to the patient. Watch each patient perform the technique at a level that is safe for them to perform when at home and not under the guidance of a healthcare professional. If a home health nurse is assigned to the patient, patient teaching continues.

Additional Patient Teaching Tips

• *Be culturally sensitive.* In the United States, it is customary to assess eye contact and to equate eye contact with interest and attentiveness in a class or activity. It is important for you to remember that this is a cultural behavior. Not all cultures believe that eye contact is a positive thing; indeed, many cultures consider direct meeting of eyes a sign of blatant disrespect for people who are older or in a position of respect or authority. Nurses and educators are typically respected in these cultural groups, and it would be a mistake on your part to assume that the lack of direct eye contact is a sign of disinterest in or disrespect for the material.

• *Incorporate teaching to family/caregivers.* This can require identifying different learning styles, which presents some challenges

• *Be honest.* Nobody said a nurse must have all the answers. If you do not know something, admit it. Then, look up the information and either bring it to the individual who asked or bring it to the next session of the class.

• *Have fun!* Teaching can be a very rewarding part of nursing. There is no better way to reinforce nursing knowledge than to teach it to someone else. It is one way in which you can keep the nursing culture alive.

> ## Evidence-Based Practice
>
> **Clinical Question:** What can you do to enhance patient teaching?
>
> **Evidence:** This study showed that effective patient teaching is audible as well as visual and does not overload the patient with information to be learned. Patient teaching was more effective when it was limited to seven items at one time. Patients also need some control of the learning materials available. Visual aids used should match the audible material being taught.
>
> **Implications for Nursing Practice:** Provide the patient a pen or pencil and paper to take notes. Provide information at the rate that is best for the patient. Have visual aids that align with the audible information you are providing. Get feedback from the patient if they understand the information being provided throughout the teaching instead of waiting until the end.
>
> Pusic, M. V., Ching, K., Yin, H. S., & Kessler, D. (2014). Seven practical principles for improving patient education: Evidence-based ideas from cognition science. *Pediatrics & Child Health, 19*(3), 119–122. https://doi.org/10.1093/pch/19.3.119

STEP 5: EVALUATION/OUTCOME

In the final step of the nursing process, the LPN/LVN plays an assisting role. The LPN/LVN's observations and documentation about the effect of the interventions on the patient and progress in attaining the goal are of great importance. Accuracy in verbal and written reporting of the patient's progress will help determine whether the interventions have been helpful or whether they need to be reevaluated and changed. In some instances, some of the interventions can be terminated, depending on the patient's progress (DeWit, 2009).

Nursing Outcomes Classification (NOC) is a standardized language that provides outcome statements, a set of indicators describing specific patient, caregiver, family, or community states related to the outcome, and a five-point measurement scale to facilitate tracking patients across care settings. NOC can help demonstrate patient progress even when outcomes are not fully met. NOC is applicable in all care settings and specialties (Doenges & Moorhouse, 2012). The NOC provides evidence if the interventions/implementations were effective for a positive patient outcome.

CRITICAL THINKING QUESTION
Select a topic to teach the class in 10 minutes (or however much time your classroom instructor chooses). This can be any topic with which you are comfortable. Develop a teaching plan, teach your topic, and evaluate your teaching. What would you do differently the next time?

Safe and Effective Nursing Care
Provide care within the LVN/LPN scope of practice
Assess each patient in a systematic manner
Create individualized care plans for patients
Collaborate with all health-care providers caring for the patient
Educate each patient regarding self-care, medication, and support groups
Advocate for providing respectful and nonjudgmental care for patients

Key Points

- The nursing process is an example of collaborative nursing practice. RNs are primarily responsible for the steps of the nursing process; LPN/LVN-prepared nurses assist in data collection and planning, implementing, and evaluating the nursing process.
- The nursing process format can be used by other health-care disciplines to create a care plan.
- Nurses conduct interviews and teaching on a daily basis. Entry-level nurses need a basic knowledge of both skills. Individual states and

- facilities set the guidelines for teaching within the scope of the nurse's practice.
- The nursing process is a helpful tool for preparing a teaching plan.
- Patient education is essential, as is including the patient in goal planning.
- The ANA sets guidelines that dictate the roles of the RN and the LPN/LVN in collaborating in the nursing process.
- New models for collaborative nursing and nursing outcome statements are being developed.

CASE STUDY

Mark is a 15-year-old student who has recently quit attending his high school classes. Mark has always been a straight A student who participated in many social and athletic activities at his school.

Today, Mark's friend Tony brings Mark to the clinic that is part of your community's hospital. Tony tells you, "Mark got in with a bad group. He's been doin' the stuff real bad. He's been doin' the needles and the smoking. He's been with me for 2 days, man, and he's real sick. Help him."

You and the health-care provider undertake an assessment of Mark and find that he has yellowing of his sclera. He has a fruity odor on his breath and is vomiting copiously. Mark's level of consciousness is lethargic; he is in and out of coherence and is not a reliable source of information about himself at this time.

The provider notifies Mark's parents and explains that Mark may have several conditions, including but not limited to serum hepatitis.

Meanwhile, you continue to admit Mark to the hospital for further testing and medical care. He is placed in enteric isolation as a precaution. An IV is started, and you begin to explain the hospital routines to Mark. After you tell him that he must remain in his room for now and that his visitors will be limited during the time of the isolation precautions, he becomes angry. He states that this is "an invasion of his privacy" and that "you nurses are all part of the conspiracy."

1. How would you start the nursing process for this patient?
2. Describe some questions you would ask as part of the mental status examination.

Review Questions

1. The nursing process is a method for:
   a. Systematically organizing and implementing patient care
   b. Documenting patient needs
   c. Differentiating the RN role from the LPN/LVN role
   d. Collecting data

2. You are assisting in collecting data on a new patient in your unit. The health-care provider suspects alcohol abuse. You want to learn the patient's history and frequency of alcohol use. Your best choice for collecting these data might be to ask:
   a. "Do you use alcohol?"
   b. "How often do you get drunk?"
   c. "How many times a week would you say you drink alcohol?"
   d. "Why do you use alcohol? It's bad for you."

3. When conducting patient teaching, the best method to evaluate understanding of the teaching is:
   a. Lecture
   b. Return demonstration
   c. Implementation
   d. Assessment

4. The mental status examination takes place during what part of the nursing process?
   a. Assessment
   b. Planning
   c. Implementation
   d. Evaluation

5. Which of the following are components of the planning part of the nursing process? (Select all that apply)
   a. Short-term goals
   b. Long-term goals
   c. Subjective data
   d. Objective data
   e. Evaluation

6. According to ANA, the RN is the primary person for developing this part of the care plan:
   a. Nursing diagnosis
   b. Implementation/interventions
   c. Evaluation
   d. Initial assessment

7. Which of the following is/are part of the principles of teaching? (Select all that apply)
   a. Being flexible
   b. Evaluating the learning
   c. Teaching without a teaching plan
   d. Knowing the patient

8. The mental health status examination includes (select all that apply):
   a. Memory
   b. Judgment
   c. Mood and tone
   d. Mood and affect
   e. Level of awareness and orientation

9. NANDA-I is responsible for:
   a. Interventions
   b. Implementation
   c. Appearance
   d. Nursing diagnoses

10. Dianne is sitting in her hospital bed holding the orange given to her to practice her insulin injections. When the nurse enters the room, Dianne asks when she is going to inject herself instead of the orange. This statement indicates that Dianne is ready for:
    a. Discharge to home
    b. More time injecting the orange
    c. Informal teaching
    d. Formal teaching

REVIEW QUESTIONS ANSWER KEY 1.a, 2.c, 3.b, 4.a, 5.a, b, 6.a, 7.a, b, d, 8.a, b, d, e, 9.d, 10.d

CHAPTER 7

Stress, Coping, and Defense Mechanisms

KEY TERMS

Adaptation
Coping
Defense mechanisms
Effective coping
Eustress
Ineffective coping
Stress
Stressor

CHAPTER CONCEPTS

Cognition
Health promotion
Stress

LEARNING OUTCOMES

1. Define coping.
2. Differentiate between effective and ineffective coping.
3. Classify defense (coping) mechanisms.
4. Identify main characteristics of various defense mechanisms.

Stress produces anxiety. Stress, which is subjective, is everywhere in today's society. Although stress is most commonly associated with negative situations, good things that happen to people, such as weddings and job promotions, can also produce stress. The stress from positive experiences, such as getting married or receiving a promotion at work, is called eustress. It can produce just as much anxiety as negative stressors. A **stressor** is any person or situation that produces anxiety responses. Stress and stressors are different for each person; therefore, it is important that you ask what the stress producers are for each patient. What is extremely stressful for one person—for example, driving in rush hour traffic—might be relaxing to someone else who goes with the traffic flow and uses that time to relax after a busy day.

Biologically, the basic stress response is called the fight-or-flight response, and it contributes to feelings of anxiety (Chapter 10). In this response to stress, the blood vessels constrict because epinephrine and norepinephrine have been released. Blood pressure rises. If the body adapts to the stress, hormone levels adjust to compensate for the epinephrine-norepinephrine release, and the body functions return to homeostasis. If the body does not adapt to the stress, many long-term health problems can be created. According to Shaw et al. (2018), most of our body systems are affected by stress (FIG. 7.1).

> ## GOOD TO KNOW
> Recent theories about the fight-or-flight response have added a third stress response: freeze. Freezing is the response of a deer in headlights. In this response to stress, a person can neither fight nor flee. In fact, they cannot even move or speak (Jacobson, 2021).

CRISIS	• "Fight or flight" • Blood vessels constrict • Norepinephrine and epinephrine are released and blood pressure is increased

ADAPTATION	• Hormone levels adjust • Body functions return to homeostasis

OR

EXHAUSTION	• Immune system becomes challenged • Lymph nodes increase in size • Potential for cardiac and renal failure • Death may occur

FIGURE 7.1 General adaptation syndrome (GAS) model of stress.

Studies are continually being conducted trying to correlate stress to physical illness. In 2019, researchers at Carnegie Mellon University in Pittsburgh, Pennsylvania, and at the University of California, San Francisco, studied the correlation between stress and physical illness (Cohen et al., 2019). One of their findings was that some stress is out of our control. According to Cohen et al. (2019, p. 16), "Chronic stressor exposure is considered to be the most toxic form of stressor exposure because chronic events are the most likely to result in long-term or permanent changes in the emotional, physiological, and behavioral responses that influence susceptibility to and course of disease."

As a nurse, you will frequently encounter stress in medical-surgical patients, as well as in patients with mental health disorders. Physical and emotional symptoms can interrelate. Therefore, it is important for you to recognize the relationship between physical and emotional responses to stress. You can provide more accurate planning and interventions for your patients by conducting accurate assessment and documentation of their symptoms as their bodies adapt to stress. Table 7.1 gives examples of medical conditions and the effects of the body's adaptation response to stress.

 COPING

Deal with it. Get a grip. Don't make a mountain out of a molehill. These are pieces of advice that most people have heard or have given at some point. But what do they mean? What is coping? Coping is the way a person adapts to a stressor psychologically, physically, and behaviorally. It is the ability a person develops to deal consciously with problems and stress.

> **GOOD TO KNOW**
> As a health-care provider, it is important to realize that coping is individualized.

Individuals have different methods of coping, or dealing, with their stressors. What makes some people very successful at handling stress and others not successful at all? What allows some

Evidence-Based Practice

Clinical Question: Is yoga an effective method to relieve stress in nurses?

Evidence: This study reviews the effects of several types of yoga on healthy people. Yoga can be used as a preventive measure for stress, especially in the workplace. There has been an increase in workplace stress for nurses with the coronavirus disease 2019 (COVID-19) pandemic. Hatha yoga has been proven to assist with whole-body relaxation. Nurses who practice yoga experienced fewer on-the-job injuries and reported improved teamwork.

Implications for Nursing Practice: Nurses should be encouraged to practice yoga. Lunchtime or after-work yoga programs can assist nurses in managing their stress, improving their health, and working better with their teams.

Ram, A. B., Kumar, P., & Rao, K. D. (2020). Stress reduction through yoga., *International Conference on Enhancing Skills in Physical Education and Sports Science 2020* (1st ed., pp. 452–454). Rubicon Publications.

Table 7.1

Stress and Its Physiological Effects on the Body

Body System	Response to Stress	Outcome
Central nervous system	• Flight, fight, or freeze response occurs. • Alterations take place in the sympathetic nervous system. • Brain signals the body to react.	• Increase in blood pressure • Increase in heart rate • Increase in blood glucose
Endocrine system	• Message sent to the brain from the hypothalamus. • Liver produces more glucose for quick energy. • Increase in thyroid stimulating hormone (TSH) boosts metabolism.	• Production of stress hormone • Increase in steroid hormone
Respiratory system	• Alteration in air flow • Alteration in gas exchange	• Increase in respiration (hyperventilation) • May create shortness of breath • Exacerbates problems for people with chronic obstructive pulmonary disease (COPD) • Asthma attack
Cardiovascular system	• Increase in blood pressure • Increase in heart rate • Constriction of coronary vessels • Increased epinephrine and norepinephrine	• Inflammation of coronary arteries • Increased risk of heart attack and/or stroke • Long-term negative effect on kidneys and endocrine system
Gastrointestinal system	• Increased stomach acid • Increased or decreased appetite • Affects peristalsis • Weakens intestinal barrier	• Diarrhea • Constipation • Gas • Bloating • Nausea and or vomiting • Heartburn • Gastroesophageal reflux
Musculoskeletal system	• Increase or decrease in muscle contraction • Affects respiratory accessory muscles	• Muscle tension • Tension headaches, migraines • Backache, muscle spasms
Reproductive system	• Alterations in menstrual/ovulation cycle • Alterations in sexual function	• Irregular menstrual periods • Increased cramping and menstrual pain • Erectile dysfunction • Decreased libido (sexual drive)
Immune system	• Interferes with effectiveness of the body's antibodies	• Increased susceptibility to bacterial and viral infections and other illnesses

people to have an occasional drink or to engage in exercise to reduce their stress and causes others to become addicted to the same behavior? The answers to these questions are, of course, complex.

Culture, religion, and an individual's belief system seem to be the primary factors in this mystery. Personal choices also play a supporting role. In addition, biological chemistry plays a role in coping in the presence of some psychiatric disorders. The short-term and long-term goals of changing a behavior emphasize the use of specific, effective coping skills. What are effective coping skills, and how do nurses observe and measure them?

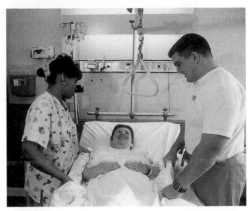

FIGURE 7.2 Involving patients and their families in the treatment plan can go a long way toward reducing the stress of hospitalization *(from Williams and Hopper [2011].* Understanding Medical-Surgical Nursing, *4th ed. Philadelphia: F.A. Davis Company, with permission).*

Tool Box

Managing Stress

For suggestions on managing stress, see www. webmd.com/balance/stress-management/ stress-management-topic-overview

---

Effective coping skills are those that are specifically identified to offer healthy choices to the patient. For example, it is very common to see patients use a variety of coping mechanisms—some effective, others ineffective—to deal with hospitalization. Hospitalization is a stressful experience for patients, families, and significant others. They will experience many unfamiliar people, things, noises, and interruptions. The patient may not understand their illness or the implications of the treatment plan. Mealtimes may be different from the routine at home, and the food served may be unfamiliar. The patient's plans are disrupted, their financial status is altered, and there is a possible temporary loss of independence. Effective coping can be even more challenging for a one-income family. Allowing the patient and their family members to be active participants in the treatment plan will increase the patient's ability to use effective coping skills (FIG. 7.2). The patient should be included in the decision making as to which new behaviors are acceptable and which ones are not. Practicing these new behaviors in a safe place, such as a hospital or organized group setting, is essential. A lifestyle change may be required for the patient, and it will be hard work. As the saying goes, "Old habits die hard." But old habits *can* die, and healthy, new ones can emerge to replace them. This process of learning effective

coping is sometimes called adaptation. Allowing the patient to practice new coping techniques will promote confidence and decrease the stress that can accompany change. The patient will adapt to stress by using the new tools. Chapters 8 and 9 will introduce you to other interventions that can be used for helping patients and health-care providers cope effectively with stress.

Clinical Activity

Before going to clinical, prepare a relaxation activity for your group to perform with each other in postconference. After completing the activity, debrief about the activity's effectiveness and evaluate the outcome.

A helpful action you can perform is to actively listen to the patient's thoughts and feelings about the stressor and then provide information that will reinforce the patient's positive feelings. Active listening will promote a sense of validation. You may privately agree or disagree with what a patient says, but validating the person allows them to be heard and accepted. Providing honest, positive feedback about the patient's progress with a given lifestyle change will let the patient know that others are noticing the hard work that they have done.

Often, the dividing line between effective and ineffective coping is in the person's degree of tension and their past experience. A little stress or anxiety can be positive thing. For example, when a bride-to-be is making preparations for her wedding, she feels stressed, but her expectation is that the outcome will be positive. Most of the time when there is a little tension, people are more alert and ready to respond. The fight-or-flight mechanism can actually help people adapt to a new situation. However, when worrying begins to cloud the consciousness, it interferes with a person's ability to make appropriate choices and recall the new adaptive tools they have learned (FIG. 7.3). For example, a different bride-to-be becomes exhausted with all the decisions to be made; she then becomes paralyzed and unable to proceed, demonstrating ineffective coping.

Ineffective coping is when the coping techniques people try are not successful or are hazardous. People often allow themselves to fall into habits that give them the illusion of coping. An example is a person having a drink every time they feel frustrated. Using drinking as a substitute for handling a frustration is an ineffective method of coping. The person who drinks when frustrated uses their frustration as a rationale for drinking. The person does not acknowledge that they are using drinking to avoid dealing with the frustration in a healthy way.

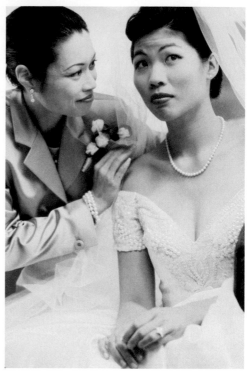

FIGURE 7.3 A little anxiety can be positive in some situations.

DEFENSE MECHANISMS

Defense mechanisms are mental "pressure valves." The purpose of defense mechanisms is to reduce or eliminate anxiety. When used in very small doses, they can be helpful. It is when they are overused that they become ineffective and can lead to a breakdown of the personality. Again, people are not born with defense mechanisms; they are learned as responses to stress. Many times, they are developed by the time people are 10 years old.

Defense mechanisms give a person the illusion that they are alleviating their stress, when in reality they mask the stress and may actually end up increasing it. The term defense mechanism comes from Freud's theory of personality and refers specifically to defense of the ego (Chapter 1). Although they appear to be very purposeful, defense mechanisms exist, for the most part, on the unconscious level. According to psychoanalyst Anna Freud, a defense mechanism is a learned behavior developed during childhood (Zhang, 2020).

Because the main purpose of defense mechanisms is to decrease anxiety, people tend to have their own repertoire of them and to use them (unconsciously) over and over. Periods of high stress are not the times to try something new, so the psyche uses the old "stand-bys" to get over yet another hump in life. Some commonly used defense mechanisms are shown in Table 7.2. A number of therapeutic techniques (Chapter 8) can offer patients and health-care providers alternative methods of reducing or eliminating ineffective defense mechanisms.

Table 7.2
Commonly Used Defense Mechanisms

Mechanism	Description	Examples
Denial	• Usually the first defense learned and used • Unconscious refusal to see reality	• The person with alcoholism states, "I can quit any time I want to." • Is not consciously lying
Repression	• An unconscious burying or "forgetting" mechanism • Excluding or withholding from the consciousness events or situations that are unbearable • A step deeper than "denial"	• Demonstrating emotions toward a person but unable to identify the specific reason why
Dissociation	• Painful events or situations are separated or dissociated from the conscious mind • Could be described as an "out-of-body experience"	• Patient who was sexually abused as a child describes the situation as if it happened to a friend or sibling. • Police visit parent to inform parent of death of child in car accident. Parent tells police, "That's impossible. My child is upstairs asleep. You must have the wrong house."
Rationalization	• Substituting acceptable reasons for the true causes for personal behavior because admitting the truth is too threatening	• "I failed the test because the teacher wrote bad questions." • "The patient kept interrupting me so I got distracted, and he caused me to make a mistake."
Compensation	• Making up for something a person perceives as an inadequacy by developing some other desirable trait	• A small boy who wants to be a basketball center instead becomes an honor-roll student. • The physically unattractive person who wants to model instead becomes a famous designer.
Reaction formation (overcompensation)	• Similar to compensation, except the person usually develops the opposite trait	• The small boy who wants to be a basketball center becomes a political voice to decrease the emphasis of sports in the elementary grades. • The physically unattractive person who wants to be a model speaks out for eliminating beauty pageants.

Continued

Table 7.2

Commonly Used Defense Mechanisms—cont'd

Mechanism	Description	Examples
Regression	• Emotionally returning to an earlier time in life when there was far less stress • Commonly seen in patients while hospitalized. Note: People do not regress to the same developmental age. This is highly individualized.	• Children who are toilet trained beginning to wet themselves • During serious illness, a patient exhibits behavior more appropriate for a younger developmental age, such as excessive dependency.
Sublimation	• Unacceptable traits or characteristics are diverted into acceptable traits or characteristics.	• Burglar teaches home safety classes. • Person who is potentially physically abusive becomes a professional sports figure. • People who choose to not have children run a day-care center.
Projection	• Attributing feelings or impulses unacceptable to oneself to others	• Wife tells patient's nurse, "My husband is worried about going home." (Wife is the one who is worried.) • Young soldier is fearful of upcoming deployment and says, "Those other guys are a bunch of cowards."
Displacement	• The "kick-the-dog syndrome" • Transferring anger and hostility to another person or object that is perceived to be less powerful	• Parent loses job without notice; goes home and verbally abuses spouse, who unjustly punishes child, who slaps the dog.
Restitution (undoing)	• Makes amends for a behavior one thinks is unacceptable. Makes an attempt at reducing guilt.	• Giving a treat to a child who is being punished for a wrong-doing • The person who finds a lost wallet with a large amount of cash does not return the wallet but puts extra in the collection plate at the next church service.
Isolation	• Emotion that is separated from the original feeling	• "I wasn't really angry; just a little upset."
Conversion reaction	• Anxiety is channeled into physical symptoms. Note: Often, the symptoms disappear soon after the threat is over.	• Nausea develops the night before a major examination, causing the person to miss the examination. • Nausea may disappear soon after the scheduled test is finished.
Avoidance	• Unconsciously staying away from events or situations that might lead to feelings of aggression or anxiety.	• "I can't go to the class reunion tonight. I'm just so tired. I have to sleep."
Scapegoating	• Blaming others	• "I didn't get the promotion because you don't like me."

Classroom Activity

- List three situations that were very uncomfortable for you. What defense mechanisms did you use to get through these situations? How could you have responded in a more effective manner to each of these situations?
- List three situations in which you observed someone else using defense mechanisms. How could you have aided that person to cope in a more effective manner?

CRITICAL THINKING QUESTION

Nurse D, licensed vocational nurse (LVN), has been routinely calling in "sick" on weekends he is scheduled to work. This has created a hardship for the patients and the staff. On Monday, Nurse D reports for the assigned work shift but is called to the nurse manager's office. The nurse manager informs Nurse D of the pattern that has developed in his attendance and gives him a chance to explain the situation. Nurse D says, "Well, I am a single parent, and I need to take care of my children. You should assign single people without families to work the weekends. If you cared a little more about your employees, we wouldn't have to call in so often."

Nurse D is quiet for a second and then says with a shaky voice, "You make me so nervous that I've started needing a couple of drinks at night so that I can sleep. I could quit drinking any time, if you'd just let me have my weekends off."

What defense mechanisms do you hear Nurse D using? How many of them have you used? If you were the nurse manager, what would you say to Nurse D? Using three of the suggested nursing diagnoses listed in Appendix E, complete a nursing process for Nurse D.

Classroom Activity

In a group, watch a newscast as assigned by the instructor. Pick one topic. Each group should watch its selected newscast at the assigned time.

1. Identify all of the defense mechanisms you can within that newscast.
2. In what ways does knowing about defense mechanisms change the way you listen to and process what you hear in the media?

Safe and Effective Nursing Care

- Support the patient emotionally.
- Assist in finding support resources.
- Identify and collect data on patient's stressors.
- Observe and identify when patient is using ineffective coping.
- Encourage self-esteem.
- Assist patient in identifying stressors.

Key Points

- Stress and people's responses to it are very individualized. People are not stressed by the same things, nor do they deal with their stress in the same ways.
- Defense mechanisms are believed to protect the ego, according to Freud's description of personality. They are based in the unconscious, for the most part, but they can appear to be very deliberate.

- Use of defense mechanisms for a short period can be helpful. The mechanisms act like a pressure valve and allow the psyche to put the stress into perspective. If the patient then deals with the problem, the outcome can be an effective coping technique; if not successful, the patient's anxiety level may increase.

Review Questions

1. A person who always sounds as though they are making excuses is displaying:
   a. Denial
   b. Fantasy
   c. Rationalization
   d. Transference

2. The person with alcoholism who says, "I don't have a problem. I can quit any time I want to; I just don't want to" is displaying:
   a. Denial
   b. Fantasy
   c. Dissociation
   d. Transference

3. Your young male patient tells you that he may not be big enough for the basketball team, but says "That's no problem because I'm a 4.0 student and on the principal's list" is displaying:
   a. Denial
   b. Transference
   c. Dissociation
   d. Compensation

4. Mr. V becomes angry that Mrs. V spent the whole day shopping with her friends. Upon her return home, he hits her and tells her, "It's your own fault. Stay home once in a while!" Mr. V is displaying:
   a. Repression
   b. Regression
   c. Dissociation
   d. Projection

5. You overhear someone jokingly repeating the social cliché "Stop smoking, lose weight, exercise; die anyway" as he orders a big burger and supersized fries. That cliché is an example of:
   a. Rationalization
   b. Repression
   c. Regression
   d. Rebellion

6. Yesterday, Tara became drunk and inappropriate at a family function. Tara's 16-year-old daughter was embarrassed and in tears. Today, Tara bought two expensive concert tickets for her daughter and a friend. This is an example of:
   a. Denial
   b. Undoing
   c. Symbolization
   d. Conversion

7. Shirley, a 70-year-old woman, went to a photo shoot for a portrait. As soon as the photographer began to photograph Shirley, she started to display signs of regression by (select all that apply):
   a. Posing as a young adolescent
   b. Posing as her mother
   c. Pouting when poses were suggested by the photographer
   d. Stopping the session to make two ponytails, one on each side of her head
   e. Posing as a 70-year-old woman

8. After receiving disappointing news about a job promotion, John stated, "I didn't get the promotion because I write with my left hand." This is an example of:
   a. Avoidance
   b. Regression
   c. Projection
   d. Denial

9. Effective coping skills are described as:
   a. Being able to make choices that are healthy and individualized
   b. Using a defense mechanism excessively
   c. Imitating the coping behavior of others
   d. Working on the problem until totally exhausted

10. The use of defense mechanisms is related to what part(s) of Freud's personality theory? (Select all that apply)
    a. Id
    b. Ego
    c. Superego
    d. Response
    e. Superid

REVIEW QUESTIONS ANSWER KEY 1. c, 2. a, 3. d, 4. d, 5. a, 6. b, 7. a, c, d, 8. c, 9. a, 10. b

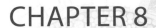

CHAPTER 8
Medications and Other Therapies

KEY TERMS

Akathisia
Antidepressants
Antimanic agents
Antiparkinson agents
Antipsychotics
Atypical antipsychotics
Behavior modification
Cognitive
Cognitive behavioral therapy (CBT)
Counseling
Crisis
Dystonia
Electroconvulsive therapy (ECT)
Hypnosis
Milieu
Monoamine oxidase inhibitors (MAOI)
Person-centered therapy
Psychoanalysis
Psychopharmacology
Rational emotive behavioral therapy
    (REBT)
Stimulants
Tardive dyskinesia
Typical antipsychotics

CHAPTER CONCEPTS

Addiction
Behavior
Cognition
Communication
Mood and affect
Safety

LEARNING OUTCOMES

1. Describe a therapeutic milieu.
2. Identify classifications of psychotropic medications.
3. Identify uses, actions, side effects, and nursing considerations for selected classifications of psychotropic medications.
4. Describe psychoanalysis.
5. Describe behavior modification.
6. Identify the nurse's role in counseling.
7. Describe three types of counseling.
8. Describe the benefits of electroconvulsive therapy (ECT) and the nurse's role in it.
9. Identify the five phases of crisis and the nurse's role in them.

When people have alterations to their mental health status or their emotional health is threatened, many of their other daily activities can be negatively affected as well. **Cognitive** ability (the ability to think rationally and to process those thoughts) can be decreased. Emotional responses can be decreased or even absent in some conditions. These alterations can be extremely frightening to patients who may already feel unable to control their lives and can lead to a deepening of the mental disorder or even to the development of another disorder.

> ### GOOD TO KNOW
> Accurate, timely observations and data collection by health-care providers may keep the patient from traveling a swift downward spiral.

Patients can develop a sense of helplessness and hopelessness about themselves and their conditions. Health-care providers help the patient regain control. Nurses may be observing the patient's treatments and therapies or may be an active part of them. Either way, making observations about the patient's reactions and participating in the plan of care are essential nursing duties. This chapter discusses some of the more frequently used methods for treating alterations in mental health.

PSYCHOPHARMACOLOGY

Since the introduction of the phenothiazines in the 1950s, the number of medications available for treating patients with mental health disorders, comprising the field of **psychopharmacology,** has increased greatly. The reasons for using medications are twofold. First, medications control symptoms, helping the patient to feel more comfortable emotionally. Second, medications are usually used with other types of therapy. The patient is generally more receptive to treatment and more able to focus on therapy if the appropriate medications are provided and taken as prescribed. Several classifications of psychoactive drugs (also referred to as *psychotropics*) exist; however, this chapter will focus on a few selected psychotropic categories. In most cases, only the most common information is presented about a medication. Medication information for mental health disorders is also provided in Chapters 10–22. Consult a pharmacist or drug reference book for more specific information before administering these medications or instructing patients on their use. This chapter will look at the following categories:

- Antipsychotics
- Antiparkinson agents
- Antianxiety/anxiolytics
- Antidepressants
- Antimanics/mood stabilizers
- Stimulants

> **Tool Box**
>
> Learn more about psychopharmacology at www. ascpp.org/resources/information-for-patients/ what-is-psychopharmacology/

Antipsychotics (Neuroleptics, Major Tranquilizers)

Action: There are two types of antipsychotic agents. **Typical antipsychotics**, or first generation agents, act on the central nervous system (CNS). Their main action is to block the dopamine receptors. Dopamine is a neurochemical that the human body produces naturally. However, if it is overproduced or utilized incorrectly, it can cause someone to exhibit psychotic behavior. **Atypical antipsychotics**, or second generation, block both serotonin (another neurochemical) and dopamine.

Uses: **Antipsychotics** are used to treat psychotic behavior in schizophrenia and other disorders that may include violent or potentially violent behavior. Typical antipsychotic agents treat the positive symptoms of schizophrenia, such as hallucinations, delusions, and suspiciousness. Atypical antipsychotic agents reduce the negative symptoms of schizophrenia, such as flat affect, social withdrawal, and difficulty with abstract thinking. See Chapter 15 for further discussion of these symptoms.

Side Effects: Antipsychotics have many unpleasant side effects. Atypical (second generation) medications have fewer side effects than typical (first generation) medications do. Side effects can be unpleasant enough to make patients reluctant to take these medications. A few of these side effects of typical psychotropics are photosensitivity (especially with chlorpromazine [Thorazine]), darkening of the skin from increased pigmentation, anticholinergic effects such as dry mouth, and a group of side effects called extrapyramidal symptoms (EPS). There is less risk of EPS with the atypical agents, but early observation and reporting of any possible EPS are crucial to minimizing these effects on the patient. EPS include:

1. ***Drug-induced parkinsonism (pseudoparkinsonism).*** Symptoms appear 1 to 8 weeks after the patient begins the medication. The major symptoms are akinesia (muscle weakness), shuffling gait, drooling, fatigue, masklike facial expression, tremors, and muscle rigidity.
2. ***Akathisia.*** Symptoms appear 2 to 10 weeks after the patient starts taking the medication. Symptoms are agitation and motor restlessness, and they seem to appear more frequently in women. The reason for this is currently unknown, but it may be due to hormonal interaction with the medication.
3. ***Dystonia.*** Symptoms appear 1 to 8 weeks after the patient starts taking the medication. Symptoms manifest as bizarre distortions or involuntary movements of any muscle group. Tongue, eyes, face, neck (torticollis), or any larger muscle group can become tightened into an

unnatural position or have irregular spastic movements. Dystonia requires immediate medical attention.

4. ***Tardive dyskinesia (TD).*** Symptoms appear within 1 to 8 weeks after the patient starts taking the medication. Frequently seen manifestations include rhythmic, involuntary movements that look like chewing, sucking, or licking motions. Frowning and blinking constantly are also common. TD used to be considered irreversible, but two drugs, valbenazine (Ingrezza) and deutetrabenazine (Austedo), have been approved to treat it.

Neuroleptic malignant syndrome (NMS) is a rare, but potentially fatal, reaction to treatment with some antipsychotic medications. Symptoms include muscle rigidity, hyperpyrexia, fluctuations in blood pressure, and altered level of consciousness. Early recognition and immediate medical care are important. Some antipsychotics, such as clozapine (Clozaril), are known to cause serious blood dyscrasias and require regular monitoring of blood counts.

Contraindications: Antipsychotics should be used carefully in patients who are hypersensitive to medications or who have brain damage or blood dyscrasias.

Nursing Considerations:

• Careful teaching by health-care providers can help the patient to understand that these are very strong medications.
• Monitor the patient's body movements using the abnormal involuntary movement (AIM) form on each shift to identify if the patient is experiencing tardive dyskinesia (see Web site listed at the end of the chapter for more information).
• Monitor the patient's blood pressure; the patient's pressure may fluctuate from very high to low.
• The possibility of seizures increases in patients who require antipsychotic medications.
• Observe for any sign of EPS or NMS and carefully monitor blood work for abnormal results.
• Observe for signs of parkinsonism.
• Carefully instruct the patient and family to wear a hat with a wide brim, cover all exposed skin, and use a broad-spectrum sunscreen when in the sun. Taking these precautions may lessen chances of the patient suffering sunburn, especially if the patient is using chlorpromazine.
• Temperature extremes should be avoided.
• Patients should be educated to avoid consuming alcohol.

• Over-the-counter (OTC) medications and supplements should not be taken without consulting a health-care provider.
• Instruct the patient not to alter the dose without first consulting with their health-care provider.
• Occasionally, the patient might experience some gastric distress with oral antipsychotics. In that case, administer the medication with food or milk.
• Encourage the patient to be compliant with the medication regimen.
• If the medication causes sedation, encourage the patient to take it at bedtime to promote sleep.
• Some antipsychotics interact with calcium-containing medications. To avoid this interaction, the patient should take antacids or calcium supplements 1 to 2 hours *after* oral administration of antipsychotics or as advised by their physician.
• Antipsychotic medication should be discontinued slowly, never stopped abruptly.

Box 8.1 lists some of the most commonly used antipsychotic agents.

Tool Box

Here is a link to a tool for determining whether a patient's movements are TD, a side effect of antipsychotic medications.
https://cpnp.org/aims
Also see Chapter 15, Table 15.4, Comparison of Side Effects Among Typical and Atypical Antipsychotic Agents.

Box 8.1

Commonly Used Antipsychotic Agents

Typical: Chlorpromazine (Thorazine), haloperidol (Haldol/Haldol decanoate), trifluoperazine (Stelazine), thioridazine (Mellaril), loxapine (Loxitane), fluphenazine (Prolixin), molindone hydrochloride (Moban), thiothixene (Serentil), perphenazine (Trilafon)

Atypical: Risperidone (Risperdal/Perseris), clozapine (Clozaril), quetiapine (Seroquel/Seroquel XR), olanzapine (Zyprexa), ziprasidone (Geodon/Zeldox), lurasidone (Latuda), paliperidone (Invega), aripiprazole (Abilify), brexpiprazole (Rexulti), cariprazine (Vraylar), pimozide (Orap)

Antiparkinson Agents (Anticholinergics)

Action: **Antiparkinson agents** (also called *anticholinergics*) (FIG. 8.1) inhibit the action of acetylcholine. Acetylcholine increases as dopamine decreases at its receptor sites (the cholinergic effect). When the amount of acetylcholine available to interact with dopamine is decreased, there is a better balance between the two neurochemicals, and the symptoms of parkinsonism decrease.

Uses: Antiparkinson agents help decrease the effects of drug-induced and nondrug-induced symptoms of parkinsonism that often occur with antipsychotics.

Side Effects: Blurred vision, dry mouth, dizziness, drowsiness, confusion, tachycardia, urinary retention, constipation, and changes in blood pressure are side effects of antiparkinson agents.

Contraindications: Patients with known hypersensitivity should not use these medications. People with narrow angle-closure glaucoma, myasthenia gravis, peptic ulcers, prostatic hypertrophy, or urine retention should not take these medications. These agents should be avoided in children under the age of 12 years and used with caution with older patients.

> **GOOD TO KNOW**
> Assess if your patient has glaucoma.

Nursing Considerations:
- Monitor blood pressure carefully (at least every 4 hours when beginning treatment).
- Monitor your patient for parkinsonian and extrapyramidal symptoms.
- Encourage using hard, sugarless candy or saliva substitute to combat the effects of dry mouth. Teach patient about possible gastrointestinal (GI) side effects if products contain sorbitol and are eaten in excess.

Box 8.2 lists some of the most commonly used antiparkinson agents.

Antianxiety Agents (Anxiolytics/ Minor Tranquilizers)

Action: Antianxiety agents depress cerebral cortex activities of the CNS (FIG. 8.2). These can be used for short-term as well as intermediate treatment goals (Vallerand & Sanoski, 2019).

Uses: Antianxiety agents decrease the effects of stress, anxiety, and mild depression. They can be used preoperatively to enhance sedation.

Side Effects: The use of antianxiety agents can cause physical and psychological dependence. Other side effects include drowsiness, lethargy, fainting, postural hypotension, nausea, and vomiting. If discontinued abruptly, severe side effects, including nausea, hypotension, and fatal grand mal seizures, can occur anywhere from 12 hours to 2 weeks after the drug is stopped.

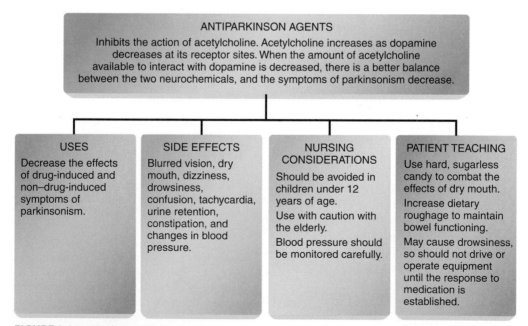

FIGURE 8.1 Antiparkinson agents

Box 8.2

Commonly Used Antiparkinson Agents

Benztropine (Cogentin), trihexyphenidyl (Artane), pramipexole (Mirapex), diphenhydramine (Benadryl)

Contraindications: Patients with known hypersensitivity should not use these medications. People with a history of chemical dependency are not good candidates for this classification of drug because of the potential for addiction. Avoid in pregnancy and during lactation and if the patient has any renal or hepatic irregularities. Some antianxiety drugs, such as buspirone, advise patients to avoid grapefruit or grapefruit juice in the diet.

Nursing Considerations:

- Nurses should monitor blood pressure before and after giving this medication and monitor for signs of orthostatic hypotension, especially if the patient is also taking other CNS depressants (Townsend, 2017).
- Assess the patient's anxiety level.
- Monitor patient's sedation level.
- During assessment, ask patient if they use any OTC medications that might affect the CNS.
- Teach the patient to rise slowly from sitting or lying positions to prevent a sudden drop in blood pressure.
- When possible, give these types of drugs at bedtime to help promote sleep, minimize side effects, and allow a more normal daytime routine.

- Administer intramuscular (IM) dosages deeply and slowly into large muscle masses, preferably using the Z-track method.
- Teach the patient and family that it is not safe for the patient to drive or use alcohol while using this classification of medication.
- Advise the patient about the possibility of drug dependence, especially if the patient has a history of drug abuse.
- Advise the patient not to stop the medication abruptly.

Box 8.3 lists some of the most commonly used antianxiety agents.

Antidepressants (Mood Elevators)

Antidepressants are divided into several subgroups, and different drug references subdivide the antidepressants differently. There are similarities and differences among the subgroups (FIG. 8.3). These subgroups are:

- Selective serotonin reuptake inhibitors (SSRIs)
- Tricyclics (TCAs)
- Tetracyclics
- Serotonin norepinephrine reuptake inhibitors (SNRIs)
- Monoamine oxidase inhibitors (MAOIs)

> **GOOD TO KNOW**
> Antidepressants generally require several weeks to effect a change in mood.

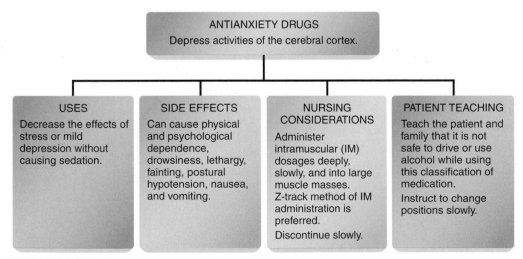

FIGURE 8.2 Antianxiety agents.

Box 8.3

Commonly Used Antianxiety Agents

Alprazolam (Xanax/Xanax SR), buspirone (BuSpar), chlordiazepoxide (Librium), oxazepam (Serax, Novoxapam), clonazepam (Klonopin), diazepam (Valium), lorazepam (Ativan), propranolol (Inderal), oxazepam (Serax), hydroxyzine (Atarax, Vistaril)

Selective Serotonin Reuptake Inhibitor (SSRI)

Action: These drugs increase the availability of serotonin, which is decreased in the brains of depressed individuals. SSRIs are a potent drug and long acting.

Uses: Treatment of depression, anxiety, obsessive disorders, impulse-control disorders, and post-traumatic stress disorder (PTSD).

Side Effects: Potential for increased suicidal tendencies, sedation, dry mouth, agitation, postural hypotension, headache, arthralgia, dizziness, insomnia, confusion, and tremors.

Contraindications: Patients with known hypersensitivity should not use these medications. People using **monoamine oxidase inhibitors (MAOIs)** or who are within 14 days of discontinuing MAOIs should not use these medications. People using certain herbal preparations and dietary supplements including, but not limited to, St. John's wort, ginseng, brewer's yeast, high-dose vitamin B_6, and ginkgo biloba should not use SSRIs without consulting their health-care provider.

Note: In October 2004, producers of SSRIs were required by the U.S. Food and Drug Administration (FDA) to place a "black box" warning on the medication container, cautioning about the danger of increased risk of suicidal tendencies in children, adolescents, and young adults while taking these medications.

Nursing Considerations:

• Do not abruptly discontinue the medication, except under the supervision of a health-care provider. Serotonin syndrome, which includes altered mental status, restlessness, tachycardia, and labile blood pressure, can occur with abrupt discontinuation as well as when SSRIs are combined with some other medications.
• Make sure that the health-care provider prescribing the SSRI is aware if the patient is taking any prescription anticoagulants.
• Teach patient and family that caution should be used with driving or other activities that require alertness.
• Instruct the patient on medication compliance.
• Inform patient a therapeutic effect may not occur for approximately 28 days or more.
• Alcohol and other CNS depressants should be avoided.

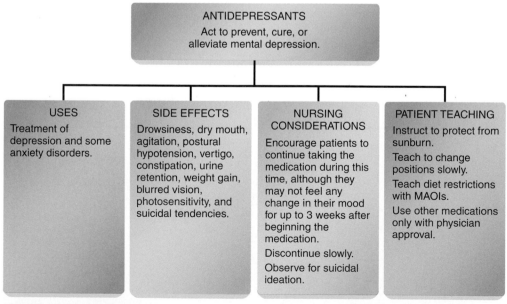

FIGURE 8.3 Antidepressants.

- Hard, sugarless candy or saliva substitute can be used to treat dry mouth.
- Teach the patient to change position slowly to avoid a sudden drop in blood pressure.
- Monitor liver function tests.
- Instruct patient to consult their health-care provider about excess bruising or nose bleeds (Siddiqui et al., 2011).
- **Monitor the patient for suicidal ideation**.

Box 8.4 lists some of the most commonly used SSRI agents.

Tricyclic Antidepressants

Action: These drugs increase the level of serotonin and norepinephrine, thereby increasing the ability of the nerve cells to pass information to each other. Patients with depressive disorders generally have decreased amounts of these two neurochemicals.

Uses: Treatment of symptoms of depression, including, but not limited to, sleep disturbances, sexual function disturbances, panic disorders, changes in appetite, and cognitive changes. Low doses of these medications can be used to treat childhood enuresis.

Side Effects: Sedation, lethargy, dry mouth, constipation, tachycardia, postural hypotension, urine retention, blurred vision, weight gain, and changes in blood glucose are possible.

Contraidications: Patients with known hypersensitivity should not use these medications. Women who are pregnant or breastfeeding and individuals with kidney disease, liver disease, or a recent myocardial infarction should not take these medications. Anyone who has asthma, seizure disorders, schizophrenia, benign prostatic hypertrophy (BPH), or alcoholism should use tricyclic antidepressants (TCAs) with extreme caution.

Nursing Considerations:

- Patients should not stop using these medications abruptly.
- Therapeutic effect may take up to 2 to 4 weeks.
- Patient may experience orthostatic hypotension.

- Men may respond better to TCAs than women do (Procyshyn et al., 2019).
- Medications (including OTC medications such as cold preparations) that contain antihistamines, alcohol, sodium bicarbonate, benzodiazepines, and narcotic analgesics can increase the effects of TCAs.
- Nicotine and barbiturates decrease the effect of the tricyclic antidepressant.
- Serotonin syndrome can occur if TCAs are combined with St. John's wort.

Box 8.5 lists some of the most commonly used tricyclic antidepressant agents.

Tetracyclic Antidepressants (Heterocyclic Antidepressants)

The actions, uses, contraindications, side effects, and nursing considerations for the tetracyclic antidepressants are similar to those for SSRIs. Tetracyclics are prescribed less frequently because of their high incidence of side effects.

Box 8.6 lists some of the most commonly used tetracyclic antidepressant agents.

Serotonin Norepinephrine Reuptake Inhibitors (SNRIs)

Action: These drugs increase the availability of serotonin and norepinephrine, which are decreased in the brains of depressed individuals.

Uses: The uses, contraindications, side effects, and nursing considerations for the SNRI antidepressants are similar to those for SSRIs.

Box 8.5

Commonly Used Tricyclic Antidepressant Agents

Amitriptyline (Elavil), imipramine (Tofranil), nortriptyline (Pamelor, Aventyl), amoxapine (Asendin), desipramine (Norpramin), clomipramine (Anafranil), doxepin (Sinequan), trimipramine (Surmontil), protriptyline hydrochloride (Vivactil)

Box 8.4

Commonly Used SSRI Agents

Citalopram (Celexa), fluoxetine (Prozac), sertraline (Zoloft), fluvoxamine (Luvox), paroxetine (Paxil/Paxil SR), escitalopram (Lexapro)

Box 8.6

Commonly Used Tetracyclic Antidepressant Agents

Bupropion (Wellbutrin, Wellbutrin SR and XL), mirtazapine (Remeron), trazodone (Desyrel, Oleptro)

Box 8.7 lists some of the most commonly used SNRI agents.

Monoamine Oxidase Inhibitors (MAOIs)

Action: MAOIs prevent the metabolism of neurotransmitters by the enzyme monoamine oxidase. Too much monoamine oxidase can lead to destructive, psychotic behaviors.

Uses: MAOIs are generally used for patients with varied types of depression who have not been helped by other antidepressants.

Side Effects: Postural hypotension, photosensitivity (sunburn potential), headache, dizziness, memory impairment, tremors, fatigue, insomnia, weight gain, and sexual dysfunction are possible.

Contraindications: Patients with known hypersensitivity should not use these medications. MAOI medications should be given carefully to patients who have asthma, congestive heart failure, cerebrovascular disease, glaucoma, hypertension, schizophrenia, alcoholism, liver or kidney disorders, or severe headaches, as well as to those who are over 60 years old or who are pregnant. Many drug–drug interactions may occur if MAOI agents are combined with other medications. Other prescriptions and OTC products should be taken only after consulting a doctor or a pharmacist. Because of the serious side effects and contraindications associated with MAOIs, these medications are seldom prescribed nowadays.

Nursing Considerations:

• Teach patients to avoid consuming the amino acid tyramine, a precursor of norepinephrine, while taking these medications. MAOIs block the metabolism of tyramine, resulting in increased norepinephrine. A hypertensive crisis may occur, so teach patients the signs of such a crisis. Foods containing significant amounts of tyramine include:
  • Aged cheese (cheddar, Swiss, provolone, blue cheese, parmesan)
  • Avocados (guacamole)
  • Yogurt, sour cream
  • Chicken and beef livers, pickled herring, corned beef
  • Bean pods
  • Bananas, raisins, and figs
  • Smoked and processed meat (salami, pepperoni, and bologna)
  • Yeast supplements
  • Chocolate
  • Meat tenderizers (MSG), soy sauce
  • Beer, red wines, and caffeine
  • Be sure patients have a list of these tyramine-containing foods and beverages.

Box 8.8 lists some of the most commonly used MAOI agents.

Alternative Treatments for Depression

Some people seek alternatives to the prescription antidepressant drugs available through traditional Western medicine. Reasons for choosing alternatives include cultural preferences, the high cost of prescription medications, lack of health insurance, and unpleasant side effects experienced with medications used in the past.

One nonprescription alternative is a chemical called SAMe ("sammy"). SAMe is a combination of an amino acid (methionine) and adenosine triphosphate (ATP). It is used as an antidepressant and sold in the United States as a dietary supplement. Other alternative forms of therapy are explored in Chapter 9.

Nurses need to be knowledgeable about these alternative choices just as they are about prescription medications. Encourage your patients to discuss their use of supplements with their physicians and provide them with as much information as possible to allow them to make safe, informed choices.

Box 8.9 provides nursing considerations for all antidepressants.

Antimanic Agents (Mood Stabilizing Agents)

Lithium carbonate and lithium citrate have been the preferred drugs for the treatment and management of bipolar mania for many years. In recent years, several other **antimanic agents** (FIG. 8.4) have

---

Box 8.7

Commonly Used SNRI Agents

Nefazodone (Serzone), venlafaxine (Effexor), duloxetine (Cymbalta)

Box 8.8

Commonly Used MAOI Agents

Phenelzine (Nardil), tranylcypromine (Parnate), isocarboxazid (Marplan), selegiline (Emsam)

Nursing Considerations for All Antidepressants

- Reinforce the teaching that these medications take several weeks to become effective. Encourage patients to continue taking the medication during this time, although they may not feel any change in their mood right away.
- All antidepressant medications should be tapered gradually rather than abruptly discontinued to prevent withdrawal symptoms.
- It is imperative that all patients receiving antidepressant medications be monitored for suicide potential throughout treatment.

become treatment options. Other medications being used as mood stabilizers include some anticonvulsants and calcium channel blockers.

Lithium Carbonate

Action: The exact action of lithium is not completely known at this time. There seems to be a connection between lithium and the constancy of sodium concentration, which might help regulate and moderate information along the nerve cells, thus preventing mood swings. Another possibility is that lithium increases the reuptake of norepinephrine and serotonin, thereby decreasing hyperactivity.

Uses: Lithium is used for the manic phase of bipolar disorder and sometimes for other depressive or schizoaffective disorders.

Side Effects: Side effects can be numerous. Some of the more common ones are thirst and dry mouth, nausea and vomiting, abdominal pain, and fatigue.

Contraindications: Brain damage, renal disease, and severe dehydration are a few of the contraindications of lithium, similar to those of the other categories listed earlier.

Nursing Considerations:

- Encourage patients to keep all appointments for blood work and evaluation of drug effectiveness. Therapeutic serum levels are between 0.5 and 1.2 mEq/L for most patients (1.0 to 1.5 in acute mania). Symptoms of lithium toxicity begin to appear at blood levels greater than 2 mEq/L (Van Leeuwen & Bladh, 2019). Signs of toxicity include flattening of T-waves, severe diarrhea, persistent nausea and vomiting, muscle weakness, tremors, blurred vision, slurred speech, and seizures.

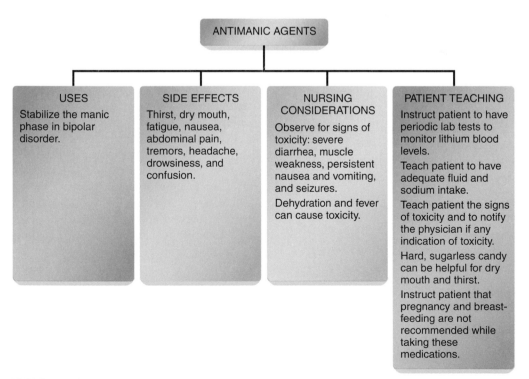

FIGURE 8.4 Antimanic agents.

- Monitor the electrocardiogram (EKG/ECG) to determine whether there is flattening of the T-wave.
- Monitor laboratory values for kidney and liver function.
- Lithium crosses the placenta and is excreted in breast milk, so women of childbearing years need to be counseled by their health-care provider regarding the effects of this drug before they become pregnant.
- Dehydration and fevers can cause increased danger of toxicity.
- Adequate fluid and sodium intake are essential. Patients should not decrease their dietary intake of salt (unless instructed to do so by the health-care provider) and should be taught to inform the physician immediately if they are ill.
- Advise patient to take lithium with food if they experience any gastric distress.
- Hard, sugarless candy can be helpful to decrease dry mouth and thirst, but patients should consult their health-care provider.

Box 8.10 lists some of the most commonly used forms of lithium.

Anticonvulsants

Action: The action of anticonvulsants in the treatment of bipolar disorder is not understood at this time.

Uses: These drugs stabilize the manic episodes in bipolar disorders.

Side Effects: Nausea, vomiting, indigestion, drowsiness, dizziness, prolonged bleeding, headache, and confusion are possible.

Contraindications: Patients with known hypersensitivity or with bone marrow suppression should not use these medications. Caution should be used in patients with renal, cardiac, or liver disease. Caution should also be used with older patients and children.

Nursing Considerations:

- Medication should not be stopped abruptly.
- The medication should be tapered when therapy is discontinued.

- Advise patients to avoid alcohol and seek professional help if needed.
- Advise patients to consult with their health-care provider or pharmacist before taking nonprescription medications and supplements.
- Patients should not drive or operate dangerous equipment until the effects of the medication on the patient are known.

Box 8.11 lists some of the most commonly used anticonvulsant agents.

Stimulants

Stimulants (FIG. 8.5) are readily available OTC as well as by prescription. Nonprescription stimulants include OTC diet preparations and pills to prevent sleep, tobacco products, and caffeinated beverages such as coffee, energy drinks, and soda with caffeine.

Amphetamines are one type of stimulant. Amphetamines can be abused, and they have many street names, including "uppers," "speed," and "bennies." Stimulants are widely available, powerful, and potentially dangerous drugs (see Chapter 17).

Action: Stimulants provide direct stimulation of the CNS. Stimulants cause increased levels of dopamine and norepinephrine to be released.

Uses: These drugs promote alertness, diminish appetite, and combat narcolepsy (a sleep disorder related to abnormal rapid eye movement [REM] sleep). They are also used in the treatment of attention deficit-hyperactivity disorder (ADHD) in children and teens.

Side Effects: Increased or irregular heartbeat, hypertension, hyperactivity, dry mouth, hand tremor, rapid speech, diaphoresis, confusion, depression, seizures, suicidal ideation, and insomnia are possible.

Contraindications: Patients with known hypersensitivity should not use these medications. Women who are pregnant or breastfeeding should not use this classification of drugs. Because these chemicals increase stimulation of the CNS and respiratory systems, they should not be given to people who are alcoholic, manic, or who display suicidal or

---

Box 8.10

Commonly Used Forms of Lithium and Other Mood Stabilizing Drugs

Lithium carbonate (Eskalith, Lithonate, Lithane, Lithobid)

Other antimanic drugs: valproic acid (Depakene), divalproex sodium (Depakote), lamotrigine (Lamictal)

Box 8.11

Commonly Used Anticonvulsant Agents

Carbamazepine (Tegretol), divalproex sodium (Depakote), valproic acid (Depakene), lamotrigine (Lamictal)

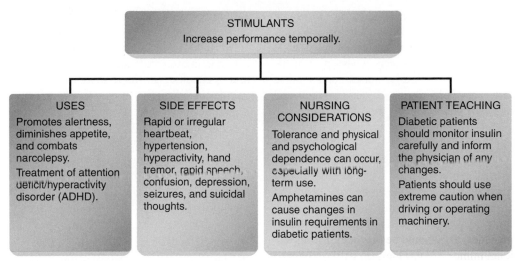

FIGURE 8.5 Stimulants.

homicidal ideations. People who have heart disease or glaucoma also should not use these drugs because of the potential effect of the medications. Older people and patients who have diabetes, hypertension, or other cardiovascular conditions should use these drugs cautiously and with careful monitoring.

Nursing Considerations:

- Tolerance and physical and psychological dependence can occur with CNS stimulants, especially with long-term use.
- Patients should not discontinue medication abruptly.
- Monitor for suicide potential.
- Diabetic patients who take amphetamines should be informed that the amphetamines may cause changes in their insulin requirements.
- These medications can also cause changes in judgment; therefore, people should be counseled to use extreme caution when driving or operating equipment and should avoid these activities if possible.
- Encourage frequent rinsing of the mouth with water or use of hard, sugarless candy or saliva substitute to relieve dryness in the mouth.

Box 8.12 provides some of the most commonly used stimulant agents.

 MILIEU

An area that nurses have some influence over is the therapeutic environment itself. In mental health, this therapeutic environment is called a **milieu** or

Box 8.12

Commonly Used Central Nervous System Stimulant Agents

Dextroamphetamine (Dexedrine), methamphetamine (Desoxyn), methylphenidate (Ritalin), dextroamphetamine/amphetamine mixtures (Adderall)

therapeutic milieu. It is believed that the environment affects behavior. Think about a person who goes to an event such as a concert or a ballgame that he does not feel excited about. That person might begin cheering or singing along and generally getting into the spirit of things shortly after arriving at the event.

CRITICAL THINKING QUESTION

You are assigned to a mental health unit to monitor a group discussing anger. You feel apprehensive and fearful about being on the same unit as these patients. Describe how you might feel after hearing how the patients' home lives relate to their anger.

The milieu is the setting that provides safety and where stress is minimized during the patient's stay. Milieu therapy is intended to combine social and therapeutic environments, creating the opportunity for a therapeutic interaction between the nurse and patient on a regular basis. The milieu must be comfortable and safe. Patients need to feel accepted while learning new behaviors. Respect is also part of the therapeutic milieu. Obviously, nurses cannot move walls and change decorating themes on a mental health unit, but you can allow the patient to choose the room for therapy or move to an area where the patient feels more comfortable. If the patient is on a psychiatric unit rather than a medical or surgical unit, they are usually allowed to walk from area to area on the unit. Nurses work to keep the area calm and quiet, arranging for roommate changes if needed. There are many things you can and must do to maintain a milieu that is conducive to a patient's progress. As the patient progresses, the milieu will be changed to allow the patient to take on more responsibility for their behavior.

 ## PSYCHOTHERAPIES

Psychotherapy (FIG. 8.6) is the term for forms of talk-therapy chosen by the psychologist, psychiatrist, or other mental health therapist to treat an individual. The goals of psychotherapy are to:

1. Decrease the patient's emotional discomfort
2. Increase the patient's social functioning
3. Increase the patient's ability to behave or perform in a manner appropriate to the situation

These goals are achieved in a variety of ways, including therapeutic relationships, open and honest venting of feelings and thoughts, allowing the patient to practice new coping skills, helping the patient to gain insight into their problem, and using consistency in the team approach to the patient's care and treatment. Positive reinforcement of progress is encouraged. Some therapies are focused on gaining insight into the reasons for current behavior, and others are more focused on changing specific behaviors.

Several types of therapy are typically used. Nurses may or may not be actively involved in the therapy, but to provide continuity in the care of the patient, they must understand the basic ideas behind the types of therapy.

Psychoanalysis

Psychoanalysis is a form of therapy originated by Sigmund Freud. In psychoanalysis, the focus is on the cause of the problem, which Freud believed is buried somewhere in the unconscious. The therapist attempts to get the patient to review their past in an effort to determine where the problem began. Chances are, according to Freud, that the current problem is related to poor parent-child relationships and ineffective psychosexual development.

During sessions, it is typical for the psychoanalyst to be positioned at the head of and slightly behind the patient so that the patient cannot see the therapist. This decreases any kind of nonverbal communication between the two people. The patient typically reclines on the couch, relaxed and ready to focus on the therapist's instruction, but the patient may request other types of seating, such as sitting on the floor.

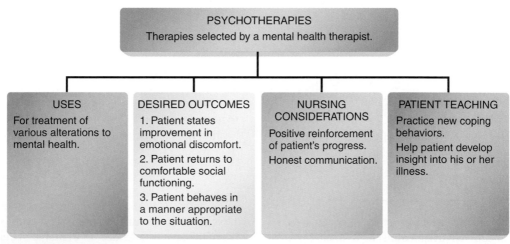

FIGURE 8.6 Psychotherapies.

Some of the techniques used in psychoanalysis are as follows:

Free Association

In free association, the patient says whatever comes to mind in response to a word that is given by the therapist. The patient can respond with any word without feeling judged. The therapist will suggest that the patient is to relax before therapy. For example, the therapist might say *mother* or *blue,* and the patient would give a response, also typically one word, to each of the words the therapist says.

The therapist then looks for a theme or pattern to the patient's responses. So, if the patient responds *evil* to the word *mother* or *dead* to the word *blue,* the therapist might pick up one potential theme. If the patient responds *kind* and *true* to the words *mother* and *blue,* the therapist might infer a completely different theme. The theme may give the therapist an insight into the patient's emotional disturbance.

Dream Analysis

Because Freudians believe that behavior is rooted in the unconscious and that dreams are a manifestation of the troubles people repress, what better way to get an idea of the problem than to monitor and interpret dreams? The patient is asked to keep a dream log. Immediately after a dream, the patient awakes and writes down as many details as possible from the dream, in a notebook kept next to the bed. Keeping a dream log is easier said than done, as many people remember only bits and pieces of a dream upon awakening. Psychoanalysts believe that dreams truly are the mirror to the unconscious and that it is possible to train patients to awaken long enough to record their dreams. The dreams are then interpreted in much the same way as free association. Significant people or situations in the dreams are explored with the patient, and possible meanings are offered by the therapist.

Hypnosis

For many years, **hypnosis** was thought to be quackery, for entertainment only, to be used in stage shows to get people to cluck like chickens. Granted, this sort of thing can happen. Fraternity and sorority members love to invite stage performers to hypnotize pledges during recruitment. Certainly, entertainers like David Copperfield have made comfortable livings with hypnosis.

However, hypno*therapy,* as professional therapists prefer to call it, is useful for certain patients in

certain instances. It is not a magic solution to problems. It takes practice on the part of the patient. It can, however, be a very effective tool for unlocking the unconscious or for searching further into memories that have been repressed. According to Alman (2001), hypnotherapy has been used successfully in patients experiencing panic attacks and phobias.

Of course, just as there are unethical people in other walks of life, a small number of therapists may abuse the hypnotherapy relationship. However, such abuse is very uncommon. People do not generally lose control when under hypnosis; they will, in most cases, still realize what is comfortable and acceptable to them personally, and they will not allow themselves to go deeper into hypnosis or to perform behaviors that they find objectionable (FIG. 8.7). Hypnosis and hypnotherapy are discussed in more depth in Chapter 9.

Catharsis

Catharsis is the "elimination of a complex (problem) by bringing it to consciousness and affording it expression" (Merriam-Webster Online, 2017). Catharsis comes from the Greek word for cleansing or purification. In psychoanalysis, the therapist helps the patient see the root of the problem and then, by talking or expressing feelings, allows

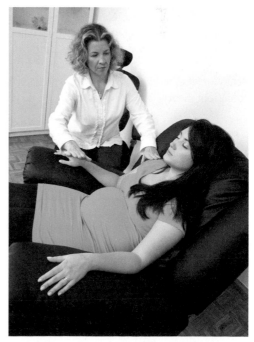

FIGURE 8.7 In hypnotherapy, a patient in a state of very deep relaxation is guided by the therapist.

the patient to learn to evacuate this problem from the psyche. This can take place in conjunction with other forms of psychotherapy.

Psychoanalysis is undertaken on a one-on-one basis between the patient and therapist. The nurse can be helpful in the treatment process by allowing the patient to talk about their experiences in therapy and by carefully documenting the patient's responses.

Behavior Modification

The treatment method known as ***behavior modification*** is based on the work of the behavioral theorists B. F. Skinner, Ivan Pavlov, and others. It is a common treatment modality used in multiple treatment settings (FIG. 8.8).

The purpose of behavior modification is to eliminate or greatly decrease the frequency of identified negative behaviors. One of the basic beliefs of behavior modification is that whenever a behavior is removed, it must be replaced by another behavior. Therefore, replacing the negative behaviors with ones that are more desirable is a major goal of this type of psychotherapy.

As Skinner and Pavlov showed, behaviors can be learned and unlearned. The process of finding the appropriate stimuli and reinforcers determines the effectiveness of the change in behavior. According to some behaviorists, it takes approximately 20 repetitions of a new behavior to make it a part of a person's lifestyle. However, anyone who has tried to lose weight or stop smoking might argue with that number.

Behavior can be changed, according to behavior modification theory, by either positive or negative reinforcement. Technically, reinforcement is anything that *increases* the likelihood of a behavior. Positive reinforcement is the *addition* of something to bring about a desired behavior. This can be as simple as the act of rewarding the patient with something pleasant when the desired behavior has been performed. For instance, if Mrs. P has the habit of demanding loudly to go outside, the desired behavior might be for her to ask quietly for what she needs. Mrs. P loves to be outside but is not allowed out except at supervised times. A suitable positive reinforcer might be to allow her 15 additional minutes outdoors when she remembers to make her request quietly. When Mrs. P exhibits the unacceptable behavior, the staff would either ignore it (because correcting it would, in itself, be a form of reinforcing the behavior) or quietly tell her that the behavior is not acceptable and then acknowledge her only when the desired change has been demonstrated.

Classroom Activity

Identify one behavior you personally would like to change, then create a care plan to direct the change. Include what a person could give you to create that change.

Negative reinforcement is the *removal* of something to increase the likelihood of a behavior. A common example is the annoying seatbelt alarm in an automobile. The alarm sounds until you fasten your seat belt, the desired behavior, increasing the likelihood that you will buckle up in the future.

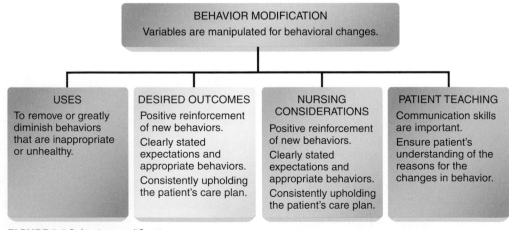

BEHAVIOR MODIFICATION
Variables are manipulated for behavioral changes.

USES	DESIRED OUTCOMES	NURSING CONSIDERATIONS	PATIENT TEACHING
To remove or greatly diminish behaviors that are inappropriate or unhealthy.	Positive reinforcement of new behaviors. Clearly stated expectations and appropriate behaviors. Consistently upholding the patient's care plan.	Positive reinforcement of new behaviors. Clearly stated expectations and appropriate behaviors. Consistently upholding the patient's care plan.	Communication skills are important. Ensure patient's understanding of the reasons for the changes in behavior.

FIGURE 8.8 Behavior modification.

Unlike reinforcement, punishment is anything that *decreases* the likelihood of a behavior.

With behavior modification, it is important to have the undesirable behaviors, desired replacement behaviors, and consequences clearly stated. In a facility, this will be incorporated into the treatment plan of care. At home, setting expectations can be done in family meetings, agreed upon orally by the family members, or made known by some other method of clear oral or written communication. For behavior modification to work, the patient must have the ability to understand the ramifications of the behavior to be changed and the purpose for the type of consequence that is chosen. If the person is not capable of understanding the situation or is not able to remember due to some other problem, behavior modification could be considered a questionable alternative to other kinds of treatment.

Cognitive Therapies
Rational-Emotive Behavioral Therapy (REBT)

Dr. Albert Ellis, a "reformed" psychoanalyst, and other cognitive therapists developed theories proposing that people teach themselves to be ill because of the way they think about their situations. *Cognitive* means "of, relating to, or involving conscious intellectual activity (such as thinking, reasoning, or remembering)" (Merriam-Webster Online, 2017). Cognitive therapy emphasizes ways of rethinking situations. The therapist confronts the patient about certain unhelpful beliefs or undesirable behaviors, and then together, patient and therapist work out ways of thinking about them differently.

Rational-emotive behavioral therapy (REBT) is one of the best-known cognitive therapies (FIG. 8.9). Ellis's theory is based on an ABCDE model:

- A is the *activating* event, or the subject of the faulty thinking.
- B is the *belief* system a person has adopted about the activating event.
- C is the *consequence* to continuing the belief system.

When behavior is thought to be related to an emotional disturbance, Ellis adds to the ABC format:

- D is *disputing* against beliefs appearing irrational.
- E is *effective* emotions and behaviors about the activating event.

Ellis invented terminology such as *musturbation* (the act of insisting that something *must* go a certain way), *awfulizing* (the belief that something is not just inconvenient or unpleasant, but "awful"), and *catastrophizing* (the point at which things are so "awful" that one loses control of a situation). In REBT, there are no "musts" or "shoulds." Feeling sad about an unpleasant experience (such as the death of a loved one) is acceptable and normal, but becoming depressed about the death is "awfulizing" and therefore considered by Ellis to be unhealthy.

Clinical Activity

Throughout your clinical experience, observe patients on the unit when they are instructed by the health-care provider that they "must" or "should" behave in a specific manner. During clinical postconferences, discuss these episodes and whether the outcome was positive or negative.

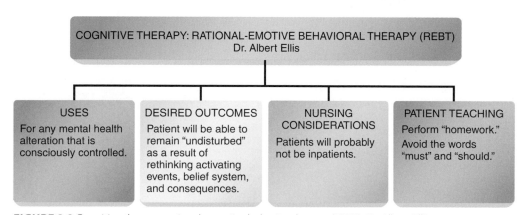

FIGURE 8.9 Cognitive therapy, rational-emotive behavior therapy (REBT), Dr. Albert Ellis.

It is common for REBT to take place in a group setting. The patients are given homework to complete in the period between sessions. The expected outcome is that patients will no longer focus on their previous thoughts.

An offshoot of REBT is known as *cognitive behavior therapy* **(CBT).** CBT is behavioral therapy that focuses on examining the relationships between thoughts, feelings, and behaviors. By exploring patterns of thinking that lead to self-destructive actions and the beliefs that direct these thoughts, people with mental illness can modify their patterns of thinking to improve coping. CBT is a type of psychotherapy that is different from traditional psychodynamic psychotherapy in that the therapist and the patient actively work together to help the patient recover from the mental illness. People seeking CBT can expect their therapist to be problem-focused and goal-directed in addressing the challenging symptoms of mental illnesses. Because CBT is an active intervention, one can also expect to do homework or practice outside of sessions.

REBT and other forms of cognitive therapy are gaining in popularity because they are significantly more short-term than psychoanalysis and therefore less costly to the patient.

Person-Centered/Humanistic Therapy

Theorists Abraham Maslow and Carl Rogers are most frequently credited with the concept of **person-centered,** or humanistic, therapy (FIG. 8.10). In this form of treatment, all caregivers are to focus on the whole person and to work in the present. It is not important in humanistic treatment to understand the cause of the problem or what happened in the person's past; what is important is the here and now. Rogers believed three conditions were required in the therapist providing services: genuineness, empathy, and unconditional positive regard (Karpiak & Spills, 2019). Although nurses may not be active participants in the actual therapy sessions with their patients, it is important to maintain these three qualities in *all* therapeutic relationships. When a patient feels betrayed, it usually results in deterioration of the nurse-patient relationship and loss of credibility for the nurse in that situation.

Unconditional Positive Regard

Unconditional positive regard is a core principle of Rogerian theory. Unconditional positive regard means full, nonjudgmental acceptance of the patient as a person. It also means that the patient must work at accepting himself or herself. Being self-aware and having feelings that are congruent (aligned) with that self-concept are some of the goals of humanistic therapy.

Counseling versus Psychotherapy

According to Schimelpfening (2020), there is a difference between a counselor and a psychotherapist. In **counseling,** the counselor usually works with their client as a guide to resolve an issue in a shorter period of time, whereas the psychotherapist has a longer relationship using a specific therapy with their client. The counselor and psychotherapist are similar in some respects. Both are professionals, but the psychotherapist will usually have a higher degree in psychology. Professional counselors are licensed

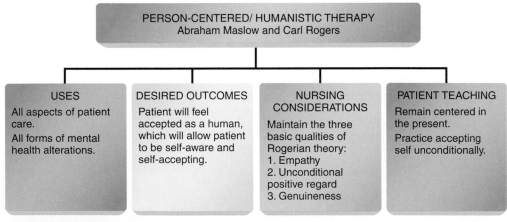

FIGURE 8.10 Person-centered/humanistic therapy.

and regulated differently, not only state by state, but also sometimes municipality by municipality (FIG. 8.11). Some states require that a person be prepared at a doctoral level to practice independently. Nurses prepared at an LPN/LVN level can counsel at a minimal level or in a support capacity. In some localities, they may practice various forms of clinical therapy. It is up to nurses who wish to counsel patients to do the appropriate research to determine their rights and responsibilities and the regulations in their locality. Nurses may be asked or required to accompany their patients to counseling sessions or to facilitate (lead) a group discussion. If you have the opportunity to observe a group session, take it. It is very interesting to see the dynamics of the group and the way the facilitator guides patients through issues.

> ## GOOD TO KNOW
> Therapy sessions are confidential, even if they are group oriented.

Pastoral or Cultural Counseling
Some people prefer to obtain assistance, guidance, or counseling from their church or spiritual leaders (FIG. 8.12). Sessions are often free or on a "free-will" or "ability to pay" status. The person who provides therapy in this time or circumstance may or may not be trained in traditional mental health theories and modalities.

In some faith-based organizations, nurses have an opportunity to serve in ways they could not in a traditional setting. For example, parish nurses are licensed registered nurses who work through their church or other religious organizations and perform tasks ranging from simply visiting a homebound church member to actually performing care and counseling or referrals for that individual. Depending on the particular religious organization, nurses who serve as parish nurses may serve in a volunteer capacity or in a paid position. Training sessions are offered in some locales for nurses who wish to provide this service, although many churches do not yet require formal training for all their nurses.

Nurses may also be in a position to counsel patients belonging to the nurse's own cultural or religious group when the patient enters the health-care system. Here are some examples:

- Jewish patients, especially those who observe kosher practices, may have concerns about dietary selections. They may refuse to have certain procedures done between sundown Friday and sundown Saturday (the Sabbath) and may insist on being admitted to a Jewish hospital if one is available.
- Muslim patients may follow rituals that may conflict with schedules and routines within the hospital. Prayer times are prescribed by traditional teachings and are strictly followed; therefore, medication times, treatment times, or attendance at therapy may meet with some conflict on the part of that patient. However, prayers can be postponed in case of a conflict in schedules. Some women of the Islamic faith wear a hijab (or head covering) that completely covers the hair. Islamic holidays and holy days fall on different days each year than the social holidays in the United States or the holidays and holy days of Christianity

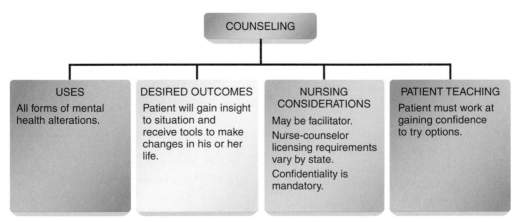

COUNSELING			
USES	**DESIRED OUTCOMES**	**NURSING CONSIDERATIONS**	**PATIENT TEACHING**
All forms of mental health alterations.	Patient will gain insight to situation and receive tools to make changes in his or her life.	May be facilitator. Nurse-counselor licensing requirements vary by state. Confidentiality is mandatory.	Patient must work at gaining confidence to try options.

FIGURE 8.11 Counseling.

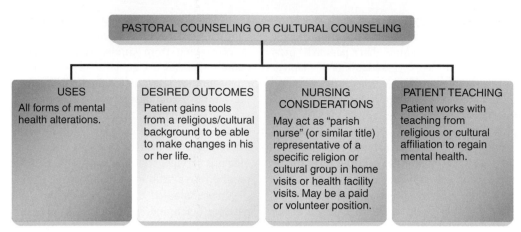

FIGURE 8.12 Pastoral or cultural counseling.

or Judaism. Also, the Muslim patient may have some dietary concerns; strict Muslims may observe halal practices, which are similar to the kosher practices of Judaism. Patients of both of these faiths may have some concerns about the contents of their medications, such as gel caps. Nurses need to be aware of the potential conflicts between hospital routines and the religious obligations of their patients.

GOOD TO KNOW

Some Native American patients may have healing traditions that conflict with traditional Western medicine. Remember that it is not appropriate to label all Native Americans as one group; different tribes have their own unique beliefs and traditions. Shamans, healers, and medicine men are examples of people who may be present in the room with a Native American patient.

CRITICAL THINKING QUESTION

A new employee on your medical floor "disappears" at odd times in addition to her assigned breaks. Today is exceptionally busy; staffing is short, and there are new patients on the floor. The patient in the private room down the hall is deteriorating; she has the potential for a stroke and is waiting to be transferred to the intensive care unit (ICU). Where is the new employee? You find her on her knees deep in prayer. You try to tell her that things are very critical right now.

She is needed; can't she pray later? She tells you she needs to pray now and that she will only be a few more minutes. What priorities must be addressed? Whose priorities are they? What potential problems could arise from this situation? What are some potential resolutions?

Group Therapy

Group therapy is a very broad topic. Groups are formed for many reasons; they can be ongoing or short-term, depending on the needs of the patients or the type of disorder. Group therapy can include formal psychotherapy groups where patients meet with a therapist regularly as part of their treatment. Self-help programs are also a form of group therapy. For example, Alcoholics Anonymous (AA) and similar 12-step groups are well-established, ongoing groups. They are held not only in the treatment facility, but also in the community. Meeting times are established and published so that people know when and how to access them. As a rule, AA meetings are "closed" meetings; that is, only alcoholics are welcome. Sometimes, maybe once a month or once quarterly, a meeting is advertised as "open," meaning that other interested persons (and students) are welcome.

TOOL BOX

Alcoholics Anonymous (AA)

For information on the concept of AA and meeting locations, see www.aa.org

Group therapy also includes family therapy. Family therapy groups assist family members in interacting with each other and identifying and resolving issues they are having. Families learn how having effective communication can reduce stress and tension in a family (Varghese et al., 2020). Family therapy sessions are often set up with individual therapists with a specialty in the problem area for that family. It is expected that the whole family attend, but there may be times when only certain members are asked to attend or when the individuals will "break out" with another therapist and then return to the family group later.

In addition to family therapy, a couple may need couples therapy to work on the way they communicate. Marriage, or couples, counseling is set up either with an individual counselor or in a group with other couples. Many times, peer counselors are used. These are people who have experienced similar obstacles in their marriage and found creative, effective ways to manage their conflicts (FIG. 8.13). Sometimes, couples choose to seek help from a spiritual leader.

Therapists and counselors are facilitators. They do not heal the patient; the patient heals himself or herself. Ideally, patients take the suggestions given by the therapist, try them, and see what works for them. Nurses can reinforce the good work patients do in learning to keep themselves healthy. Nurses can also remind patients gently that they are doing their own healing. Sometimes, when the road to healing gets rocky, patients may use the therapist as a scapegoat. Rather than agree or disagree with the patient, remember to use therapeutic communication skills, empathize with the hard work the patient is doing, and encourage the patient to discuss their frustration with the therapist.

Other Types of Therapy
Electroconvulsive Therapy

Electroconvulsive therapy (ECT), or electroshock therapy as it is sometimes still called, is a form of

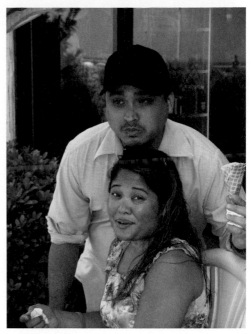

FIGURE 8.13 This obviously happy couple is a reminder that people can find creative, effective ways to manage conflicts within their relationships. A therapist may help them with suggestions, but they must try those suggestions themselves and find what works for them *(courtesy of Robynn Anwar).*

treatment that can be frightening to some patients. ECT delivers a small electrical charge to the brain that creates a change in nerve impulses. ECT is an alternative treatment for certain mental disorders when nothing else works.

Because of patients' misconceptions, it is important for health-care providers to educate them about ECT (FIG. 8.14). After informed consent is obtained, patients are generally given a sedative before the treatment. Nurses carefully monitor blood pressure and pulse before and after treatment. The amount of electricity used is individualized to the patient, and a treatment usually lasts only a few minutes. If an observer is slow to look, they might miss seeing a patient's so-called "seizure." Often, only a toe or a finger may twitch slightly; gone are the days of uncontrolled seizures on the treatment table.

ECT has a few side effects that can be fairly unpleasant. The patient may feel confused and forgetful immediately after the treatment. This can be from a combination of the ECT and the pretreatment medication. If there has been a stronger seizure, the patient may have some muscle soreness. Patients are secured with restraints during the treatment, however, so

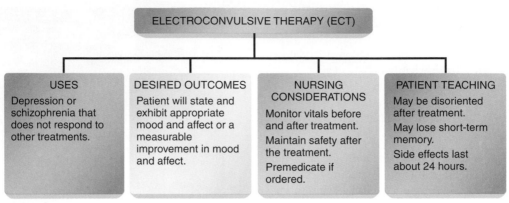

FIGURE 8.14 Electroconvulsive therapy.

movement is minimal. Because of the possibility of confusion and forgetfulness, it is common to restrict the patient's activity for 24 hours after a treatment, and it is recommended that the nurse stay with the patient until the patient is oriented and able to care for himself or herself. ECT is not used indiscriminately as it once was. Today, it is used when other therapies have not been helpful. According to Murphy (2013), ECT treats "major depression, bipolar disorders, and schizophrenia" when other treatments have not produced positive outcomes, and ECT can be used in all three trimesters of pregnancy.

Nursing Responsibilities

Before the ECT, ensure that informed consent with the patient's signature is present. The nurse taking care of the patient should be competent in providing care for a patient receiving ECT. The nurse's responsibilities include careful monitoring of vital signs and accurate documentation relating to the patient's subjective and objective responses to the treatment. This is especially important if the patient has any cardiac disorders. The patient should have nothing by mouth (NPO) for at least 4 to 8 hours before a treatment. Before ECT, remind the patient to empty their bladder and to remove dentures, contact lenses, hairpins, and items that may create a safety issue. Monitor the amount of hypnotics and sedatives given the night before ECT. Finally, ensure that the patient is kept safe after therapy.

Humor Therapy

Many studies have been done over the years showing the effects of smiles, hugs, and laughter on mental health as well as on physical conditions such as cancer (FIG. 8.15). The movie *Patch Adams,* based on a

real-life doctor, demonstrated the potential of humor therapy. In it, viewers saw breakthroughs take place in patients previously thought untreatable.

> **GOOD TO KNOW**
> The downside of humor therapy is that what some people find funny, others find offensive. Be sensitive to varied reactions and cultural differences. Remember that some people are fearful of clowns.

Humor therapy uses many modalities, from clowns to movies to just 10 good "belly laughs" daily. Whatever the medium, laughter alters outlooks and neurochemical production. Patients can show remarkable progress. In fact, this kind of intervention has brought responses such as singing, hand clapping, and laughter from patients with dementia who do not usually respond to other programming. Laughter may not be a cure for a disease or disorder, but it may release endorphins.

Smiles are always appropriate along with congruent behavior. Wearing a red rubber nose when walking into the room of an appropriate patient might allow you to ease that person's pain—either mental or physical—even if only for a short while. Humor is important for nurses as well as for the patient, because caring for others on a daily basis creates a great deal of stress.

Animal-Assisted Therapy

Animal-assisted therapy (AAT) has been found to reduce stress in patients. If the patient has a pet, they may be missing their pet during their confinement in a facility. In some facilities, pets reside with patients

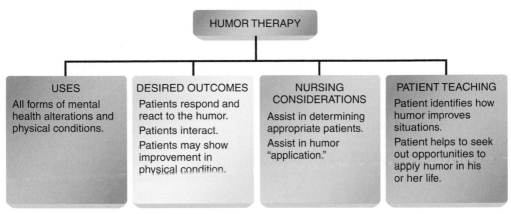

FIGURE 8.15 Humor therapy.

or come as visitors to meet with patients. Most are specially trained. According to Perkins (2020), pet therapy can reduce patients' blood pressure, stress, and anxiety.

According to the National Institutes of Health (NIH), pets can be used in several health-care settings, including mental health units and long-term care facilities. Studies have shown that AAT has therapeutic effects, including reducing anxiety in children, adolescents, and adults (Murphy, 2015). In addition, service animals can be trained to recognize when the person is having a mania episode or serve as a reminder to take medication. These service animals often have ways to calm the person.

Crisis Intervention

A crisis can happen at any time to anyone. It can involve one's child, the next-door neighbor, or a patient. *Crisis* is defined in several ways. In the health fields, a crisis is a sudden, unexpected event in a person's life that drastically changes their routine. *Crisis* has been defined as a state in which the body is out of homeostasis. It is thought of as a situation in which a person may feel out of control and feel in turmoil (Shives & Isaacs, 2002).

A person in crisis is at risk for physical and emotional harm inflicted by self or by others. Examples of people who may be experiencing a crisis are those who have lost a job suddenly, have divorced recently, are in an abusive relationship, have experienced the death of a loved one, or are contemplating or attempting suicide. An important concept to remember is that each person has a different set of stressors and a different way of dealing with stress. What is a crisis for one person may be simply a minor nuisance for another.

Many employers recognize the potential for crisis and offer some type of employee assistance

Evidence-Based Practice

Clinical Question: What is the role of AAT in the treatment of mental health disorders?

Evidence: Koukourikos et al. studied the effects of AAT on patients diagnosed with autism, depression, dementia, and schizophrenia. Patients in facilities that provided AAT experienced fewer episodes of anxiety and depression. Research has also shown positive results introducing this type of therapy to facilities. For some patients, it helped with their self-image, developing social skills, and being less negative.

Implications for Nursing:
- Train staff in recognizing zoonotic (animal-borne) diseases.
- Recognize signs of when the therapeutic animal is stressed.
- Team the patient with the appropriate AAT for a positive outcome.
- Document therapeutic interactions and patient responses.

Koukourikos, K., Georgeopoulou, A., Kourkoutaz, L., & Tsaloglidou, A. (2019). *Benefits of Animal Assisted Therapy in Mental Health.* ResearchGate. https://www.researchgate.net/publication/336810495_Benefits_of_Animal_Assisted_Therapy_in_Mental_Health.

program (EAP). The service is confidential, and usually the initial call is free to the employee. EAPs vary in what they are able to provide and may act as a referral service for the employee. Ask the patient if their employer provides this benefit.

Although crisis is highly individualized, most experts agree that people experiencing a crisis pass through the four stages identified by Gerald Caplan in 1964: initial threat, increase in threat, continual failure to reduce threat, and a major breakdown if the crisis is not resolved (Poal, 2015). Refer to Table 8.1.

Goals of Crisis Intervention

Nurses often have the unique opportunity of being present for the first three phases of the crisis and not for the outcome (FIG. 8.16). In many agencies, nurses are not involved with longer-term treatment, but they may very easily be the ones who walk into the room during a suicide attempt or who take the call at the nursing station from a distraught parent who is about to hurt their child.

The goals of crisis intervention change according to the degree of treatment in which the nurse will be involved. Crisis intervention for the health-care provider is obviously provided at a different level than it would be from a law enforcement or emergency-dispatch viewpoint. Because this text is meant to be an overview to prepare nurses at an entry level of practice, we will look at the goals of crisis intervention from a health-care perspective.

Nursing Responsibilities

1. *Ensure safety:* Assess the situation. If you or the patient is in physical danger, signal for help. *Do not* leave the patient unless danger to you is imminent. It may sound harsh, but you will be no good to anyone if you are injured or worse. Take care of your own safety and then take care of the patient's safety.

2. *Diffuse the situation:* Do this verbally, when at all possible. A person in crisis is most likely not in control of their thoughts, feelings, or actions. Physical attempts at restraining or calming the patient are best left until all verbal attempts have been made and only when there is enough help to ensure the safety of the patient and the staff.

3. *Determine the problem:* Attempt to find out the patient's viewpoint and the cause of the crisis. It is very important *not to push* the patient for any reason and *to remain calm* during the intervention. The last thing a patient in crisis needs is a nurse in panic. There will be time to talk about your feelings when the patient is safe.

4. *Decrease the anxiety level:* Your adrenaline level will probably be at an all-time high, but it will not be even close to that of the person in crisis. Make every attempt to reassure the patient that they are in a safe place. Gently but firmly tell the patient you are concerned and will do whatever is possible to make the situation more comfortable but that the patient's help and cooperation

Table 8.1

The Four Phases of Crisis

Phase	Behaviors
Initial exposure to stressor	Person feels "fine"; will often deny stress level and, in fact, state a feeling of well-being.
Crisis	Person denies problem is out of control; withdraws or rationalizes behaviors and stress; uses defense mechanism of projection frequently. This may last varied amounts of time.
Adaptive	Crisis is perceived in a positive way. Anxiety decreases. Person attempts to regain self-esteem and is able to start socializing again. Person is able to do some positive problem-solving.
Postcrisis	Surprisingly, both positive and negative functioning may be seen. Person may have developed a more positive, effective way of coping with stress *or* may show ineffective adaptation, such as being critical, hostile, depressed, or using food or chemicals, such as alcohol, to deal with what has happened.

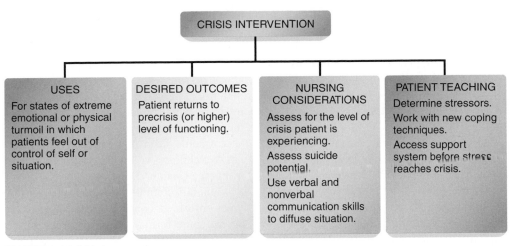

FIGURE 8.16 Crisis intervention.

are needed. *Caution:* Be very careful with physical contact at this point. Touch as a nonverbal communication skill may be interpreted inaccurately as aggression or sexual innuendo by a patient whose thoughts and feelings are in turmoil.

5. *Return the patient to precrisis (or better) level of functioning:* You may or may not be able to calm the patient to the point that they are able to understand what just happened. It might take a longer-term session of treatment to help the patient gain that kind of insight. No matter what level of intervention the patient requires, the ultimate goal is for the person to learn the skills necessary to cope with stress in a more positive way than before the crisis. Much of that learning will come from the role modeling provided by nurses. **Quite often the most effective techniques are nonverbal, where actions speak louder than words.**

CRITICAL THINKING QUESTION

With a student partner, role play one or more of the following potential crises (or think up your own). Think about your communication techniques. Do they change when dealing with a crisis? If so, how? What about your nonverbal communication techniques?

- A parent whose child has been abducted at the mall
- A man who calls the clinic, stating he has just killed his wife

- A woman who is frantically seeking shelter from an abusive relationship
- A friend of your adolescent daughter who is slashing her own wrists
- An alcoholic, the main wage earner for the family, who has just been fired from his job

Classroom Activity

Conduct an internet search for agencies that handle crisis intervention. Contact one agency in person. Inform the agency that this is a school project and you wish to ask them a few questions: Whom does the agency service? What are its hours of operation? How is the agency funded? What does the emergency care cost the patient? How is the agency staffed? Write a short report of your findings. If possible, appoint someone to compile all the information so that each student nurse has a "starter set" to be able to help others.

Crisis, if treated in an appropriate and timely way, is usually temporary. Crisis intervention theories are changing to try to keep up with the current concepts of illness. The Center for Disease and Control Prevention (CDC) has an online manual, *Crisis and Emergency Risk Communication* (CERC), which is frequently updated with vital crisis information. When crisis happens, it is important that the person who is there to help understands that this is a very frightening time for the person in turmoil. Nurses must understand that they are in a special position as they have some knowledge of crisis and communication skills and are able to help, yet they must always be aware of the legal ramifications of intervention.

Legal Considerations in Crisis Intervention

Today's society is a litigious one, meaning that people are quick to sue one another in court. As a result, it is tempting to stay uninvolved when people call out for help. In some states, nurses, physicians, and anyone else in the health field are required by law to help. Some localities even require health-care professionals to post identifying insignia on their vehicles. Most states do not require this yet, but many are considering it. What is an entry-level nurse to do? Nurses want to help, but nursing curriculum at the entry level provides very little training in hands-on crisis-intervention techniques. What if something goes wrong? Crisis intervention literature suggests that nurses risk a higher liability if they fail to try to help. In other words, it is safer legally for a nurse to do something to help than to do nothing.

Exactly what a nurse is able to do depends greatly on their locale, level of preparation, state's nurse practice act, and comfort level. Staying within the legal parameters of one's nursing licensure is of major importance; nurses should do only what they know how to do and what is legal. The truth is that anyone can sue anyone for anything. The good news is that most states will find in favor of the medical professional who has acted in good faith and in accordance with their licensure to help a person in a crisis situation. "Good Samaritan" laws protect nurses as well as physicians and other health-care providers. However, Good Samaritan laws *do not* generally cover nurses within the confines of their employment, only when they are acting to assist in a crisis or emergency situation.

GOOD TO KNOW
Crisis intervention can be compared with cardiopulmonary resuscitation (CPR): Once a nurse starts and makes that commitment to help, they cannot quit until physically unable to continue. Starting to provide help and then changing one's mind can be interpreted as neglect or abandonment, and in such an instance the nurse could be found at fault.

What happens to the patient experiencing the crisis? Because of the nature of crisis, the patient probably does not have a valid insight into the situation. The patient is very likely to be concerned about personal safety. On top of that, fear and inability to perceive the situation as it really is will interfere with communication. In most instances, the medical staff will encourage the patient to accept some form of treatment. The patient then has two choices: voluntary or involuntary commitment (see Chapter 3).

Voluntary commitment happens when the patient gives informed consent to be hospitalized or to accept some formal treatment program. *Informed* consent means that the patient has been made aware of their behaviors, the implications of the behaviors, and the expected effects of treatment. Informed consent can be oral, nonverbal, or written. *Implied* consent allows people who are unconscious to be treated in such a way as to preserve life. If the patient is an adult of legal age who is considered to be competent in the eyes of the law (or an adolescent who has acquired legal emancipation), this patient can also sign himself or herself out of the hospital or facility at any time.

Involuntary commitment varies somewhat from state to state. Many states have the capability to place a "hold" on the patient, usually for 48 to 72 hours. During this time, the patient is confined to the treatment setting. Usually, a social worker is assigned to visit the patient and act as an advocate for them. The goal of the hold period is for the patient to see the need for help with their crisis and then consent to voluntary treatment. If, at the end of the hold period, the patient does not consent to treatment, they are free to leave the facility, as long as no other manifestation of crisis has surfaced during the hold.

In either instance, patients maintain all civil rights while in the treatment setting. The patient is covered under the Patient's Bill of Rights, and most often the patient is given a copy of these rights.

The Community Mental Health Centers Act made provisions for community-based treatment. Communities are supposed to develop mental health centers and provide treatment according to the needs of the area; not all centers provide all types of treatment or 24-hour service. However, the community is supposed to provide some method of emergency psychiatric treatment to help people in crisis as well as those who are chronically mentally ill. These centers can be in the form of freestanding crisis centers or walk-in clinics, and many are connected with the community hospital. In reality though, many communities have minimal resources to provide these services, so nurses should know what is available in their communities.

 SUMMARY

Table 8.2 summarizes treatment modalities that may be used alone or in conjunction with medications to treat a wide variety of mental health issues. The common uses and desired outcomes are covered.

Table 8.2
Summary of Commonly Used Treatment Modalities

Treatment Modality	Uses	Desired Outcomes
Psychotherapy	For treatment of various alterations to mental health	Patient states improvement in emotional discomfort. Patient returns to comfortable social functioning. Patient behaves in a manner appropriate to the situation.
Behavior modification	To remove or greatly diminish behaviors that are inappropriate or unhealthy	Former undesirable behaviors have been replaced by new, healthy behaviors.
REBT/CBT	Short-term, problem-focused therapy for any mental health alteration that is consciously controlled	Patient will be able to remain "undisturbed" as a result of rethinking activating events, belief system, and consequences.
Person-centered/ humanistic	All aspects of patient care; all forms of mental health alterations	Patient will feel accepted as a human, which will allow patient to be self-aware and self-accepting. Patient will gain insight into the situation and receive tools to make changes in his or her life.
Pastoral counseling or cultural counseling	All forms of mental health alterations	Patient gains tools from a religious/cultural background to be able to make changes in his or her life.
Group therapy	Many uses, including family, couples, self-help	Patient gains knowledge that there are others with similar problems. Patient learns from peers and helps others.
ECT	Depression or schizophrenia that does not respond to other treatments	Patient will state and exhibit appropriate mood and affect or a measurable improvement in mood and affect.

Continued

Table 8.2
Summary of Commonly Used Treatment Modalities—cont'd

Treatment Modality	Uses	Desired Outcomes
Humor therapy	All forms of mental health alterations and physical conditions	Patients respond and react to humor. Patients interact. Patients may show improvement in physical condition.
Crisis intervention	For states of extreme emotional or physical turmoil in which patients feel out of control of self or situation	Patient returns to precrisis (or higher) level of functioning.

Safe and Effective Nursing Care

Education on injury prevention
AIMS documentation
Administering psychotropic medications with awareness of dosage, side effects, adverse effects, and contraindications
Monitoring diagnostic laboratory values
Responses to therapy
Ability to recognize chemical dependency characteristics
Crisis interventions

Key Points

- Psychopharmacology is very important to the effective treatment of the patient. There are many classifications of psychoactive medications and many individual medications within each classification. It is the nurse's responsibility to consult a drug reference regarding all the psychotropic medications given to patients. It also is part of the nurse's role to teach the patient about their medications.
- Milieu is a word used to describe a therapeutic and safe environment for treatment.
- Psychotherapy, sometimes provided in conjunction with medications, is often used to treat patients. There are several methods of psychotherapy, including psychoanalysis, behavior modification, REBT, and humanistic, or person-centered, therapy.
- Counseling is carried out in different ways, depending on the patient's needs and type of illness. Counselors may be licensed, and the nurse's role in counseling regulated differently

from state to state and municipality to municipality. Counseling is given individually or in group settings, according to the situation.
- ECT is used for specific situations and requires the patient's signed informed consent. Premedication is usually ordered. It is the role of the nurse to monitor vital signs, maintain safety, and document post-treatment observations.
- Gerald Caplan identified the four phases in any crisis.
- Crisis intervention is very individualized, and each person experiences crisis differently.
- EAPs are becoming more accessible through employers. They are confidential and free or reasonably priced.
- Pastoral or cultural counseling may be the treatment of choice for an individual. Nurses must do all they can to help the patient receive care that is personally meaningful.

CASE STUDY

Andrea, an emergency department nurse, has just entered a major theme park with her friend and two children. Andrea and her friend are alerted that the theme park has just experienced an active shooter. Details are sketchy, but there are numerous injuries. Many of the park's exits have been barricaded. Andrea and her friend suddenly witness many individuals running, injured, and crying. Police, park security, and other first responders are directing Andrea and her friend away from the site. Andrea tells them she is a nurse and offers to help. At this moment, her help is not wanted, but all are directed to a "holding" area. The children, whose ages are 4 and 13, are crying and asking Andrea questions about what they are seeing, such as people with bloody clothes and some people lying on the ground and motionless. If you were Andrea, what would your emotional response be? How would you answer and calm the children? After a few minutes, the police accept Andrea's offer to help the wounded. The children become hysterical at Andrea's leaving them, yet Andrea feels responsible to help. What should Andrea do? What stages of crisis is she experiencing?

Review Questions

1. Which of the following is not a behavior noted in the crisis phase?
   a. Denial
   b. Feeling of well-being
   c. Projection
   d. Rationalization

2. One of the first comments a nurse might make to a person who has been abused might be:
   a. "Why didn't you leave the first time you were attacked?"
   b. "Do you want to prosecute or not?"
   c. "What do you think made that person hit you?"
   d. "You're safe here. I would like to help you."

3. A therapeutic environment (milieu) is *best* defined as:
   a. An environment in which a patient is under a 72-hour hold
   b. An environment that is locked and supervised
   c. An environment that is structured to decrease stress and encourage learning new behavior
   d. An environment that is designed to be home-like for persons who are hospitalized for life

4. Which of the following is *false* regarding ECT?
   a. It is used to treat depression and schizophrenia.
   b. It is used to stop convulsive seizures.
   c. Fatigue and disorientation are immediate side effects.
   d. Memory will gradually return.

5. Psychopharmacology (psychotropic drug therapy) is used:
   a. As a cure for mental illness
   b. Only to control violent behavior
   c. To alter the pain receptors in the brain
   d. To decrease symptoms and facilitate other therapies

6. Avoiding such foods as bananas, cheese, and yogurt should be emphasized to patients who are taking:
   a. Fluoxetine (Prozac)
   b. Lithium
   c. MAOIs
   d. TCAs

7. The goals of crisis intervention include all of the following *except:*
   a. Ensuring safety
   b. Increasing anxiety
   c. Taking care of the precipitating event
   d. Returning to precrisis or better level of functioning

8. In order for psychotherapy to be effective, it is necessary to do all of the following *except:*
   a. Encourage the patient to repress feelings.
   b. Reinforce appropriate behavior.
   c. Establish a therapeutic patient-staff relationship.
   d. Assist patient to gain insight into the problem.

9. Your patient, Mrs. L, is on your unit for bowel resection. She is exhibiting signs of nervousness and anxiety, which she attributes to the upcoming surgery. You note from her record that she has a history of ethyl alcohol (ETOH) abuse. Which of the following classification of drugs would be potentially addictive for her?
   a. Lithium salts
   b. Antianxiety drugs
   c. Antipsychotic drugs
   d. Anticholinergics

10. James is a 13-year-old who has been transferred to your medical-surgical unit after being stabilized in the emergency department (ED). He slit both wrists and took an overdose of his bupropion (Wellbutrin). You know medications such as Wellbutrin:
    a. Are antidepressants and should have stopped his suicidal impulse
    b. Have no particular nursing considerations for children and adolescents
    c. Are antidepressants and may cause an increase in the suicidal ideation for children and adolescents
    d. Are not effective as antidepressants for children or adolescents

REVIEW QUESTIONS ANSWER KEY 1.b, 2.d, 3.c, 4.b, 5.d, 6.c, 7.b, 8.a, 9.b, 10.c

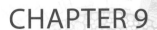

CHAPTER 9
Complementary and Alternative Treatment Modalities

KEY TERMS

Alternative medicine
Aromatherapy
Ayurveda
Beliefs
Biofeedback
Complementary medicine
Dietary supplement
Herbal supplement
Holistic
Hypnotherapy
Integrative medicine
Mind-body connection
Mindfulness
Models
Placebo
Presupposition
Rapport
Reflexology
Reiki
Traditional chinese medicine
Trance
Yoga

CHAPTER CONCEPTS

Cognition
Comfort
Health promotion
Safety

LEARNING OUTCOMES

1. Differentiate between complementary and alternative medicine.
2. Define integrative medicine.
3. Identify the concept of the mind–body connection.
4. Identify support for patient beliefs and models.
5. Identify three alternative and complementary treatment modalities.
6. Describe three types of massage.
7. Differentiate between trance and sleep.
8. Identify the three primary channels of experience.
9. Define key terms.

Many factors affect a patient's choice of treatment: the patient's education, experience, economic status, belief system, environment, and culture are a few of those factors. Many health-care providers prefer to prescribe conventional medications. Yet for some patients, conventional Western medicine is not the only course for treatment. In 2010, the World Health Organization (WHO) estimated that about 75% of the world's population depends on traditional treatments (Ansari & Inamdar, 2010).

Complementary and **alternative medicine** (CAM) present additional options in health promotion. In general, alternative medicines *replace* those of conventional/Western medicine, whereas complementary medicine methods are *used together* with conventional treatments. Many traditional practices and remedies have been used for centuries, and they offer patients different choices from the medications dispensed at the local pharmacy and traditional physical therapies. Often, these unconventional practices or treatments differ considerably from what is considered "acceptable" medical care in Western culture. Complementary or alternative methods may lack extensive scientific research to prove their effectiveness, or even their safety, according to the standards of conventional medicine. Those practices that do have at least some research validating that they are safe and effective comprise **integrative medicine**, which provides the best of both worlds.

An alternative practice, for example, would be to use an herbal preparation to treat depression instead of a prescription medication ordered by a health-care provider. A complementary treatment might consist of using biofeedback to reduce the symptoms of anxiety associated with mental illness while the patient continues to participate in psychotherapy and take antianxiety medications. Both approaches address a key concept in alternative and complementary medicine: the **mind-body connection**.

 ## THE MIND-BODY CONNECTION AND MINDFULNESS

The ways in which people's minds and bodies connect stretch beyond the obvious physical world in which people live. First, there is the brain, an organ directly connected to the body by tissue such as nerves and blood vessels. The *brain* is contained within the bony cavity of the skull, which constitutes its protection and support. The *mind* represents the cognitive, emotional, and logical responses that make people individual human beings. The mind is clearly more than just the brain, the sum of its cells, chemicals, electrical activity, and connections. **Mindfulness** is an awareness of what is going on at

the present time and realizing the mind-body connection (Greenland et al., 2019).

It may seem strange to think that there was ever a question about the interconnectedness of the mind and the body. It has long been known that physical disease can affect the mind, but conventional medicine has only recently started to accept that the reverse is also true—that the mind affects physical disease. People's thoughts and emotions often affect the way their bodies function, even on a cellular level. This **holistic** view makes complementary and alternative medicine increasingly popular choices for the treatment of all types of illness, including mental health disorders.

Important to the effectiveness of any type of treatment are the patient's **beliefs**. Nursing asserts that respect for the beliefs and values of other people and cultures is fundamental to good practice. It is useful to remember that everyone has a different way of viewing the world. Everyone forms **models** of the world based on their unique beliefs, values, education, environment, and experience. Models are pictures or ideas that people form in their minds to explain how things work. Models help people to understand and interact with others and their environment and to formulate beliefs.

To a large extent, a person's beliefs will determine the success of a given treatment. This can be plainly seen when a **placebo** medication is given and is effective in relieving symptoms like severe

---

Evidence-Based Practice

Clinical Question: What are the effects of health-care providers practicing mindfulness at work?

Evidence: Mindfulness exercises can benefit the health-care provider as well as patients, especially if the health-care provider is having a stressful day. Researchers reviewed 14 studies with a total of 833 participants, the majority female. Physicians, nurses, and nursing students were included in the studies. Participants were taught several types of mindfulness interventions. Results indicate that using mindfulness practices at work allows health-care providers to be more aware and to improve their decision making.

Implications for Nursing Practice: To increase their awareness and improve decision making, nurses should consider

• learning different types of mindfulness exercises
• finding a setting at work where they could briefly practice mindfulness (e.g., an empty room or classroom or a lounge).
• scheduling time for mindfulness before or during work
• scheduling a time for mindfulness at home
• journaling about which mindfulness techniques benefited them

Gilmartin, H., Goyal, A., Hamati, M. C., Mann, J., Saint, S., & Chopra, V. (2017). *(PDF) Brief Mindfulness Practices for Healthcare Providers …* ResearchGate. https://www.researchgate.net/publication/318201540_Brief_Mindfulness_Practices_for_Healthcare_Providers_-_A_Systematic_Literature_Review.

pain, even though the placebo contains no actual medication. Clearly, what the patient believes the placebo can do and expects the placebo to do can be more important than the actual composition of the tablet. The downside of using placebos is the potential loss of the patient's trust in the nurse if the patient becomes aware of the ruse (Micozzi, 2015). According to the American Medical Association (AMA) Code of Medical Ethics Opinion 2.1.4, before giving a placebo a nurse must explain and get permission from their patient to administer a placebo (AMA, 2021).

Even though you might not be directly providing a complementary or alternative treatment, supporting the patient's cultural and belief systems is important in helping the patient to move forward on a path to wellness. Each patient will have a different level of acceptance of various complementary and alternative approaches. You must remain nonjudgmental, open, and accepting and at the same time be aware of any safety concerns for the patient.

As always, the boundaries of legal and acceptable nursing practice vary from state to state. Check with your state board of nursing or other regulating agency to determine acceptable standards of practice regarding alternative, integrative, and complementary therapies.

COMMON COMPLEMENTARY AND ALTERNATIVE TREATMENTS

Biofeedback

Stress-related anxiety is a common element of mental health disorders. The direct effects of sustained stress can be devastating (see Chapter 7, Coping and Defense Mechanisms). In a critical moment or progressively over time, the biological response to stress can impair cognitive function and cloud a person's thinking. Prolonged stress can lead to emotional anguish that is experienced as fear, anxiety, anger, and depression. Prolonged stress can also lead to exhaustion and possible death. Anxiety contributes to physical symptoms, many of which can be reduced or controlled by biofeedback techniques. **Biofeedback** is a training program designed to develop one's ability to control the autonomic nervous system. Biofeedback has been widely accepted in the West because of its use of scientific measuring devices and proven techniques.

The primary purpose of biofeedback training is to teach patients to be aware of tension within the body and to respond with relaxation (FIG. 9.1). Typically, training for patients takes place in a series of 1-hour sessions, sometimes spaced 1 week apart. The patient is taught to obtain a deep level of relaxation as a means to control a light, buzzer, image, or a video game, to which he or she is attached by electrodes and cables. The machine is then gradually adjusted to greater sensitivity, and the patient learns improved control. When training is completed, all the patient needs to do to obtain relaxation and symptom resolution at any time or place is to recall the particular thought and feeling that worked in the clinic.

Biofeedback has been used with good results for conditions including insomnia, migraines, some types of seizures, functional nausea and vomiting, tinnitus, and phantom-limb pain. As with other forms of therapy, biofeedback practitioners must be aware of functional or even psychological symptoms that are actually caused by organic problems and require different treatment. For example, it may not be appropriate to use biofeedback to treat extreme or acute states of mental illness, like severe depression, mania, agitation, schizophrenia, paranoia, obsessive-compulsive disorder (OCD), delirium, and identity or dissociative disorders. Critics of biofeedback have pointed out that relaxation training can provide similar effects and is more economical and easily obtained.

Patients who believe they can influence their own health outcomes are the most likely to be successful at mastering biofeedback. The experience of gaining control of one's physical reactions can have a tremendous effect on how the person will view

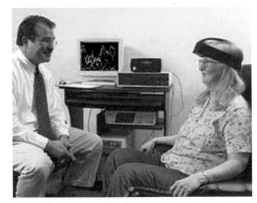

FIGURE 9.1 Biofeedback training teaches patients to recognize tension and respond with relaxation *(courtesy of Santé Rehabilitation Group, Euless, TX).*

stressful situations in the future. The most common form of biofeedback is breathing exercises. For more skeptical patients, learning biofeedback can demonstrate that they have a great deal more control over their responses and symptoms than they first expected. Biofeedback is done without drugs, is noninvasive, and involves learning techniques and relaxation exercises (Nordqvist, 2018).

Aromatherapy

Aromatherapy may well be one of the oldest methods used to treat illness in people. Related to herbal therapy, aromatherapy provides treatment by both the direct pharmacological effects of aromatic plant substances and the indirect effects of certain smells on mood and affect. Throughout human history and in many cultures, there have been accounts of the use of aromatics to treat varying forms of illness. Aromatherapy may be applied as a warm compress; used to scent a room; inhaled; massaged into the skin via salves, ointments, or essential oils; used in incense; or administered in a diffuser. It can be a cost-effective approach to healing.

Smells have strong significance in peoples' lives. People associate certain aromas with particular situations, conditions, and emotional states. Many individuals are able to relive particularly strong memories when exposed to an aroma that was present when the remembered event occurred. For example, the fragrance of baking cookies or apple pie reminds some people of being at home and even experiencing some of the emotions connected to that memory. The ability of a particular smell to create positive alterations in mood makes aromatherapy attractive to many people and has created a large market in everyday products designed to evoke calm and well-being. Scented candles and personal care products like bath oils, shampoos, and body lotions are especially popular.

Treatment for anxiety-based mental illness and depression using aromatics like lavender, thyme, gardenia, and other botanicals is becoming a more acceptable adjunct to conventional methods. Farrar and Farrar (2020) observed that the use of lavender has benefited those feeling anxious about being an inpatient as well as being an outpatient. It is important to be aware that the oils and plant matter used in aromatherapy can be toxic if improperly administered and should be kept out of the reach of children and people with cognitive impairments. Many concentrated plant oils, or essential oils, are caustic and must be diluted with other oils before

being applied to the skin. In addition, plant oils can trigger an allergic reaction in some people. Observe and assess patients to determine whether the aromatherapy products used are effective and be sure to note any negative side effects. As with all alternative treatments, it is advisable for patients to find a competent and knowledgeable practitioner so they can benefit fully from the potential of aromatherapy.

Classroom Activity

Bring several different aromatic herbs, such as thyme, rosemary, basil, and mint, to class. Pass them around, allowing your classmates to sniff them. Afterward, discuss your feelings after inhaling each herb. Are people's emotional responses similar or are they highly individual?

Herbal and Dietary Supplements

In the United States today, the use of herbal and dietary supplements to treat illness is growing steadily. To differentiate between herbal and dietary supplements, the National Center for Complementary and Integrative Health (NCCIH, 2020) makes the following distinction:

- **Dietary supplements** are products that are taken by mouth, are made to supplement the diet; contain one or more dietary ingredients such as vitamins, amino acids, or herbs; and are labeled as being dietary supplements.
- **Herbal supplements** are a type of dietary supplement containing one or more herbs.

Because dietary supplements can be purchased online and at stores, many people assume they are safe. However, persons using a dietary supplement should purchase these supplements only from reputable sources. Although the Food and Drug Administration (FDA) regulates conventional foods, dietary supplements fall under a different set of regulations, and the FDA is not responsible for evaluating supplements for efficacy and safety. Because certain herbs and dietary supplements may interact with prescribed medications, it is essential that patients' medication records also include any supplements they take.

The popularity of self-treatment with herbs is in large part due to the desire of many people to return to a simpler lifestyle and to avoid costly prescription medications. These products are also perceived by the public to be better, or safer, than pharmaceuticals because they can be purchased over the counter (OTC) and do not require an appointment with a health-care provider. But not all supplements are harmless. Some can have dangerous side effects. For example, ginkgo is taken to increase cognitive functioning; however, ginkgo can cause excessive bleeding, so precautions must be taken if the patient who uses ginkgo is having surgery. Countless products are available to consumers seeking relief through herbal and nutritional means, but not all of these products are safe and effective for every patient. Patients who choose to use supplements need to educate themselves about the possible side effects, interactions, and complications associated with the supplements they plan to take.

> ### GOOD TO KNOW
> Belief plays a considerable role in the acceptance and use of herbal and dietary supplements.

In a world full of processed food, the quality of modern nutrition has come into question, and there is a growing conviction that artificial additives lack the ability to provide the basics needed for good health.

Daily, people are assured in the news and on social media that the solution to many of their problems can be found in dietary and herbal supplements. Low cortisol has been blamed for weight loss, and taking compounds rich in human growth hormone (HGH) has been credited with reversing aging. Infomercials tout the benefits of taking coral calcium and improving sexual performance with herb-based preparations. The internet is flooded with ads for supplements that promise to improve people's lives by making them healthier and stronger. But most of these claims about "miracle" cures lack research to back them up.

On the other hand, some herbs have been researched and proven effective in treating disease conditions. This should not be surprising, for many modern medications were developed from herbs and other botanical origins. For example, Native Americans knew the value of the inner bark of the willow tree, gathered and used for its ability to reduce fever and ease pain. They also used foxglove in their sweat lodges to energize people who were frail and restore vitality to older people. They did not know that the salicylate in willow bark and digitalis in foxglove were the reasons for the effectiveness of these botanical preparations. They just knew these preparations worked.

Europe also has a long tradition of using herbal and dietary supplements to treat disease. For example, Germans routinely plant and harvest herbs in their garden plots to create remedies for common ailments. In Europe, some herbal preparations are available only by a doctor's prescription, and others can only be obtained through a licensed pharmacist. In the United States, the use of fresh or garden-grown herbs is discouraged because of the difficulty in determining the strength of the active compounds produced by plants under different growing conditions. Europeans are guided by generations of experience and practice to safely use available botanicals.

The public's belief in the safety of herbs concerns health-care providers. Deciding on an appropriate dose is difficult because herbal preparations are not regulated for strength or purity. People tend to think that if a small amount is effective, more could be better. Some herbs are toxic, particularly in their pure form. Moreover, many herbs interact negatively with prescription medications. As a result, it is vital that nurses ask direct questions about a patient's use of any CAMs. Teach your patients the importance of consulting with a health-care provider or pharmacist before beginning any sort of herbal therapy. Table 9.1 describes the most often used herbal and dietary supplements in the treatment of mental illness in this country.

Traditional Chinese Medicine

Another form of CAM, which is thousands of years old, is **traditional Chinese medicine** (TCM). The underlying principle of TCM is that balance is essential to maintain optimal health. TCM uses herbs as well as many therapies (Fais et al., 2015). Acupuncture is one popular TCM therapy; others include cupping, massage, and moxibustion, the application of heat on or near the body's energy meridians and acupuncture points. Diagnosis in TCM looks for imbalances among the five elements (wood, fire, metal, water, and earth), which refer to certain properties in the body. TCM practitioners also pay close attention to the tongue when examining the patient.

> ### Tool Box
> Traditional Chinese medicine techniques:
> https://www.practicalpainmanagement.com/
> patient/treatments/alternative/6-traditional-
> chinese-medicine-techniques

Ayurveda

Another ancient therapeutic practice, Ayurveda was first developed more than 5,000 years ago and is known in Sanskrit as the "science of life" (Lad, 2006). Ayurveda originated in India and continues to be widely practiced there. In the United States, there is no formal licensing body for practitioners, but some states have approved schools for learning Ayurveda (John Hopkins, 2021). Like TCM, **Ayurveda** is based on the principle of healthy balance. Ayurvedic practitioners assess three energies, vata, pitta, and kapha, which exist in different proportions in each person and regulate the body (Ratini, 2021). These energies are formed from earth, fire, water, air, and space (Ratini, 2021). When an imbalance in a person's energies occurs, this manifests as illness. Another belief in Ayurveda is that there is a common connection between the mind, spirit, and body.

GOOD TO KNOW

During admission interviews, ask patients if they take any dietary or herbal supplements, including teas and salves or ointments. Some of these may be contraindicated with medications ordered by the health-care provider.

Tool Box

A division of the National Institutes of Health, the National Center for Comprehensive and Integrative Health (NCCIH), is an excellent resource for obtaining information on a specific CAM, including scientific data if available.

nccih.nih.gov/

Table 9.1

Common Herbal and Dietary Supplements

Specific Therapy	Uses	Side Effects	Contraindications	Drug/Food Interactions	Patient Teaching
Ginkgo biloba (herb)	Short-term memory loss, though research is conflicting as to benefits. Problems with concentration. Depression, dementia, anxiety disorders. Used with antipsychotics for schizophrenia	Bleeding; contact dermatitis; nausea, vomiting, diarrhea, headache; rarely, subdural hematoma; seizures (especially in children)	Pregnant or breast-feeding, children; use cautiously for patients taking anticoagulants, MAOI medications because ginkgo biloba can act as an MAOI	May increase the effects of anticoagulant and antiplatelet drugs. Avoid foods containing large amounts of tyramine: aged meat and cheese, red wine, pickled herring, yogurt, raisins, sour cream, and other foods high in tyramine; also OTC cold and flu preparations.	Do not use if on warfarin (Coumadin), aspirin, or other blood thinner. Works well for people over 50 as well as younger adults. May take 6–8 weeks to experience benefits. Use with some fruits and nuts can cause a poison ivy–like reaction.

Table 9.1

Common Herbal and Dietary Supplements—cont'd

Specific Therapy	Uses	Side Effects	Contraindications	Drug/Food Interactions	Patient Teaching
Kava kava (herb)	Antidepressant, antianxiety, antipsychotic, sleep aide. Used for premenstrual syndrome (PMS).	Drowsiness, changes in reflex and judgment, nausea, gastric problems, muscle weakness, blurred vision, decreased platelet counts, decreased urea and bilirubin levels, dry skin, is a dopamine antagonist. Liver toxicity.	Pregnancy, breastfeeding. Skin yellowing from accumulation of plant pigment can occur in chronic use. Liver disease.	Do not use with: Alcohol: increases risk of kava toxicity. Alprazolam (Xanax): risk for coma exists. Central nervous system (CNS) depressants: kava potentiates these. Levodopa: can increase parkinson-like symptoms. Phenobarbital (Luminal): can increase effects.	Symptom relief may occur in as little as 1 week. Potential for significant adverse reactions when using kava. Alcohol and CNS medications are enhanced with kava.
St. John's wort (herb)	Mild to moderate depression; anxiety disorders	Severe photosensitivity, dry mouth, constipation, gastrointestinal (GI) upset, sleep disturbances, restlessness, fatigue, possible inducement of hypomania.	Consult with health-care provider if taking other medications. Pregnant or breastfeeding, children; use cautiously for patients taking anticoagulants, MAOI medication.	MAOIs, antidepressants, digoxin, birth control pills	Avoid prolonged exposure to sunlight. Use high sun protection factor (SPF) sunscreen. May increase the effects of MAOIs, OTC flu and cold medications, alcohol; do not use with these types of chemicals.

Continued

Table 9.1

Common Herbal and Dietary Supplements—cont'd

Specific Therapy	Uses	Side Effects	Contraindications	Drug/Food Interactions	Patient Teaching
Omega 3 fatty acids (dietary supplement)	Depression, postpartum depression, bipolar disorder, anxiety, dementia, ADHD, Alzheimer disease, schizophrenia	Loose stools with higher doses; "fishy" reflux, increase in bleeding with high dosages	Use cautiously for patients taking anticoagulants	May increase effects of anticoagulants Taking medication for hypertension may decrease drug effect, may increase cholesterol levels	If taking anti-coagulant drugs or high doses of aspirin, practice good safety. The oils may increase clotting time.
Sam-E (dietary supplement)	Depression	Mild and transient anxiety, insomnia, heartburn, loose stools	Can cause mania in patients with bipolar disorder; rule out before beginning treatment	Antidepressant medications	Patients with bipolar disorder should not use except under supervision of physician. Enteric-coated preparations may reduce gastric upset. Can be found in proteins foods.

Venes, D. (2017). *Complementary and alternative medicine.* Retrieved from http://resources.fadavis.com/5904/appendices/ComplementaryandAlternativeMedicine.pdf
National Center for Complementary & Alternative Medicine at http://nccam.nih.gov

Massage, Energy, and Touch

Massage in one form or another has probably been used since before the dawn of history. Massage is the manipulation of the body using methodical pressure, friction, and kneading. Touch and movement are essential to life and well-being in both physical and psychological ways. People are affected almost literally by their childhood experiences of touching. An infant has limited sensory discrimination but will react positively to being cuddled and held and even to the feel of a snugly wrapped blanket.

Tool Box

Types of massage therapy: www.massagetherapy.com/glossary/index.php

Massage has many different variations (FIG. 9.2). The use of touch is common to many different treatment approaches that diverge in their philosophical, theoretical, and practical ideas about how touch is applied. Western variations of massage include Swedish, which was developed in the early

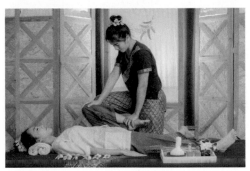

FIGURE 9.2 Massage can be an effective tool for relieving tension *(courtesy of everything-jersey.com)*.

nineteenth century and is the type most Americans are familiar with. It is characterized by long, smooth strokes that go toward the heart.

The manipulation of specific body sites to relax muscle groups is known as *trigger-point massage.* Conventional medical science has generated a similar trigger-point therapy in which injections of steroids are applied at these key areas in place of massage to both relax the muscle group and reduce local inflammation.

Of course, there are also other means of massage available. Rolfing is a therapy designed to realign the body with gravity through fascial manipulation,

a vigorous form of bodywork that is finding increasing acceptance. Eastern massage traditions have followed a different path.

Among Eastern CAM treatment methods are modalities centered on manipulating the body's energy fields. It is widely believed among Eastern practitioners that the body is governed by energy paths, called *meridians*. This energy is perceived as the life force, called *chi, ki,* or *prana.* When the life force is obstructed, emotional and physical illnesses result. Various types of pressure, massage, and other techniques are employed along these meridians to release the flow of chi, restore balance, and improve health. Shiatsu is a Japanese form of acupressure that uses pressure from the fingers to free energy flow. **Reflexology** is also based upon the belief that energy pathways and zones cross the body, connecting vital organs and body parts (FIG. 9.3). Reflexologists use massage of the feet to act upon these pathways, unblocking and renewing the energy flow.

Therapeutic touch also deserves mention. **Reiki** is representative of methods of touch healing that are often associated with massage. Reiki is a term that means "universal life energy" and refers to the process whereby this energy is drawn along the body's meridians. Unlike methods that use physical movement, pressure, or massage to unblock these

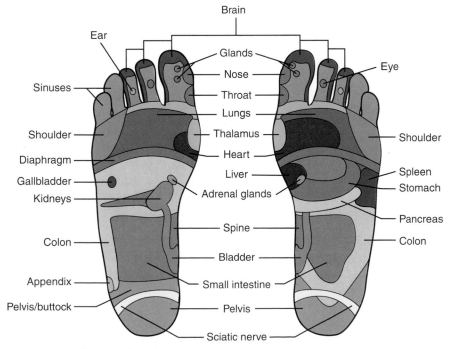

FIGURE 9.3 Reflexology foot diagram.

channels, Reiki uses the flow of life energy itself to accomplish the task. Practitioners are "attuned" to the energy channels and can manipulate them hands-on, hands just above the body, or even at a distance. Reiki techniques can even be employed as part of a more traditional massage session to enhance the physical benefits of the massage. Reiki has been demonstrated to increase warmth in the areas being treated and also to produce relaxation in the subject.

Before providing any type of touch or massage therapy, explain the procedure and receive permission from the patient. You also need to know whether the patient has a history of being sexually abused. Knowing about a patient's history of abuse allows the nurse to identify any type of interaction that may trigger a flashback of the abuse incident.

Yoga

Yoga, which has been in existence for over 5,000 years, is a mind-body connection method of healing that uses body positions to facilitate balance and flexibility. Benefits of yoga are that it creates body relaxation, slows breathing, and reduces stress. Once the yoga poses, called *asanas,* have been mastered, yoga can be practiced in a group, in the privacy of the home, or in the workplace. Ganpat, Ishwar, and Ishwara (2015) provide evidence that yoga can be used to treat patients with irritable bowel syndrome (IBS). In a group of patients with IBS, the practice of yoga resulted in the need for less prescription medication and reduced stress.

Hypnotherapy

Hypnotherapy is one of the most controversial CAM treatment modalities. Hypnosis is a means for entering an altered state of consciousness, and in this state, using visualization and suggestion to bring about desired changes in behavior and thinking. Called a **trance**, this state of focused attention is one people enter every day. The English language even contains references to this common experience of "zoning out." A trance is not sleep, but rather a state of mind wherein a person is less aware of what is going on around and instead is very focused on an internal experience, like a memory or an imagined event.

Everyone responds to unconscious suggestions to some extent. A person who is watching television and wants a snack after seeing commercials for a favorite fast-food restaurant has responded to suggestion. Fortunately, people's minds filter out suggestions that are unacceptably dangerous so that they are not persuaded to imitate some of the more unsafe things seen on TV.

> **GOOD TO KNOW**
> A hypnotherapist uses suggestion, both direct and indirect, to help the patient create change.

The general public has been subjected to an enormous amount of misinformation about hypnosis by stage hypnotists, movies, and books. Picture the scene where a hypnotist makes a volunteer from the audience cluck like a chicken, and everyone laughs. As a result of such displays, hypnotherapy is widely misunderstood and wrongly feared by many people. It is very hard for some people to overcome these fears, especially the stubborn belief in the myth that hypnosis is somehow "mind control" exercised for evil (or entertainment) purposes by the therapist.

Whereas some researchers and practitioners contend that hypnosis cannot stand on its own as a treatment modality, others are equally convinced that even lay practitioners can deliver effective therapy with a minimum of training and practice. No doubt this controversy will continue, as there are at present few regulations governing the use of hypnosis. In some states, a therapist must be certified or licensed to use hypnotherapy, and in others, no one but a psychologist, psychiatrist, medical doctor, or other professional may practice these techniques.

Hypnosis is very deep relaxation. A person who has listened to a relaxation tape and felt the effects of it or who has driven a car and noticed that 20 minutes have passed that cannot be accounted for has been hypnotized.

In hypnotherapy, a therapist who has been trained in techniques of trance formation guides the relaxation process. The therapist asks certain questions of the patient or uses guided imagery to help the patient picture the situation in an effort to find the cause of the problem. At the end of the session, the therapist leaves some helpful hints, called *posthypnotic suggestions*, for the patient. These typically include positive, affirming statements for the patient to think about as well as instructions to help the person accomplish self-hypnosis.

Milton H. Erickson (1901–1980) was one of the best-known figures in the development of hypnosis for modern therapeutic purposes. As a child, Erickson had polio, which left him partially paralyzed. He had little strength in his arms and upper body and used a wheelchair. In addition, he had dyslexia, tone deafness, color blindness, and heart problems. Left alone during long periods of illness, Erickson became a master of observation and learned that subtle changes in facial expression, skin color, nuance of voice, and physical posture could tell him much about a person's inner state.

Erickson structured his therapeutic approach to patients in a new way. Just as he refused to allow his own disabilities to prevent him from living life to its fullest, he refused to let old problems get in the way of his patients' enjoyment of living. Erickson ignored patients' histories, preferring instead to focus on their present and future outcomes. In one classic case, Erickson gave the task of tending violets to a woman with depression. Through this and other therapeutic suggestions, she was kept too busy and involved in her community to remain depressed.

Traditional hypnotherapy and psychotherapy centered on diagnosing problems and treating symptoms. In contrast, Erickson promoted well-being, and his methods have challenged a new generation of hypnotherapists to do the same. John Grinder and Richard Bandler, who developed the field of neurolinguistic programming (NLP), based their work in large part upon their study of the extraordinary sensory acuity of Milton Erickson.

Neurolinguistic Programming

Investigating the techniques and methods of many successful therapists, Bandler and Grinder searched for ways to make psychotherapy more consistently effective. It was through these explorations that they realized language cues could be used to understand how an individual experiences their world. Using these cues, a practitioner can help patients change their experiences and respond to problems in a different way. Unlike traditional hypnosis, NLP does not use lengthy trance sessions but instead requires patients to take an active part in their treatment. When Grinder and Bandler began developing NLP, they based this extraordinary new type of therapy on a basic set of ideas, or **presuppositions**.

Presuppositions are the assumptions people make when forming communication. These assumptions are most often not spoken or written but understood within the context of what is being communicated. For example, if someone states, "I am so happy today!" the presupposition, or unspoken assumption, is that the speaker is not normally happy. People's daily communications are filled with such assumptions, things that they take for granted. NLP differs from other therapies in that there is no presupposition that the patient is somehow "broken" and requires "fixing." Instead, practitioners are taught that patients are whole individuals who already possess the internal resources they need to recover from their illness. All that is required is to direct the patient to those resources and enable their use.

Another key aspect of NLP is understanding how patients receive information about their world. People observe their world through distinct channels of experience, tending to prefer one channel over another, but eventually using them all for important cues and sensory information about their environment and other people.

PRIMARY SENSORY REPRESENTATION

The three primary methods of sensory representation are the visual, auditory, and kinesthetic channels (seeing, hearing, and touching). Of course, people also use taste and smell to gather information, but these paths are rarely the most important channels, and they are generally ignored.

Paying attention to speech patterns gives the practitioner a starting point for meaningful communication with the patient. The most obvious way to do this is to listen to the predicates, the language patterns, a person uses while describing thoughts and ideas. The practitioner can then establish positive **rapport** by using the same language patterns to create a starting point for meaningful communication. Recognizing these patterns can help improve communication with patients. Table 9.2 illustrates types of word patterns, or predicates, people use.

Of course, just about everyone uses all three learning styles (forms of predicates) at one time or another. The most important thing to remember is to match the dominant, or most used, form. In the following examples, the words in italics show how the nurse's sensory language reflects the sensory language used by the patient.

Table 9.2

Learning Style Predicates

Visual (Seeing)	Auditory (Hearing)	Kinesthetic (Touch)
An eyeful	Clear as a bell	All washed up
Appears to me	Clearly expressed	Boils down to
Beyond the shadow of a doubt	Call on	Chip off the old block
Bird's-eye view	Describe in detail	Come to grips with
Catch a glimpse of	Earful	Control yourself
Clear cut	Express yourself	Cool, calm, collected
Dim view	Give an account of	Firm foundations
Eye to eye	Give me your ear	Get a handle on
Get a perspective on	Grant an audience	Get in touch with
Scope out	Heard voices	Hand in hand
Hazy idea	Hidden message	Hang in there
Horse of a different color	Hold your tongue	Hold on
In light of	Idle talk	Hold it
In view of	Inquire into	Keep your shirt on
Make a scene	Keynote speaker	Know how
Mental image	Loud and clear	Lightheaded
Mind's eye	Manner of speaking	Moment of panic
Naked eye	Pay attention to	Pain in the neck
Paint a picture	Power of speech	Pull some strings
Memory	Outspoken	Sharp as a tack
Plainly seen	Rings a bell	Slipped my mind
Pretty as a picture	To tell the truth	Start from scratch
Sight for sore eyes	To announce displeasure	Underhanded

Examples

(VISUAL) *Mary:* "I can't picture myself getting any better."

Nurse: "In *light* of your progress, *see* yourself going back to school. How does that *look* to you?"

(AUDITORY) *James:* "I've *heard* that the doctor is *tuned in* to the newest treatments."

Nurse: "He can *describe* those in detail to you. I'll *tell* him you want to *hear* about them."

(KINESTHETIC) *Diane:* "I couldn't *come to grips* with the situation. I was *under too much pressure* all the time."

Nurse: "It is hard to get in *touch* with what's important when you *feel* that way."

These exchanges demonstrate communication on more than one level. By using the same language patterns used by the patient, health-care providers can establish that they are listening closely to the message that is being sent. NLP is a powerful tool in creating and maintaining rapport, the foundation of a therapeutic relationship.

Clinical Activity

Interact with a patient to determine their primary method of sensory representation—sight, hearing, or touch. Afterward, communicate with the patient using their preferred language patterns. In postconference, share with fellow students if using the patient's preferred language patterns enhanced your rapport with the patient.

SUMMARY

Nursing practice is evolving and is incorporating complementary and alternative therapies into conventional care-delivery systems. State boards of nursing determine at what level and scope of practice nurses can and should provide alternative therapy.

Tool Box

In 2003, the Minnesota Board of Nursing adopted guidelines for the appropriate use of complementary therapy in Minnesota, which they reaffirmed in 2010.

https://mn.gov/boards/nursing/practice/
nursing-practice-topics/integrative-therapies.jsp

Safe and Effective Nursing Care

Identify evidence-based findings for CAM treatments in journals.

Identify during initial interview with patient the use of CAM modalities.

Ensure safety when combining complementary treatments and prescriptions ordered by the health-care provider.

Acknowledge the patient's cultural and spiritual beliefs.

Key Points

- Alternative and complementary treatments provide options for patients other than those offered by conventional (Western) medicine. Alternative modalities are used instead of and complementary treatments are used in addition to conventional practices.
- The mind-body connection is an important concept in all types of medical treatment. Disease and wellness affect the whole person. Holistic treatments address both the illness and the person.
- An individual has beliefs based upon their model of the world. Nurses must respect these beliefs. However, health-care providers must be aware of

any safety issue related to these beliefs, which may harm the patient or put others in harm's way.

- Anxiety is common to disorders relating to mental illness. Prolonged stress and anxiety lead to physical as well as mental and emotional afflictions.
- Biofeedback is a technique that teaches the patient to recognize and control stress responses in the body. It is widely accepted because of its use of scientific measuring devices to demonstrate the effectiveness of the treatment.

- Aromatherapy uses a person's emotional response to smell as well as the pharmacological effects of various fragrant botanical and other substances to treat illness.
- Herbal and dietary supplements are becoming more prevalent as the public embraces "natural" healing. Many modern medications have evolved from botanical products. Relative safety and effectiveness of herbal preparations are still in question, as the industry is largely unregulated, with no set standards for these products.

- Other types of alternative and complementary therapy focus on manipulation, strengthening, and removing blockage from the free flow of energy in the human body. Massage and therapeutic touch modalities can be both stand-alone and adjunctive treatment for disease.
- Hypnotherapy and NLP are two prominent modalities that address mental and bodily illness by empowering change in the patient's thought patterns. Both tightly focus on communication patterns and the patient-therapist relationship.

Review Questions

1. Alternative therapy modalities are used:
   a. Infrequently, as they have no value to patients today
   b. In combination with conventional therapies
   c. In place of conventional therapies
   d. Only when there is no hope for recovery

2. A treatment modality used with conventional medical therapies is:
   a. A medical approach
   b. An alternative approach
   c. A holistic approach
   d. A complementary approach

3. When traditional medicine is combined with less traditional methods, it is called:
   a. Integrative medicine
   b. Alternative medicine
   c. Hypnotherapy
   d. Biofeedback

4. The mechanism that describes thoughts and expectations affecting health is:
   a. A complementary therapy
   b. A misconception that is dangerous to the patient
   c. An integrated therapy
   d. The mind-body connection

5. Mrs. Lucas is telling you about her ideas for curing her depression by taking an herbal medication. She is convinced that because St. John's wort is a natural product, it is better for her than her prescription therapy. You should:
   a. Quickly get the drug handbook and show her she is wrong.
   b. Remain open and supportive.
   c. Point out to her that herbal therapy is contraindicated.
   d. Suggest some available brands for her to use.

6. Of the following, which are either complementary or alternative modalities? (Select all that apply.)
   a. Electroconvulsive therapy (ECT)
   b. Hypnotherapy
   c. Psychotherapy
   d. Aromatherapy
   e. Reiki
   f. Massage

7. Mr. Douglas wants to know more about massage therapy. Which one of the following is *not* a massage modality?
   a. Reiki
   b. Trigger point
   c. Rolfing
   d. Swedish

8. Which of the following statements about trances is *false*?
   a. They are an altered state of consciousness, just like sleep.
   b. Humans move in and out of trance states during the day.
   c. They are a state of relaxed awareness.
   d. Trance is a common experience, even if you are not aware of it.

9. Which of the following statements indicates a visual channel preference for information?
   a. "That really feels good! My gut feeling is that it will work!"
   b. "It sounds good to me; this idea is worth paying attention to."
   c. "I can see the solution, and clearly it will work."
   d. "I smell a rat. I think the whole thing stinks."

10. Which of the following should be *avoided* when communicating with a mentally ill patient?
    a. Having an expectation that the patient will get better
    b. Making the presupposition that the patient will not improve
    c. Taking the time to convey respect for the patient
    d. Demonstrating through your expression and posture that you are listening

REVIEW QUESTIONS ANSWER KEY 1.c, 2.d, 3.a, 4.d, 5.b, 6.d, e, f, 7.a, 8.a, 9.c, 10.b

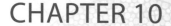

CHAPTER 10
Anxiety, Somatic Symptom Disorders, and Post-Traumatic Stress Disorder

KEY TERMS

Agoraphobia
Amygdala
Anxiety
Conversion
Free-floating anxiety
Generalized anxiety disorder
Hypochondriasis
La belle indifférence
Malingering
Panic disorder
Post-traumatic stress disorder
Primary gain
Secondary gain
Signal anxiety
Somatic symptom disorder
Somatization
Somatoform disorder
Specific phobia
Stressor
Survivor guilt

CHAPTER CONCEPTS

Cognition
Health promotion
Mobility
Mood and affect
Safety
Trauma

LEARNING OUTCOMES

1. Define anxiety disorders.
2. Describe the causes of anxiety and stress.
3. Identify the classifications of anxiety disorders.
4. List some of the differential diagnoses for anxiety.
5. State physical and behavioral symptoms of anxiety disorders.
6. Identify treatment modalities for anxiety disorders.
7. List several nursing interventions for anxiety disorders.
8. Define the difference in diagnosing somatic symptom disorder (SSD) and diagnosing somatic symptoms.
9. Identify medical treatments for people with somatic symptoms and related disorders.
10. Identify nursing interventions for people with somatic symptoms and related disorders.
11. Identify medical treatments for a person with post-traumatic stress disorder (PTSD).
12. Identify nursing interventions for patient with PTSD.

ANXIETY DISORDERS

Anxiety can be defined as an uncomfortable feeling of dread that is a response to extreme or prolonged periods of stress. According to Gorman and Sultan (2008), anxiety is an unpleasant feeling of tension, apprehension, and uneasiness or a diffuse feeling of dread or unexplained discomfort. A person's level of anxiety needs to be assessed in order to treat it effectively.

The four commonly accepted levels of anxiety are:
Mild

• anxiety that is a normal part of one's everyday life.
• person is usually aware of what is creating the anxiety.
• person displays some mild noticeable behavior.

Moderate

- displays noticeable behavior
- has difficulty remaining focused
- displays nervous habits; nail biting
- has increased heart rate

Severe

- episodes of nausea
- chest discomfort
- difficulty following directions

Panic

- unable to problem solve
- has distorted perceptions
- has impaired rational thinking

Hildegard Peplau taught that a mild amount of anxiety is a normal part of being human and that it is necessary for people to develop ways of coping with stress (FIG. 10.1).

The experience of anxiety may also be influenced by one's culture. It may be acceptable for some people to acknowledge and discuss stress. Others may believe that one should keep personal problems to oneself. This can be a challenge to the nurse during an assessment.

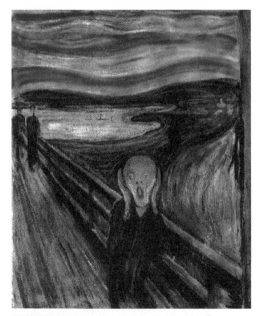

FIGURE 10.1 Anxiety ranges in severity from mild through panic. *The Scream*, a famous painting by Norwegian artist Edvard Munch, depicts a person in a very high state of anxiety.

Anxiety is usually referred to in one of two ways: **free-floating anxiety** or **signal anxiety**. Free-floating anxiety is described as a feeling of impending doom. The person might say something like "I just know something bad is going to happen if I go on vacation" without knowing what the dreaded event is or when or where it might occur. Signal anxiety, on the other hand, is an uncomfortable response to a known **stressor** (e.g., "Finals are only a week away, and I know I am going to fail even if I study, because studying doesn't work"). Both types of anxiety are involved in the various anxiety disorders.

Nurses working with children and adolescents must be aware that young people also experience anxiety and stress. They may not be able to or may not want to verbalize their feelings, and they may display symptoms differently than adults do. Some indicators of stress and anxiety in these age groups include decline in school performance, changes in eating habits or sleeping patterns, and withdrawal from friends and usual activities. Nurses can be instrumental in screening children and adolescents for signs of anxiety.

According to the *Diagnostic and Statistical Manual,* 5th edition-*TR* (2013), anxiety disorders include the following: generalized anxiety disorder, separation anxiety, specific phobias, panic disorders, and agoraphobia.

ETIOLOGY AND SYMPTOMS OF ANXIETY

According to Freud's psychoanalytic theory, anxiety is caused by conflict between the id and the superego, or the unorganized and the organized parts of the personality. At some time in the individual's development, this conflict was repressed, but it emerges again in adulthood. When conflict emerges, patients realize they have "failed," and the manifestations of anxiety are felt once again. Sukel (2018) notes that the amygdala plays a part in anxiety. The **amygdala** may be involved when a person experiences the "fight or flight" response. The amygdala does play a role in memory and thus how fear is processed. Once fear has been triggered, the amygdala then places it into a person's memory.

Symptoms of anxiety:

- muscle aches
- shaking or tremors

- palpitations
- dry mouth
- nausea
- vomiting
- diarrhea
- hot flashes
- chills
- polyuria
- insomnia
- difficulty swallowing

Tool Box

State-Trait Anxiety Inventory (STAI) is a tool used to determine a patient's anxiety level and to evaluate the stress level of the caregiver. https://www.apa.org/pi/about/publications/caregivers/practice-settings/assessment/tools/trait-state

DIFFERENTIAL DIAGNOSES

Differentiating normal anxiety from an anxiety disorder can be challenging. Because so many symptoms are associated with anxiety disorders (see the section Types of Anxiety and Anxiety-Related Disorders in this chapter), it is important for patients to have a complete physical and mental status examination on admission before diagnosis can be made. Symptoms of anxiety disorders can mimic those seen in patients with diabetes, cardiac problems, endocrine disorders, medication side effects, and electrolyte imbalances, and also in patients with a history of alcoholism or physical trauma. For example, in one analysis, Siegmann et al. (2018) reviewed studies of 44,388 participants with autoimmune thyroiditis. Of these patients, 34,094 experienced depression and 43,382 experienced anxiety. The health-care provider must rule out systemic infection or an allergy that might be related to chills or swallowing difficulty. Hot flashes, which can occur in some anxiety states, could be related to a fever or to menopause. The health-care provider must always consider the possibility of drug or alcohol abuse as partial causes for the symptoms. Certainly, more than one condition can occur simultaneously. A psychiatric evaluation is often needed to confirm a diagnosis of an anxiety disorder.

Diagnostic Studies

Several diagnostic studies may be ordered on admission into a facility or as an outpatient to determine whether a medical condition is related to the patient's anxiety. The initial patient work-up may include an electrocardiogram (ECG), complete blood count (CBC), electrolyte study, and a thyroid-function test.

Treatments

Anxiety can be treated by combining psychotropic and psychotherapy treatments. It is important that the anxiety-related disorder be diagnosed correctly to provide the best therapies. Drug therapies for anxiety are listed in Chapter 8 (Box 8.3, Commonly Used Antianxiety Agents). Among the psychotherapies, behavioral therapy and cognitive behavioral therapy (CBT) have provided positive outcomes for anxiety.

TYPES OF ANXIETY AND ANXIETY-RELATED DISORDERS

Generalized Anxiety Disorder (GAD)

In **generalized anxiety disorder** (GAD), the anxiety itself (also referred to as *excessive or persistent worry* or *severe stress*) is the expressed symptom. GAD is diagnosed when excessive worry is related to three or more of the six symptoms listed and lasts 6 months or longer:

- restlessness
- fatigue
- difficulty focusing or not being able to think momentarily
- irritability
- tensed muscles
- sleep difficulties (e.g., not sleeping continuously though the night, restlessness, difficulty falling asleep)

These symptoms become pervasive and debilitating, as they affect all aspects of a person's life. These symptoms are more common in people in their 30s and occur more frequently in females. Patients with GAD experience worry daily.

GOOD TO KNOW
GAD can be paralyzing and can affect all areas of a person's life.

Etiology
According to Munir and Takov (2020), causes of GAD can include genetics, environmental factors, and drug abuse. They also indicate that there is some evidence that neurotransmitters (low serotonin and raised noradrenergic system) play a part in a person's response to stress.

Differential Diagnoses
Before diagnosing GAD, it is important to rule out other conditions that mimic GAD. DSM-5 (American Psychiatric Association, 2013) suggests the following conditions be ruled out:

- other medical illnesses that create anxiety
- medications or substance abuse
- obsessive-compulsive disorder (see OCD in Chapter 14)
- post-traumatic stress disorder
- psychotic disorders

Treatment
Treatment that can assist in managing GAD episodes includes pharmacotherapy (see Pharmacology Corner) and cognitive behavior therapy (CBT).

Panic Disorder
Panic disorder, a recurrent condition, is an abrupt surge of extreme fear or discomfort that cannot be controlled and that reaches a peak in a short period of time. This disorder can lead to intense fear and worry about it happening again. Panic disorder is also referred to as panic attack, and people may not consider it to be a serious disorder initially. In the past, panic disorder was linked to agoraphobia; however, the DSM-5-TR

distinguishes between panic disorder (recurrent panic attacks) and panic attack. The DSM-5 identifies the following 13 symptoms, of which 4 or more need to be present for a diagnosis of panic disorder:

- fear of being out of control or going crazy
- fear of dying as the 13th
- dissociation (a feeling that events are happening to someone else or not happening at all) or out-of-body experience
- nausea or gastrointestinal upset
- a feeling of choking (being unable to speak or swallow)
- diaphoresis
- chest pain
- palpitations, increase in heart rate
- chills or feeling flushed
- numbness or tingling
- shaking or tremors
- unsteadiness or feeling faint
- a feeling of being suffocated or unable to catch one's breath

GOOD TO KNOW
Panic symptoms develop suddenly and unexpectedly in the susceptible person. Because of this, people with a history of panic disorder need to be prepared to identify early signs in the hope that they can gain some control before the symptoms are out of control.

Etiology
Burke (2018) identifies three sources of panic disorder: genetics, dramatic changes in lifestyle (e.g. retirement), and major life transitions (e.g. COVID-19).

Differential Diagnoses
- medication reaction
- other related anxiety disorders
- use of central nervous system (CNS) stimulants
- medical conditions (hyperthyroidism, seizure disorders, asthma, pulmonary and cardiac disorders)

Diagnostic Tests
In order to treat the panic disorder, the health-care provider may need to order diagnostic tests such as ECG, pulse oximetry, a thyroid-stimulating test, and cardiac monitoring to rule out any medical condition.

Specific Phobia

This is the most common of the anxiety disorders. Phobia can be defined as an "irrational fear." The person is very aware of the fear and even of the fact that it is irrational, but the fear continues. In specific phobias these feelings of fear are extreme. People develop specific phobias to many different things—approximately 700 different things, in fact (Box 10.1). Snakes, spiders, enclosed spaces, and the number 13 are some of the more common phobias (FIG. 10.2). People also develop phobias of things such as caring for their children (because they fear they might hurt them) and eating in places other than their own home. The mere thought of confronting these fears can produce anxiety.

The psychoanalytic view of phobias is that the fear is not necessarily of the object itself, but rather that an unconscious fear has been displaced onto the object or event, such as snakes or heights. Learning theory views phobias as learned responses. When the person avoids the phobic object, they avoid the fear, and that is a powerful reward. Most phobias start in childhood, sometimes related to a traumatic event, but people can also develop them later in life. In older people, fear of falling or choking is common. It is common for more than one phobia to develop in a person.

The DSM-5 identifies three main types of phobias: agoraphobia, social phobia, and specific phobias.

Agoraphobia has been removed from specific phobias and has its own diagnostic criteria. **Agoraphobia** is the irrational fear of being in open spaces and being unable to leave or being very embarrassed if leaving is required. For a diagnosis of agoraphobia, the patient must present with

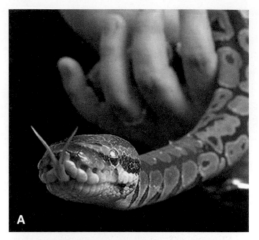

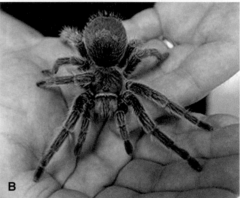

FIGURE 10.2 A, Fear of snakes (ophidiophobia) and B, fear of spiders (arachnophobia) are two of the most common phobias *(courtesy of the University of Texas Libraries, The University of Texas at Austin).*

fear of a minimum of two of the following five situations:

- using any public transportation vehicle (e.g., buses, trains, planes)
- being in open spaces
- being in walled or sealed off spaces
- standing in a crowd
- being outside alone

Example
- *People who fear shopping in large malls or going to sporting events may actually fear the possibility of being unable to leave when they wish to.*

Social phobia is another phobia, which has its own set of diagnostic criteria. Social phobias are also known as social anxiety disorder. People with these phobias avoid social situations because of fear of humiliation or being judged negatively. This reaction is out of proportion to the situation. People

---

Box 10.1

Some Common Specific Phobias

Acrophobia: fear of heights
Ailurophobia: fear of cats
Carcinomatophobia: fear of cancer
Decidophobia: fear of making decisions
Nyctophobia: fear of darkness
Odontophobia: fear of teeth or dental surgery
Scoleciphobia: fear of worms
Thanatophobia: fear of death

Source: Adapted from Townsend (2017). *Essentials of Psychiatric Mental Health Nursing,* 7th ed. Philadelphia: F.A. Davis Company, with permission.

with this type of phobia may self-medicate with alcohol and/or drugs.

Social phobia diagnostic criteria are as follows:

- displaying notable anxiety and fear in a social situation
- avoiding social circumstances
- avoiding any circumstances that will provoke any fear or anxiety
- avoiding any encounters that will subject the person to humiliation

Example
- *The fear of speaking in public and the fear of using public restroom facilities are two examples of social phobias.*

Specific phobias are related to specific situations or entities, such as heights, animals, and blood. These are the classic phobias that most people are familiar with.

Tool Box
For a comprehensive list of phobias, go to http://phobialist.com/#A-

Clinical Activity
When your hospitalized patient has a phobia, such as agoraphobia, anticipation of the patient's reaction to leaving their room for testing must be addressed with the patient to prevent distress.

Example
- *Claustrophobia (fear of enclosed places), hematophobia (fear of blood), and acrophobia (fear of heights) are examples of specific phobias.*

MEDICAL TREATMENT OF PEOPLE WITH ANXIETY AND ANXIETY-RELATED DISORDERS

Treatment is individualized to the patient and may include one or more of the following: psychopharmacology, individual psychotherapy, CBT, group therapy, systematic desensitization, hypnosis, guided imagery, relaxation exercises, exposure therapy, and/or biofeedback.

Evidence-Based Practice
Clinical Question: Which psychotherapy effectively treats specific phobias?

Evidence: This 5-year study followed 33 adults experiencing different specific phobias. Study participants included more females than males. Several types of psychotherapy, such as exposure therapy, relaxation, applied muscle tension, and CBT, were used. Other therapies included technology-assisted therapy and pharmacotherapy. The most effective therapy for treating specific phobias was CBT.

Implications for Nursing Practice:
- Communicate with the patient about their fears and negative thoughts.
- Encourage patient to journal thoughts.
- Instruct patient in relaxation techniques.
- Encourage patient to engage in positive self-talk.

Thng, C. E. W., Poh, B. Z. Q., Lim, C. G., & Lim-Ashworth, N. S. J. (2020, March 19). Recent developments in the intervention of specific phobia among adults: A rapid review. F1000*Research*. https://www.ncbi.nlm.nih.gov/pmc/articles/PMC7096216/.

ALTERNATIVE INTERVENTIONS FOR PEOPLE WITH ANXIETY AND ANXIETY-RELATED DISORDERS

Aromatherapy
Essential oils such as lavender and bergamot are popular aids in relaxation. Methods of application include using diffusers (machines that turn the oil into droplets that diffuse into the air), placing a drop on a piece of clothing, or applying directly to the skin, such as the temple area. Patients can purchase these essential oils and equipment at specialty stores, some bath oil supply stores, or even in some pharmacies. There are online resources as well. Prescriptions are not needed, but patients should be cautioned to use essential oils in very small amounts (drops at a time) and to observe for allergic responses, especially if the oils are applied directly to the skin.

Biofeedback
Biofeedback, a form of behavior modification, is a system of progressive relaxation. There are many products on the market to assist patients in this "do-it-yourself" method of relaxation. Biofeedback done effectively alters the brain to a slower wave

Pharmacology Corner

Medications can be used effectively to control anxiety disorder, including GAD, panic disorders, and specific phobias. The most common are antianxiety medications, such as benzodiazepines, which are effective in most cases. See Table 10.1 for a list of common antianxiety medications. Use of antianxiety drugs is short-term whenever possible because of the strong potential for dependency. Individuals with anxiety disorders who are also chemically dependent are managed with other medications having calming qualities but not the same high potential for addiction as the antianxiety drugs. Hydroxyzine hydrochloride (Atarax) and clonidine (Catapres) are examples.

The antidepressant class of selective serotonin reuptake inhibitors (SSRIs) is used as primary treatment in many cases of GAD, panic disorders, social phobias, and PTSD. Sometimes higher doses of the drugs than are used with depression are needed, so close monitoring of side effects is important. Panic disorders have been successfully treated with paroxetine, fluoxetine (Prozac), and sertraline. Dosing increases must be done slowly, as these patients are especially sensitive to overstimulation from these medications. Research is underway to identify more effective medications for these conditions.

Psychotherapy includes individual treatment as well as group therapy and may include systematic desensitization. This technique causes the patient to experience the anxiety-producing situation in a controlled environment and helps them integrate the painful feelings associated with the anxiety. Patients concentrate on esteem needs and reality.

---

frequency and can actually increase the immune response for humans. The patient should discuss with the doctor if biofeedback is appropriate. The nurse may assist with providing information and resources.

Hypnotherapy

Hypnosis, done by a qualified, licensed therapist, may be helpful. It will assist the patient in relaxation. Some people joke about "going to their happy place," but there is validity in finding pleasure in a light-hearted memory. Patients need to continue to do the relaxation as directed by the therapist. Hypnosis is not a "one-time" therapy. It, like biofeedback, needs to be practiced routinely to be effective. The nurse's role may be as simple as reminding the patient to find quiet time for this. If the patient is being seen as an outpatient, the nurse may ask the patient how frequently they have been able to do the self-hypnosis and what kind of results the patient has experienced thus far.

Additional Alternative Interventions

The following may provide additional relief:

- stress-reduction and relaxation techniques
- yoga
- acupuncture
- kava (an herbal supplement)

NURSING CARE FOR PEOPLE WITH ANXIETY AND ANXIETY-RELATED DISORDERS

Common nursing diagnoses for people with anxiety and anxiety-related disorders are as follows:

- anxiety, coping, ineffective
- fear
- thought process, disturbance
- violence, risk for
- knowledge deficit related to disorder

General Interventions

1. *Maintain a calm milieu:* Patients who have anxiety disorders need to have a calm, safe treatment

Table 10.1

Commonly Used Antianxiety Medications

Alprazolam (Xanax)
Buspirone (BuSpar)
Chlordiazepoxide (Librium)
Clonazepam (Klonopin)
Clonidine (Catapres)
Diazepam (Valium)
Hydroxyzine (Atarax)
Lorazepam (Ativan)
Oxazepam (Serax)

area. Minimizing the stimuli helps the patient to keep centered and focused.

2. *Maintain open communication:* Encourage the patient to verbalize all thoughts and feelings. Honesty in dealing with patients helps them learn to trust others and increases their self-esteem. Patients will feel the value that nurses place on the relationship. Observe the patient's nonverbal communication. As previously stated, affect and body language often reveal more about a patient's thoughts and feelings than the words that are spoken.

3. *Observe for signs of suicidal thoughts:* Patients with anxiety disorders, as well as those with PTSD, are at risk for suicide as a result of feelings of low self-esteem or decreased self-worth. Nurses must be alert to this possibility and should observe and confront the patient and document any suspicions the nurse has or any statements the patient expresses.

4. *Document any changes in behavior:* Any change, no matter how small, can be significant to the patient's care. Positive or negative alterations in

the way a patient responds to the nurse, to the treatment plan, or to other people and situations should be documented. The data collected and documented will allow the nurse to provide accurate feedback.

5. *Encourage activities:* Activities that are enjoyable and not stressful can help the patient in several ways. Activities provide a diversion, giving the patient time to concentrate on something other than the anxiety-producing situation and an opportunity to provide positive feedback to the patient about the progress they are making. These activities should be purposeful, not just "busy work." The patient should not be put in competitive situations. Competition could increase anxiety and be counterproductive to treatment.

Table 10.2 summarizes the types of anxiety and anxiety-related disorders, the general symptoms, and common nursing actions for them. Table 10.3 outlines a nursing care plan for a patient with anxiety. See also Figure 10.3, a concept map for panic disorder and GAD.

Table 10.2
Nursing Care for Patients With Anxiety and Related Disorders

Disorders	Symptoms	Nursing Actions
Generalized anxiety disorder	Muscle aches, shakes, palpitations, dry mouth, nausea, chills, vomiting, hot flashes, polyuria, difficulty swallowing, feeling of dread	• Provide calm milieu. • Communicate calmly and clearly. • Focus on brief messages. • Teach early signs of escalating anxiety. • Implement suicide precautions if the person indicates any self-destructive thoughts. • Document behavior changes. • Encourage activities. • Promote deep breathing and other relaxation methods. • Offer reassurance.
Panic disorder	Fear, dissociation, nausea, diaphoresis, chest pain, increased pulse, shaking, unsteadiness, paralysis	Same as above • Stay with patient during attack.
Specific phobia	Irrational fear of a particular object or situation	Same as above • Focus on nonthreatening topics. • Reassure patient about their safety.

Continued

Table 10.2

Nursing Care for Patients With Anxiety and Related Disorders—cont'd

Disorders	Symptoms	Nursing Actions
Post-traumatic stress disorder	Flashbacks, social withdrawal, low self-esteem, change in relationships or difficulty forming relationships, irritability, anger seemingly for no reason, depression, chemical dependency	Same as above • Keep patient oriented to the present. • Encourage patient and significant others to attend groups for patients with PTSD. • Encourage patient to talk about traumatic events if he or she is able.

Table 10.3

Nursing Care Plan for Patient With Anxiety

Assessment/Data Collection	Nursing Diagnosis	Plan/Goal	Interventions/ Nursing Actions	Evaluation
Patient is: • restless • irritable • pacing • hyperventilating • verbalizing negative thoughts and expecting a calamity	Anxiety	Demonstrate a sense of increased comfort	• Provide a calm environment. • Promote relaxation techniques including deep breaths. • Play soothing music. • Verbalize reassurance about current situation resolving.	Patient appears more relaxed and verbalizes more positive outcomes.

SOMATIC SYMPTOM AND RELATED DISORDERS

Somatic Symptom Disorder (SSD)

Somatic refers to the body. **Somatic symptom disorder** (SSD) is characterized by bodily symptoms that are either very distressing or that result in significant disruption of functioning and are accompanied by excessive and disproportionate thoughts, feelings, and behaviors regarding those symptoms. To be diagnosed with SSD, an individual must be persistently symptomatic (typically for at least 6 months). SSD is both a category of disorders in the DSM-5 as well as a specific diagnosis.

The term **somatoform disorders** is no longer used and was associated with physical symptoms having no organic cause. This condition may be present in SSD, but it is not required. A prominent feature of SSD is excessive focus on one's physical symptoms that interferes with daily functioning. These symptoms may or may not be associated with an actual medical condition. For example, a patient with a small sore seeks multiple opinions out of fear of skin cancer. Despite negative biopsies, the patient keeps checking the sore, talking about it, and seeking other possible providers who might offer other tests despite great financial burden. In SSD, high levels of worry about one's health become the central focus in the person's life, even to the point of becoming the person's identity. These patients, heavy users of the health-care system, often seek out different specialists and testing. As a result, nurses typically encounter these patients

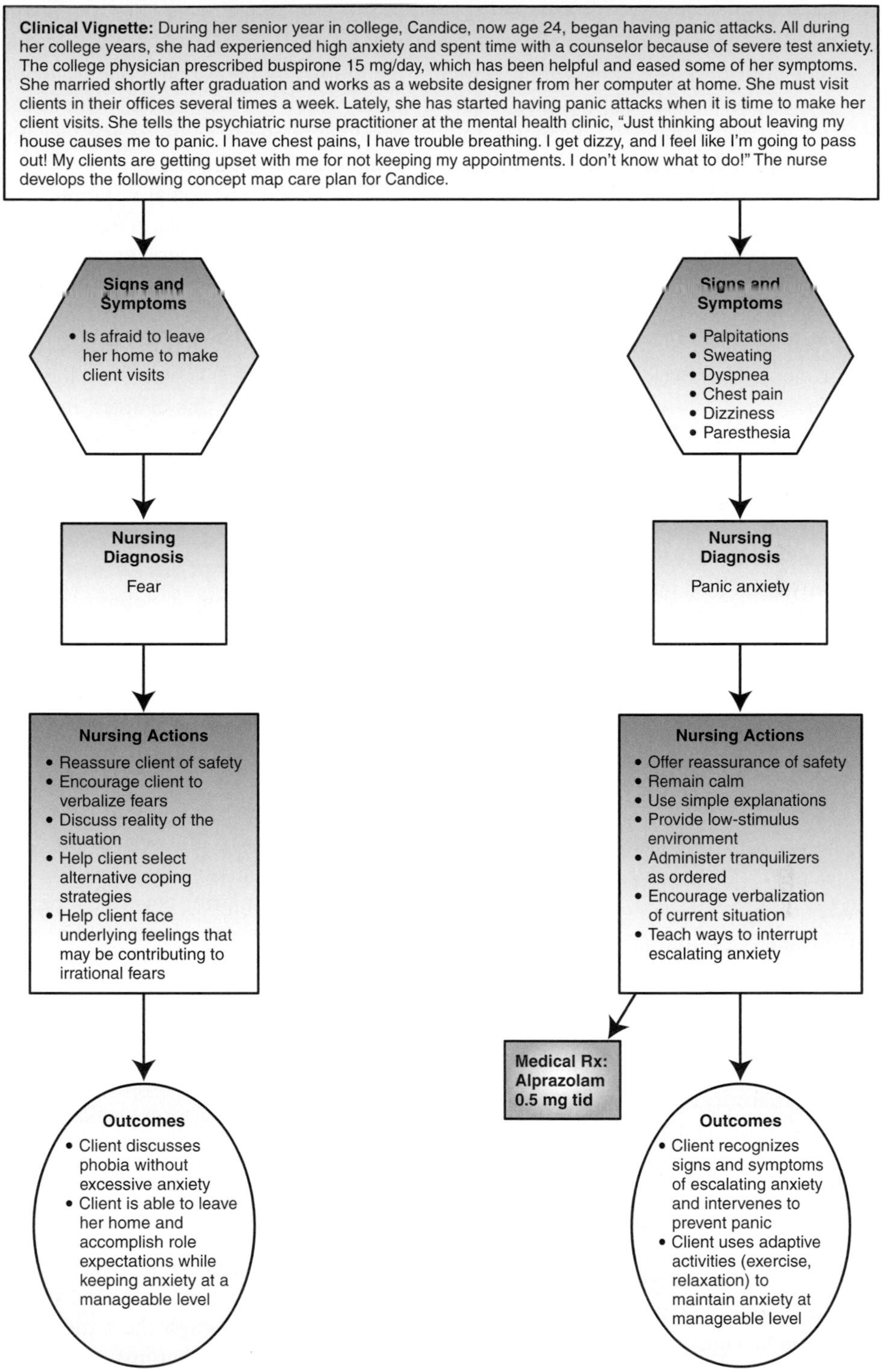

Clinical Vignette: During her senior year in college, Candice, now age 24, began having panic attacks. All during her college years, she had experienced high anxiety and spent time with a counselor because of severe test anxiety. The college physician prescribed buspirone 15 mg/day, which has been helpful and eased some of her symptoms. She married shortly after graduation and works as a website designer from her computer at home. She must visit clients in their offices several times a week. Lately, she has started having panic attacks when it is time to make her client visits. She tells the psychiatric nurse practitioner at the mental health clinic, "Just thinking about leaving my house causes me to panic. I have chest pains, I have trouble breathing. I get dizzy, and I feel like I'm going to pass out! My clients are getting upset with me for not keeping my appointments. I don't know what to do!" The nurse develops the following concept map care plan for Candice.

Signs and Symptoms

- Is afraid to leave her home to make client visits

Signs and Symptoms

- Palpitations
- Sweating
- Dyspnea
- Chest pain
- Dizziness
- Paresthesia

Nursing Diagnosis

Fear

Nursing Diagnosis

Panic anxiety

Nursing Actions

- Reassure client of safety
- Encourage client to verbalize fears
- Discuss reality of the situation
- Help client select alternative coping strategies
- Help client face underlying feelings that may be contributing to irrational fears

Nursing Actions

- Offer reassurance of safety
- Remain calm
- Use simple explanations
- Provide low-stimulus environment
- Administer tranquilizers as ordered
- Encourage verbalization of current situation
- Teach ways to interrupt escalating anxiety

Medical Rx: Alprazolam 0.5 mg tid

Outcomes

- Client discusses phobia without excessive anxiety
- Client is able to leave her home and accomplish role expectations while keeping anxiety at a manageable level

Outcomes

- Client recognizes signs and symptoms of escalating anxiety and intervenes to prevent panic
- Client uses adaptive activities (exercise, relaxation) to maintain anxiety at manageable level

FIGURE 10.3 Concept map care plan for client with somatic disorder *(from Townsend [2017]. Essentials of Psychiatric Mental Health Nursing, 7th ed. Philadelphia: F.A. Davis Company, with permission).*

in a nonpsychiatric setting. Anxiety is definitely a component of this disorder, as the individual worries excessively. Although distress is normal with a new symptom, exaggerated responses before a diagnosis would be a factor in considering SSD diagnosis. In the past, the term **hypochondriasis** might have been used to describe someone with SSD. A patient who focuses extensively on physical symptoms is sometimes referred to as suffering from **somatization** or somatizing. Although the patient on a mental health unit expresses discomfort such as chest pain or difficulty breathing, you will need to assess this patient as if they were on a medical-surgical floor.

Etiology of Somatic Symptom Disorder

Biologically, research has looked for a genetic or biological predisposition to somatic difficulties. For example, some individuals may have increased sensitivity to pain. Early childhood traumatic experiences are also associated with SSD. Psychological theories include physical symptoms rooted in unconscious mechanisms that develop to deny, repress, or displace anxiety.

Cultural Considerations

How an individual experiences a bodily sensation can be linked to their cultural perspective. Some symptoms may be more or less acceptable to acknowledge in different cultures.

Differential Diagnoses

People with somatic disorders present many challenges to obtaining an accurate diagnosis. You must be alert to any physical illness that may actually be causing the symptoms. Multiple sclerosis, for example, can present with many and varied symptoms. Discuss with the patient's health-care provider all possibilities for physical illness. These patients can end up being subjected to many tests, procedures, and even surgeries with no improvement in symptoms. However, it is important to avoid labeling a person with SSD just because a physical basis for symptoms has not been found yet.

For a diagnosis of SSD, the following criteria must be present:

• More than one somatic symptom that is related to a substantial disruption in activities of daily living.

• Extreme thoughts, behaviors, and feelings related to the somatic complaint producing at least one of the following: persistent thoughts about the symptoms, which are inconsistent with its seriousness; being overly anxious; and focusing on these symptoms for long periods.

• "Although any one somatic symptom may not be continuously present, the state of being symptomatic is persistent" (American Psychiatric Association, 2013, p. 311) for at least 6 months.

Somatic Symptom Related Disorders

In addition to SSD, several somatic-related disorders are covered in this chapter, including conversion disorder, illness anxiety disorder, and factitious disorder.

Conversion Disorder (Functional Neurological Symptom Disorder)

Conversion reaction, a defense mechanism (see Chapter 7), is converting anxiety into a physical symptom. Conversion disorder is the illness that emerges from overuse of this mechanism. In conversion disorder, the patient experiences a loss or decrease in physical functioning that cannot be explained by any known medical disorder or pathophysiological mechanism. Paralysis and blindness are two examples of this disorder. It is common for the dysfunction to somehow be deeply connected to denial and to a prior negatively perceived experience (e.g., someone who loses the sense of vision after watching a pornographic movie). Age of onset is usually adolescence or young adulthood, but it can occur later in life as well. Conversion disorder is also referred to as *functional neurological symptom disorder*, which refers to the fact that persons diagnosed with this disorder will likely be seen by a neurologist.

The symptoms, although not supportive of organic disease, are very real to the patient. Do not, by word or action, imply to a patient that you think the patient is "faking" the illness; it is real to the patient. The patient is truly experiencing the symptoms. Even though the patient is concerned enough about the symptoms to consult a physician, they may give the impression of really not caring about the problem. **La belle indifférence** is the clinical term used to describe this lack of concern.

The accepted understanding of this disorder is that the symptom, such as paralysis or blindness, allows the patient to avoid a situation that is unacceptable to them. This unacceptable situation is the source of extreme anxiety, which is converted into the dysfunction. The dysfunction, then, relieves the anxiety. This is called **primary gain** and it is believed to be the function of the paralysis or blindness. **Secondary gain** is the extra benefits one may acquire because of staying ill. Secondary gain includes extra emotional support, such as sympathy and love or financial benefits. These gains occur at the unconscious level.

Malingering, the use of a nonexistent medical condition for achieving personal gain, is not an SSD. Malingering is a conscious effort to avoid unpleasant situations. The patient "fakes" or pretends to have the symptoms.

Illness Anxiety Disorder
In this disorder, somatic symptoms are not present, or if present, are only mild in intensity. The person's distress is not from the physical complaint itself but rather from their anxiety about the meaning, significance, or cause of the complaint. These patients are popularly referred to as hypochondriacs or as professional patients.

A major difference between illness anxiety disorder and conversion disorder is that the person with conversion disorder focuses on the symptoms of the illness, whereas the person with illness anxiety disorder is afraid he or she will *get* a serious disease.

CRITICAL THINKING QUESTION
Is the term *illness anxiety disorder* less socially negative than the term *hypochondriac*? Why or why not?

Factitious Disorder
Falsification of medical or psychological signs and symptoms in oneself or others is called a factitious disorder. This diagnosis requires demonstrating that the individual is taking secretive actions to misrepresent, simulate, or cause signs or symptoms of illness or injury in the absence of obvious external rewards. When the individual falsifies information for another, as in a child or pet, the diagnosis is factitious disorder imposed on another or by proxy.

CRITICAL THINKING QUESTION
Penny is a 35-year-old married mother of three children, ages 2 years, 3 years, and 4 months. She works as a clerk in a large office. She has been visiting the clinic regularly since her last pregnancy. She is experiencing severe, intermittent pain in her right arm and left foot. The pain does not interfere with her life as a wife and mother, and she is not able to detect any kind of pattern to the pain. She tells you that she is not especially concerned about the pain. "When it gets too bad for me, my husband cooks and cleans the kitchen."

Penny says that she thinks the source of her pain is related to "the day I banged my right hip real hard on the door of the copy machine." She also has begun expressing concern that things are going so well for her that she "just has the feeling that something terrible is about to happen." What is your preliminary impression of Penny's illness? What other information might you want to obtain from Penny?

Medical Treatment of Patients With Somatic Symptom and Related Disorders
Patients with these disorders are usually admitted to a medical unit rather than a psychiatric unit. Treatment focuses on the symptoms, which more than likely are medical in nature. The patient does not generally display unusual or unmanageable behavior that indicates the need for mental health unit admission.

Treatment is, of course, individualized for each patient. Once a somatic disorder is diagnosed, the ongoing involvement of a psychiatrist is helpful to give insight on managing this patient. Some approaches that may be used to treat these disorders include individual and group psychotherapy, hypnosis, and relaxation techniques. It is beneficial for the therapist to help the patient express the underlying cause of their anxiety. Hypnosis can be very effective in allowing the patient to explore such underlying issues. Behavior modification can be effective if the patient is prone to secondary gains from the somatic symptoms. Methods of stress management are also taught as the person learns new ways to handle anxiety. Patients may resist accepting that their problem has a strong psychological or emotional component and refuse to understand how a paralyzed limb or pain has anything to do with anxiety. People who have an SSD may feel insulted, become resistive to treatment, and search for other ways to explain the physical problem.

Pharmacology Corner

Medications are used sparingly with SSDs because these patients typically have a history of being overprescribed. When medications are ordered for a patient, the classifications of choice are usually selective serotonin reuptake inhibitors (SSRIs) (e.g., fluoxetine); other antidepressants, particularly the tricyclics, such as imipramine (Tofranil); antianxiety drugs; or combinations of these medications. At this time, if medications are considered, SSRIs are considered the first line of treatment, greatly preferred over the other classes of antidepressants. See Table 10.4 for medications commonly used to treat somatic symptom and related disorders.

Alternative Interventions for Patients With Somatic Symptom and Related Disorders

Alternative treatments of choice are related to the particular condition or symptom set a patient has. Choices may include the following treatments in addition to biofeedback, hypnosis, relaxation, and guided imagery.

Table 10.4

Commonly Used Medications for Somatic Symptoms and Related Disorders

Medications are ordered judiciously for these disorders. When a medication is used, it is generally an antidepressant or an antianxiety agent.
Amitriptyline (Elavil)
Bupropion (Wellbutrin)
Doxepin (Sinequan)
Fluoxetine (Prozac)
Paroxetine (Paxil)
Sertraline (Zoloft)
Trazodone (Oleptro; Desyrel)

Massage

Massage therapies are believed to not only relieve tension and discomfort in the musculoskeletal system but to also assist with blood and lymph flow. Massage may be effective, especially with medication, to assist the patient to overcome physical symptoms. Caution should be used, however, not to actually emphasize the body complaint and reinforce the illness.

Herbal/Nutritional Supplements

It is possible that a patient is experiencing a nutritional deficiency or possibly a condition such as arthritis along with the SSD. Herbs or supplements geared to the specific pain issue may help the patient to experience less pain, either physically or psychologically.

Nursing Care of the Patient With Somatic Symptom and Related Disorders

Common nursing diagnoses used with somatic symptom and related disorders include the following:

• anxiety
• coping, ineffective
• sensory perception, disturbed
• thought processes, disturbed

Table 10.5 summarizes the symptoms and nursing interventions for the SSDs discussed previously. FIGURE 10.4 is a concept map of SSD.

Communication Skills

Honesty in dealing with the patient is very important. Gaining trust that will encourage the patient to verbalize thoughts and feelings about the physical and emotional aspects of this type of disorder is crucial. Do not discount the patient's disorder.

Example

Nurse: "Ms. P, your health-care provider can find no physical or life-threatening conditions to explain your symptoms at this time. We will continue to observe and examine you. We will make every attempt to help you improve."

In this way, the patient understands that nothing is showing up in the tests that have been made to this point. The person hears that nothing life-threatening is causing the symptoms. The nurse has said that the staff is attempting to help the patient but has stopped short of promising to "cure" the patient.

Table 10.5

Nursing Care for Patients With Somatic Symptoms and Related Disorders

Type	Symptoms	Nursing Interventions
Somatic symptom disorder	• high level of anxiety about health • excessive time and energy devoted to symptoms • may or may not have an organic disorder	• Listen to patient's concerns but then focus on other issues. • Promote trust. • Encourage patient to express self about issues other than the symptoms.
Conversion disorder	• loss or decrease in physical functioning that seems to have a neurological connection (paralysis, blindness) • indifference to the loss of function • primary and secondary gain	• Use therapeutic communication skills. • Encourage therapy (occupational therapy, physical therapy, etc.). • Provide emotional support. • Respond to the patient's symptoms as real.
Illness anxiety disorder	• "professional patient" • intense fear of becoming seriously ill • preoccupation with the idea of being seriously ill and not being helped—may be concerned about not being taken seriously or evaluated properly	• Do not reinforce the symptom. • Be nonjudgmental. • Continue to focus on trusting relationship.

Socialization and Group Activities

Keeping the patient focused on other topics may help in the recovery. Involve the patient in goal setting and interventions of the care plan. Aiding the patient in learning assertive communication skills can be helpful. Working with other health-care staff in occupational therapy, recreational therapy, and social activities can also act to divert the patient's focus from the dysfunction.

Support

It is important for the nurse caring for patients with SSD to remember to pay attention to the patient but not to reinforce the symptom(s). Always make a thorough head-to-toe assessment, but do not focus on the area of dysfunction or reinforce the problem. This shows the patient that you are concerned for their health. Document all findings in a matter-of-fact way. Patients need to know that they are being taken seriously, even though they may not agree with the medical findings of their illness.

Post-Traumatic Stress Disorder

Although PTSD is no longer categorized as an anxiety disorder by the DSM-5, it will be covered in this chapter.

Post-traumatic stress disorder (PTSD) is a person's response to an unexpected emotional or physical trauma that could not be controlled. A person with PTSD will probably have reoccurring, intrusive, disturbing memories of the incident that may last over a period of time. This disorder was once viewed as an anxiety problem, but the current view is that it belongs in a new category—Trauma and Stress or Related Disorders (American Psychiatric Association, 2013)—and is related to physical and emotional responses to a trauma. People suffering from PTSD often are more troubled by pervasive sadness, aggressive behaviors, and dissociative symptoms such as flashbacks than they are by anxiety symptoms. Young children can also suffer from PTSD.

People who have fought in wars, who have survived rape, who have survived violent storms or other actual or threatened traumatic events are susceptible to this disorder. Police, fire, and rescue personnel are also at risk for PTSD when they see victims of violence and destruction whom they cannot help. In the United States, the terrorist attacks on September 11, 2001, brought new attention to the condition of PTSD. Nowadays, the horror of such violence reaches anyone with a television or a smartphone and can affect a person who suffers

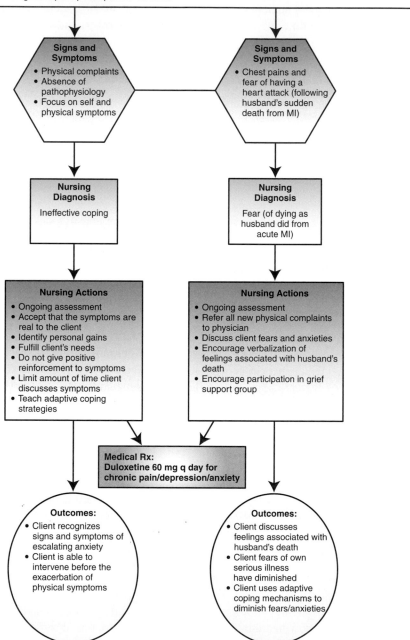

Clinical Vignette: Veronica, age 51, has a long history of "doctor shopping" for numerous complaints of gastrointestinal distress, daily headaches, and abdominal pain. She has undergone numerous tests that show no evidence of pathophysiology. Her husband of 25 years recently died of a myocardial infarction (MI). Yesterday, she began having chest pains and was certain she was having a heart attack. Her daughter called 911, and Veronica was transported to the emergency department. The staff performed diagnostic studies and laboratory tests, which were all negative for pathophysiology. She was admitted to the psychiatric unit with a diagnosis of Somatic Symptom Disorder. The nurse develops the following concept map care plan for Veronica.

Signs and Symptoms
- Physical complaints
- Absence of pathophysiology
- Focus on self and physical symptoms

Signs and Symptoms
- Chest pains and fear of having a heart attack (following husband's sudden death from MI)

Nursing Diagnosis

Ineffective coping

Nursing Diagnosis

Fear (of dying as husband did from acute MI)

Nursing Actions
- Ongoing assessment
- Accept that the symptoms are real to the client
- Identify personal gains
- Fulfill client's needs
- Do not give positive reinforcement to symptoms
- Limit amount of time client discusses symptoms
- Teach adaptive coping strategies

Nursing Actions
- Ongoing assessment
- Refer all new physical complaints to physician
- Discuss client fears and anxieties
- Encourage verbalization of feelings associated with husband's death
- Encourage participation in grief support group

Medical Rx:
Duloxetine 60 mg q day for chronic pain/depression/anxiety

Outcomes:
- Client recognizes signs and symptoms of escalating anxiety
- Client is able to intervene before the exacerbation of physical symptoms

Outcomes:
- Client discusses feelings associated with husband's death
- Client fears of own serious illness have diminished
- Client uses adaptive coping mechanisms to diminish fears/anxieties

FIGURE 10.4 Concept map care plan for client with somatic symptom disorder *(from Townsend [2017]. Essentials of Psychiatric Mental Health Nursing, 7th ed. Philadelphia: F.A. Davis Company, with permission).*

from PTSD. People in countries far away are able to experience tragedy in "real time." In 2020, the COVID-19 pandemic affected health-care providers and first responders globally seeing patients dying and facing jeopardy daily. The effects of PTSD on this population will likely be felt for years.

GOOD TO KNOW

PTSD is not limited to combat veterans or survivors of rape. "Trauma is any type of distressing event or experience that can have an impact on a person's ability to cope and function. Trauma can result in emotional, physical, and psychological harm" (Tull, 2020).

CRITICAL THINKING QUESTION

Think for a moment about what you felt when you heard about schools and businesses being shut down because of COVID-19. Recall watching the death toll grow. Then, discuss how you felt after returning back to school or to work post COVID-19.

A term associated with PTSD is **survivor guilt**. Sometimes, survivors of a traumatic event are haunted by a feeling of guilt that they survived and someone else did not. The person may have experienced the trauma or may have been a witness. Either can scar a person's memory. A military veteran may say, "Why me? Why did my buddy get blown away, and I lived? He didn't deserve that." Another concern associated with PTSD is suicide. Since the Afghanistan war began, there has been a rise in suicide among military veterans, suggesting that PTSD is a factor. This population continues to need more mental health services (Drummond, 2012).

The diagnostic criteria for PTSD in an adult, an adolescent, or a child 6 years or older are the following, along with additional subcategories.

PTSD symptoms may appear immediately or may be repressed until years later and can include the following:

- difficulty sleeping/restless
- negative feelings (e.g., low self-esteem as a result of the event)
- depression
- memories that are unwanted and upsetting

Criterion A. Exposure to an actual or potential death, life-threatening injury, or any type of sexual violence.

Criterion B. Reliving the traumatic occurrence (having flashbacks); memories, dreams, acting out, reacting to external and internal episodes that resemble the trauma (lasting more than 1 month).

Criterion C. Avoiding anything that resembles the traumatic event (lasting more than 1 month).

Criterion D. Noticeable change in mood and alteration in cognitive thinking at unpredictable times, which either started or worsened after the incident (lasting more than 1 month).

Criterion E. Alterations in reaction either at the beginning or end of a traumatic event.

Criterion F. Persistence of symptoms in criteria B, C, D, and E lasting more than 1 month.

Criterion G. Impaired relationships with others. Social withdrawal and having lack of trust.

Criterion H. The impaired relationships with others are not related to abusing drugs or to medical conditions.

DIFFERENTIAL DIAGNOSES

The patient may display symptoms of other disorders that resemble PTSD, which need to be ruled out before the actual diagnosis of PTSD is established. Ruling out the differentials will permit the patient to receive treatment that is appropriate for PTSD. A few disorders that resemble PTSD are acute stress disorder, dissociative disorders, depression, GAD, panic disorder, specific phobias, substance abuse, and psychiatric appearance of medical conditions.

Pharmacology Corner

The most common medications for PTSD are antidepressants: venlafaxine (Effexor XR), sertraline, fluoxetine, and paroxetine. Sertraline and paroxetine both have received FDA approval (Vallerand et al., 2019).

Psychotherapeutic Treatments (APA, *Clinical*, 2017)

- CBT
- cognitive processing therapy (CPT)
- prolonged exposure therapy
- brief eclectic psychotherapy

Complementary and Alternative Therapies for PTSD

The recent surge in the number of people diagnosed with PTSD has led to wider use of conventional medication and therapies to treat this condition. In addition, studies have found some complementary therapies to be beneficial, including recreational therapy, animal-assisted therapy, and yoga. Yoga is the most popular complementary therapy of the three, especially because yoga can be practiced in a facility/fitness center or at home (Wynn, 2015). Yoga is beneficial in both medical and mental health disorders. Acupuncture is another popular alternative therapy. Studies have shown the benefits of acupuncture in treating anxiety and substance abuse (Wynn, 2015).

Diagnostic Test

Before a patient is diagnosed with PTSD, be sure thyroid labs have been drawn to rule out other conditions. Abnormal thyroid levels could be related to the patient's depression and inappropriate thinking (Van Leeuwen & Bladh, 2019).

Nursing Interventions

Trust, communication, and listening skills are very important tools for nurses who have patients with PTSD. Expressing thoughts and feelings surrounding the experience and the survivor guilt is an important first step in the patient's ability to begin the process of healing (FIG. 10.5). Validate the patient's feelings regarding the situation and provide time to actively listen. Honesty and genuineness in communicating with your patients will help to build a working rapport. Advise patients of the importance of taking their medications.

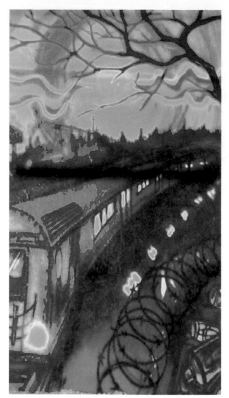

FIGURE 10.5 Encouraging the patient's expression of thoughts and feelings about the traumatic experience, as in this painting, is an important first step in identifying the problem and beginning the healing process (*courtesy of the National Institute of Mental Health, Bethesda, MD*).

Classroom Activity

- Watch the movies *Coming Home* and *The Best Years of Our Lives* to get a veteran's perspective of returning to civilian life after war.
- Watch the movie *Nuts*, which is about trauma after rape and incest.
- *Welcome to Marwen* is about a person who was physically assaulted and left for dead. After coming out of a coma, he suffers with PTSD.

CRITICAL THINKING QUESTION

Jeanne is a 21-year-old single woman admitted for pneumonia. Her social history indicates that she survived a house fire when she was 10 years old and that her twin sister died in that fire. Today is the day for the monthly fire drill at the hospital. During the drill, you note that Jeanne is not in her bed. After the drill, you search her room and find her sitting on the floor of her closet. She is wrapped in a blanket and is crying. She does not respond to your verbal cues. What do you think is happening to her? What illness might she have? How will you get her out of the closet? What can you do to help her?

Family members and significant others can suffer from the effects of PTSD as well as the person who experienced the traumatic event personally, even though they were not present for the original event. The term *vicarious trauma* may apply in this situation.

Safe and Effective Nursing Care

Update the plan of care according to changes in the patient's anxiety level.
Provide safe and ethical care.
Participate in interdisciplinary meetings concerning patient.
Involve the patient in their plan of care.
Promote self-esteem.
Provide the patient with support resources in their community.
Use therapeutic communication.
Suggest complementary and alternative therapies.
Explore etiology of patient's anxiety.

Key Points

- Anxiety disorders have many common characteristics. Psychoanalytic theories propose that it is important to find the underlying cause of the anxiety. Medications and therapies should be individualized for the patient.
- Trust and communication techniques are important tools for the nurse caring for a patient with an anxiety disorder. Maintaining a calm milieu is also essential.
- SSD is characterized by somatic symptoms that are either very distressing or that result in significant disruption of functioning, as well as excessive and disproportionate thoughts, feelings, and behaviors regarding those symptoms. The symptoms may or may not have an organic cause.
- Treatment and nursing care for patients with SSD may be difficult and long term, as these are chronic disorders. Patients may use the defense mechanisms of denial and conversion reaction.

CASE STUDY

A patient comes for his scheduled appointment with Dr. Caldwell. The patient is a well-known politician who has been the subject of negative press in recent months. His main symptoms are general malaise, sneezing, chronic headache, and "feeling like I have a constant cold." Dr. Caldwell orders blood work and a chest x-ray and does a complete physical examination of the patient. You collected vital signs and the health history when you roomed the patient. The patient is on the road campaigning and meeting his constituents almost daily. He believes he has become infected with something serious because his symptoms do not seem to subside. Dr. Caldwell tells the patient that his examination and laboratory work do not show any physical illness and suggests that the symptoms are "most likely viral in nature and probably stress and anxiety related." Dr. Caldwell suggests the patient take over-the-counter medications for his symptoms and find methods to reduce his stress. Dr. Caldwell leaves the room. The patient expresses his extreme disappointment at not being given "something to take" and asks you to explain to him how stress can give him a cold.

1. How will you respond to the patient's request for medication?
2. What are your thoughts about the patient's expectation for receiving medications? How will you discuss that with him?
3. What alternative remedies (for example, dietary changes, herbal supplements, meditation) can you discuss with him or ask the health-care provider to discuss with him?

Review Questions

1. Audrey is a veteran who served in Afghanistan. It is very difficult for her to drive through a parking ramp because "There are people hiding behind the pillars! They have guns! Be careful!" Audrey is most likely experiencing:
   a. Auditory hallucinations
   b. Flashbacks
   c. Delusions of grandeur
   d. Free-floating anxiety

2. Ms. T complains of headaches and body pains whenever her husband mentions that the house needs to be cleaned. This has been a reoccurring problem for more than 6 months. Ms. T probably is suffering from what kind of disorder?
   a. GAD
   b. Phobia
   c. PTSD
   d. SSD

3. Mr. L, who has a severe fear of needles, is hospitalized on your medical unit. The laboratory technician enters to draw blood for the routine CBC, and Mr. L begins to cry out "Get away from me! I can't breathe! I'm having a heart attack!" Your first response to Mr. L would be:
   a. "I'll take your vital signs and call my supervisor."
   b. "Why do you think you're having a heart attack, Mr. L?"
   c. "Don't worry. She's done this many times before."
   d. "Mr. L, relax. Take a few deep breaths. I'll stay with you."

4. Which of the following is *not* an anxiety disorder? *(Select all that apply.)*
   a. Panic disorder
   b. Depressive disorder
   c. Multiple personality disorder
   d. Agoraphobia

5. A patient with PTSD is:
   a. Suspicious and hostile
   b. Flexible and adaptable to change
   c. Extremely frightened of something
   d. Likely to avoid any stimuli associated with the traumatic event

6. Which of the following is *true* regarding a phobic disorder?
   a. It involves repetitive actions.
   b. It involves a loss of identity.
   c. It results in sociopathic behavior.
   d. It is an irrational fear that is not changed by logic.

7. Agoraphobia is:
   a. Fear of speaking
   b. Fear of shopping in a large mall
   c. Fear of heights
   d. Fear of blood

8. The medication(s) of choice for the treatment of anxiety is (are) *(select all that apply)*:
   a. Alprazolam (Xanax)
   b. Diazepam (Valium)
   c. Lorazepam (Ativan)
   d. Venlafaxine (Effexor)
   e. Buspirone (Buspar)

9. The three subcategories of phobia include all of the following *EXCEPT*:
   a. Agoraphobia
   b. Social phobia
   c. Acrophobia
   d. Specific phobia

10. Which of the following are NOT nursing interventions for people with anxiety disorders? *(Select all that apply.)*
    a. Maximize stimuli to create diversion from the anxiety.
    b. Encourage the patient to verbalize all thoughts and feelings.
    c. Observe the patient's nonverbal communication for data on the patient's thoughts and feelings.
    d. Observe for signs of suicidal thoughts.
    e. Document only positive changes in behavior.
    f. Discourage activities; activities might only increase a patient's anxiety level.

REVIEW QUESTIONS ANSWER KEY 1. b, 2. d, 3. d, 4. b, c, 5. d, 6. d, 7. b, 8. a, b, c, e, 9. c, 10. a, e, f

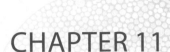

CHAPTER 11
Depressive Disorders

KEY TERMS

Anhedonia
Depression
Dysthymic disorder
Major depressive disorder
Mood
Persistent depressive disorder
Postpartum depression
Pseudodementia

CHAPTER CONCEPTS

Behaviors
Caring
Communication
Grief and loss
Mood and affect
Self
Stress and Coping

LEARNING OUTCOMES

1. Define depressive disorders.
2. Identify three types of depressive disorders.
3. Describe common physical and behavioral symptoms of major depressive disorder.
4. Identify treatment modalities for depressive disorders.
5. Describe key nursing care interventions for depressive disorders.

Feeling down, discouraged, and depressed is something all people experience at some time in their lives. Periods of emotional highs and lows are normal. However, depressive disorders are very different from a transient bout of the "blues" or depressed **mood**. Mood is an individual's sustained emotional tone, which influences behavior, personality, and perception. **Depression** is a painful and debilitating illness that affects all areas of one's life. There are several types of depressions that are collectively called *depressive disorders*. These can change or distort the way people see themselves, their lives, and those around them.

People who suffer from depression usually see everything with a more negative attitude. They cannot imagine that any problem or situation can be solved in a positive way. Depression can take a variety of forms and can affect all age groups. Depressive disorders all have similar symptoms that vary by duration, timing, and presumed etiology. These disorders are more common in women, but men with depression may be underdiagnosed (FIG. 11.1). See Box 11.1 for a list of general facts about depressive disorders.

Depressive episodes can occur with other disorders such as bipolar disorder, schizophrenia, and dementia. It is estimated that 50% of all depression diagnoses may actually be bipolar illness (Akiskal, 2017; for more about bipolar disorder, see Chapter 12). In addition, depression is often seen in people with diabetes and heart disease.

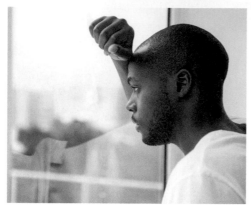

FIGURE 11.1 Depression is less reported in the male population, but this may be caused by the male tendency to mask emotional disorders with behaviors such as alcohol abuse.

GOOD TO KNOW

The coronavirus disease 2019 (COVID-19) pandemic led to an increase in the incidence of depressive disorders. In fact, these disorders were diagnosed at a more than threefold higher rate during the COVID-19 pandemic than before. Factors associated with greater risk of depression during COVID-19 were having a lower income, having less than $5000 in savings, and having exposure to more stressors (Ettman et al., 2020; Vahratian et al., 2021).

TYPES OF DEPRESSIVE DISORDERS

Major Depressive Disorder

Major depressive disorder, or major depression, is characterized by a combination of symptoms that severely interfere with a person's ability to work, sleep, study, eat, and enjoy once-pleasurable activities. To be considered a major depressive disorder, these symptoms must last at least 2 weeks and very often last much longer. Major depression is disabling and prevents a person from functioning normally. Some people may experience only a single episode of major depression within their lifetime, but more often a person has multiple episodes. Major depression is one of the most common mental disorders in the United States. Worldwide, it is a major cause of disability (World Health Organization, 2020). In 2020, 8.4% of Americans had at least one major depressive episode in the past year (Substance Abuse and Mental

Box 11.1

General Information About Depressive Disorders

- Common not only in the United States but also internationally
- Most common reason for seeking out a mental health professional
- Nearly twice as many women as men are affected by depressive disorders annually. However, men frequently suffer from depression that may be masked.
- First episode often occurs between ages 18 and 29, but depression can start at any age, including childhood. Highest occurrence is in age group 18–25.
- Prevalence highest among individuals reporting being of 2 or more races
- Older adults are prone to depression often related to multiple losses and decline of health, among other variables. They may have less obvious symptoms and may be less likely to admit feelings of sadness.
- Depressive disorders are being diagnosed earlier in life than they were in previous generations, including in children and adolescents.
- Because symptoms can be hidden and vague, the primary care provider is often the first to identify depression.
- Symptoms often go unrecognized and can be a factor in poor work performance, family conflict, and substance abuse.
- Once one is diagnosed with a depressive disorder, there is a high probability of recurrence.

Source: Adapted from American Psychiatric Association, 2022.
    Kessler et al. (2005).
    Morgan & Townsend (2021).
    National Alliance on Mental Illness (2017). https://nami.org/About-Mental-Illness/Mental-Health-Conditions/Depression.

Cultural Considerations

Depression crosses all cultures and socioeconomic groups. However, depressive disorders may be misdiagnosed or underdiagnosed in some cultures due to language barriers and lack of access to mental health services. This is particularly true in cultures that are more fearful of being labeled with a psychiatric diagnosis. Some cultures may express depressive symptoms as physical symptoms, such as fatigue and headache, whereas others may be more prone to speak in psychological terms of sadness and guilt.

Health Services Administration, 2020; National Institute of Mental Health, 2022). A person has a 16.6% chance of developing a major depressive disorder in their lifetime (Kessler, 2005).

Major depressive disorder is characterized by a classic cluster of symptoms. Behavioral and physical symptoms include five or more of the following for at least a 2-week period that represents a change in functioning (American Psychiatric Association, 2022):

- sad mood
- sleep pattern disturbances
- increased fatigue
- increased agitation
- feelings of guilt or worthlessness
- weight loss or gain
- decreased interest in pleasurable activities **(anhedonia)**
- decreased ability to think, remember, or concentrate
- recurrent thoughts of death or suicide
- These symptoms are often the same ones someone experiences in a low period in their life such as after a loss of job or end of a relationship, but the duration and intensity are increased in major depression (FIGS. 11.2 and 11.3).

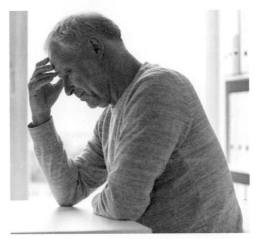

FIGURE 11.2 Sadness becomes depression when it lasts a long time and interferes with day-to-day functioning.

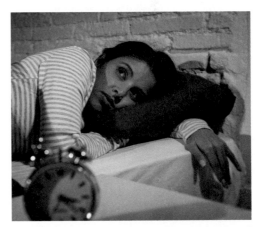

FIGURE 11.3 Insomnia is a common symptom of depression.

Tool Box

Clinicians use a number of depression scales to follow the severity of the patient's symptoms over time. These include:

1. Beck depression inventory:
   https://www.ismanet.org/doctoryourspirit/pdfs/Beck-Depression-Inventory-BDI.pdf
2. Hamilton depression rating scale:
   http://www.assessmentpsychology.com/HAM-D.pdf

Differentiating a grief response to a major life loss from a major depressive disorder can be difficult, as some of the symptoms, such as sadness, insomnia, and poor appetite, may resemble a depressive episode.

Prolonged Grief Disorder

In 2022, the American Psychiatric Association added a new diagnosis category to the Diagnostic and Statistical Manual 5th edition text revision (DSM-5-TR, 2022). Prolonged grief disorder is an intense response to grief that is beyond what is expected. The disorder is characterized by intense longings for the individual who died (within 6 months for adults and 12 months for children and adolescents); and preoccupation with thoughts of this person may manifest for most of the day and nearly every day for at least a month. Other symptoms include intense yearning for the deceased most days, marked sense of disbelief, and increased suicidal ideation. The duration of the person's bereavement exceeds expected social, cultural, or religious norms and the symptoms are not better explained by another mental disorder. Prolonged grief disorder is classified under trauma rather than depression in DSM-5-TR.

See Table 11.1 for tips to differentiate grief from depression.

Table 11.1

Differentiating Grief From Depression

	Uncomplicated Grief	*Major Depression*
Reaction	• Labile • Heightened when thinking of loss	• Mood consistently low • Prolonged, severe symptoms
Behavior	• Variable, shifts from sharing pain to being alone • Variable restriction of pleasure	• Completely withdrawn or afraid to be alone • Persistent restriction of pleasure
Sleep patterns	• Periodic episodes of inability to sleep	• Early morning wakening
Anger	• Often expressed	• Turned inward
Sadness	• Varying periods	• Consistently sad
Cognition	• Preoccupied with loss • Self-esteem not as affected	• Focused on self • Feels worthless; has negative self-image
History	• Generally no history of depression	• History of depression or other psychiatric illness
Responsiveness	• Responds to warmth and support	• Hopelessness • Limited response to support • Avoids socializing
Loss	• Recognizable, current	• Often not related to an identified loss

Source: Adapted from Ferszt (2006): How to distinguish between grief and depression? *Nursing, 36*(9), 60–61.
    Brown-Saltzman (2018). Transforming the Grief Experience. In: Bush and Gorman (eds.). *Psychosocial Nursing Along the Cancer Continuum,* 3rd ed. Oncology Nursing Press: Pittsburgh, PA.

GOOD TO KNOW

A period of depression after the death of a loved one is normal. When this response goes on longer than expected and interferes with a person's self-esteem, it may indicate a depressive disorder.

GOOD TO KNOW

The classic image of a depressed person does not fit all patients. Some may have more of the physical signs, such as loss of appetite, insomnia, and early morning wakening, but they do not display the outward sadness that is usually associated with depression.

Persistent Depressive Disorder

Persistent depressive disorder is a less severe form of depression that is characterized by its chronic nature. It was previously referred to as **dysthymic disorder**. It affects approximately 5% to 6% of the U.S. population age 18 and older at some point in their lifetimes (Kessler, 2005). It often begins in childhood, adolescence, or early adulthood. About 40% of adults with persistent depressive disorder also meet criteria for major depressive disorder or bipolar disorder at some point in their lives. In earlier versions of the American Psychiatric Association's Diagnostic and Statistical Manual (DSM), chronic depression was viewed as more of a personality disorder, but that thinking has changed to its current definition of a depressive disorder rather than a personality style (American Psychiatric Association, 2013).

Persistent depressive disorder is characterized by a depressed mood for most of the day, for more days than not, as indicated by either subjective account or observation by others, for at least 2 years in adults and 1 year in children. These symptoms are less severe than those of major depressive disorder but go on for long periods (American Psychiatric Association, 2022).

Symptoms often include:

- poor appetite or overeating
- insomnia or hypersomnia
- low energy or fatigue
- low self-esteem
- poor concentration or difficulty making decisions
- feelings of hopelessness

CRITICAL THINKING QUESTION
Describe the behaviors that would differentiate persistent depressive disorder from major depressive disorder.

Postpartum Depression
Depression during pregnancy is called perinatal depression. The postpartum "blues" is a common response a few days after giving birth and may be related to fatigue, hormone changes, and anxiety. It resolves in a short time with rest and support. Post partum blues is not depression. **Postpartum depression,** also called postpartum-onset depression, occurs up to 1 year after childbirth and is a much more serious condition. Postpartum-onset depression is classified as a major depressive disorder with the same classic cluster of symptoms as previously mentioned, with the addition of lack of interest in the baby. It can progress to rejection of the baby and lead to a psychotic state. A patient suffering from this disorder needs intensive treatment with medications and psychotherapy. See Chapter 20 for more information about postpartum-onset depression.

Substance/Medication-Induced Depressive Disorder
Substance/medication-induced depressive disorder is depressed mood from the physiological effects of withdrawal from, intoxication with, or exposure to a substance. This can include drugs of abuse such as alcohol, opioids, sedatives, and antianxiety medications as well as exposure to toxins. See Box 11.2 for drugs that cause depression.

Box 11.2
Drugs That Can Cause Depression
- alcohol
- amphetamine or cocaine withdrawal
- anabolic steroids
- some antibiotics, including some antifungals and antivirals
- antihypertensive agents including:
  - beta blockers
  - calcium channel blockers
- barbiturates
- benzodiazepines
- HIV drugs, including:
  - zidovudine (Retrovir)
- opioids
- oral contraceptives
- smoking cessation agents, e.g., varenicline (Chantix)
- corticosteroids

Adapted from: Morgan & Townsend (2021). *Psychiatric Mental Health Nursing,* 10th ed. Philadelphia: F.A. Davis.
Rogers, D. & Pies, R. (2008). General medical drugs associated with depression, *Psychiatry* (Edgmont). Dec;5(12):28-41.

Depressive Disorder Due to Another Medical Condition
This condition is characterized by a prominent and persistent depression that is judged to be the result of direct physiological effects of a general medical condition. See Box 11.3 for medical conditions associated with depression.

Clinical Activity
Review your depressed patient's risk factors, including medications and medical conditions that could contribute to their depression.

CRITICAL THINKING QUESTION
Your patient with stage II lung cancer shows signs of depression. Besides the emotional stress of having cancer, what other factors could be contributing to their depression?

Premenstrual Dysphoric Disorder
This form of depressive disorder was added to the DSM-5 in 2013 (American Psychiatric Association, 2017). The features include a consistent pattern of

Box 11.3

Medical Conditions Associated With Depression

- vascular brain disease including stroke
- myocardial infarction (MI), congestive heart failure (CHF)
- adrenal disorders
- dementia
- diabetes
- cancer
- thyroid disorders
- brain tumors

- systemic lupus erythematosus (SLE)
- Parkinson's disease
- multiple sclerosis (MS)
- nutritional deficiencies
- chronic pain
- hormonal disruption
- chronic kidney disease
- traumatic brain injuries (TBI)

Source: Morgan & Townsend (2021). *Psychiatric Mental Health Nursing,* 10th ed. Philadelphia: FA Davis.
Morgan & Townsend (2020). *Essentials of Psychiatric Mental Health Nursing,* 8th ed. Philadelphia: FA Davis.
Wisel & Alici (2015). Special considerations in older adults with cancer. In: J.C. Holland, W.S. Breitbart, P.N. Butow, P.B. Jacobsen, M.J. Loscalzo, & R. McCorkel (eds). *Psycho-Oncology,* 3rd ed. (pp. 549-53). New York: Oxford University Press.

markedly depressed mood, excessive anxiety, and mood swings during the week before menses, which start to improve after the onset of menses and then become minimal or absent after menses.

Depressive Disorder With Seasonal Pattern

Previously called seasonal affective disorder (SAD), some depressions may have a seasonal pattern. Symptoms generally are exacerbated during the winter months and subside during the spring and summer. This type of depression is thought to be related to the hormone melatonin. During months of longer darkness, there is increased production of melatonin that seems to trigger depressive symptoms in some people. It is associated with loss of energy, weight gain, hypersomnia, overeating, and craving for carbohydrates (American Psychiatric Association, 2017). The DSM-5 no longer lists this as a major depressive disorder category.

DIFFERENTIAL DIAGNOSES FOR DEPRESSIVE DISORDERS

- bipolar disorders
- adjustment disorder with depressed mood (depression associated with a psychosocial stressor when all symptoms of major depressive disorder are not met)
- grief reaction
- medication side effect
- prolonged grief disorder

ETIOLOGY OF DEPRESSIVE DISORDERS

Depressive disorders are complex and may have multiple etiologies. Biochemical theories have become more important with the identification of insufficiency of neurotransmitters, especially norepinephrine and serotonin, as a cause of depression. These insufficiencies may be the result of inherited or environmental factors. The effectiveness of antidepressants seems to result from enhancing levels of these neurotransmitters, giving strong credibility to these theories. Family history remains an important risk factor, indicating the existence of genetic links. Psychological theories have focused on personal histories of deprivation, trauma, or significant loss. Classic psychoanalytic theory views depression as the reaction to the loss of a significant person who was both hated and loved. Cognitive theory suggests that learned negative and defeated attitudes contribute to depression. An individual can also be prone to low self-esteem and a sense of helplessness due to environmental factors and have a tendency toward depression. Physical illness and medications are also frequent contributors to depressive symptoms.

TREATMENT OF DEPRESSIVE DISORDERS

Treatment involves a combination of pharmacological and psychotherapeutic approaches. This approach has better outcomes than either approach used alone does. The advent of many new antidepressants has provided more opportunities for successful treatment (see Pharmacology Corner). Individual psychotherapy to address past losses and stressors, short-term cognitive behavioral therapy (CBT) to develop new strategies to alter negative thinking, and group therapy to address socialization and poor self-esteem can all be helpful.

For the patient with severe depression who does not respond to drugs or psychotherapeutic approaches, electroconvulsive therapy (ECT) is sometimes suggested. It can be used in conjunction with other modalities such as medication. People may have therapeutic sessions of 6 to 10 ECT treatments over 4 to 8 weeks. Patients are given sedation before the treatment. The side effect of memory loss is frequently seen. See Chapter 8 for more information on nursing management for the patient receiving ECT.

Transcranial magnetic stimulation (TMS) is a non-invasive procedure that uses magnetic fields to stimulate nerve cells in the brain to improve symptoms of depression. TMS is typically used when other depression treatments have not been effective. This procedure is sometimes used as an alternative to ECT.

Alternative Treatments
Light Therapy
Light therapy is being prescribed and is used successfully in the treatment of depression associated with a seasonal pattern. It consists of special lights to be used for certain amounts of time during the day. Also, exposure to natural light has been shown to reduce depression and increase alertness.

Herbal and Nutritional Therapy
General dietary changes such as avoiding caffeine, sugar, and alcohol or adding servings of whole grains and vegetables may help a person with mild depression. Supplements such as St. John's wort, gingko biloba, fish oil, and SAMe have been shown to provide antidepressant effects in some patients with mild depression. St. John's wort should not

---

Pharmacology Corner

Antidepressants are the medications of choice in treating depressive disorders. See Table 11.2 for the categories of antidepressants. They are also used to treat depression associated with bipolar disorder, schizophrenia, and dementia. Selected agents may be used to treat other disorders including anxiety disorders, obsessive compulsive disorders, and bulimia. Some of the target symptoms that antidepressants may treat include sadness, inability to experience pleasure, change in appetite, insomnia, restlessness, poor concentration, and negative thoughts. These medications work to increase the concentration of neurotransmitters such as serotonin and norepinephrine. The early antidepressants were called tricyclics and monoamine oxidase inhibitors (MAOIs). The newer antidepressants, including selective serotonin reuptake inhibitors (SSRIs), serotonin norepinephrine reuptake inhibitors (SNRIs), and heterocyclics (also called *tetracyclics*), have fewer side effects. The anticholinergic actions of tricyclics and the rigid dietary restrictions needed for MAOIs often limit the use of these medications, but these older medications can still be effective for some patients who are resistant to the other categories.

All of these medications require several weeks of use before some improvement in depression can be expected; they should not be stopped abruptly. These medications are all oral preparations. Patients may need to try different antidepressants or combinations with other medications such as some antipsychotics to achieve better outcomes. Genetic studies are sometimes done on patients to determine which antidepressants would have improved side-effect profiles. Safety of antidepressants during pregnancy and lactation is a concern, and the patient should discuss potential risks with their health-care provider. Serotonin syndrome is a complex of symptoms including restlessness, tachycardia, and altered mental status that can occur when SSRIs and SNRIs are discontinued abruptly. See Chapter 8 for more information on these medications.

As noted earlier, antidepressants take several weeks to improve symptoms, but new categories of medications that work more quickly and have different mechanisms of action are being researched. One of these is esketamine (Spravato), which provides some relief of symptoms in 24 hours. This drug is only available for patients with treatment-resistant depression. It is administered by nasal spray in a treatment-approved center under supervision by health-care professionals because of the side-effect profile, which includes potential for sedation and disassociation.

Table 11.2
Antidepressants

Drug Category	Examples	Important Considerations
Tricyclics (TCAs)	amitriptyline (Elavil) nortriptyline (Pamelor) desipramine (Norpramin) doxepin (Sinequan) trimipramine (Surmontil)	Major side effects are anticholinergic symptoms requiring close monitoring. Symptoms include dry mouth, urinary retention, constipation, blurred vision, sedation. Use with extreme caution in the elderly. Smoking can increase metabolism of tricyclics.
SSRIs (selective serotonin reuptake inhibitors)	paroxetine (Paxil) sertraline (Zoloft) fluoxetine (Prozac) escitalopram (Lexapro) citalopram (Celexa) fluvoxamine (Luvox)	SSRI withdrawal syndrome can occur with sudden discontinuation; includes dizziness, nausea, cholinergic rebound (salivation, loose stool).
SNRIs (serotonin norepinephrine reuptake inhibitors)	duloxetine (Cymbalta) venlafaxine (Effexor) desvenlafaxine (Pristiq)	Monitor for insomnia, restlessness.
Heterocyclics (tetracyclics)	bupropion (Wellbutrin) mirtazapine (Remeron) trazodone (Oleptro)	Monitor for dizziness, headache, tachycardia.
MAOIs (monoamine oxidase inhibitors)	phenelzine (Nardil) tranylcypromine (Parnate) isocarboxazid (Marplan) selegiline transdermal system (Emsam)	Serious, potentially fatal hypertensive crisis may occur in presence of foods high in tyramine (aged cheeses, red wine, smoked and processed meats). Special diet must be followed.

Source: Adapted from Morgan & Townsend (2021).
  Pederson & Leahy (2010)

Evidence-Based Practice

Clinical Question: What factors contribute to improvement of depression in patients with chronic health problems?

   Discussion: Patients with heart failure experience high rates of depression.

   Evidence: In a research study published in the *Journal of Advanced Nursing,* patients with heart failure completed a series of tools that found a high rate of depression (over 18% with symptoms of severe depression) as well as malnutrition. The researchers found that improving functional status was an important factor in improving nutritional status and depressive symptoms.

   Implications for Nursing Practice: To relieve depressive symptoms in patients with heart failure, it is important to improve their functional status, especially for those with poor nutritional status. It is important to screen patients with heart failure as well as patients with diabetes for depression.

Zhang, X., Zou, H., Hou, D., He, D., Fan, X. (2020). Functional status mediates the association of nutritional status with depressive symptoms in patients with heart failure. *J Adv Nurs.* 2020 Sep 15. Doi: 10.1111/jan.14522. Epub ahead of print. PMID: 32932558

be used with selective serotonin reuptake inhibitors (SSRIs) or monoamine oxide inhibitors (MAOIs) (Skidmore-Roth, 2010).

NURSING CARE OF THE PATIENT WITH DEPRESSIVE DISORDERS

Common nursing diagnoses with this population include the following:

- hopelessness
- self-care deficit
- self-esteem, disturbed, deficit
- social interaction, impaired
- thought processes, disturbed
- violence to self, risk for

General Nursing Interventions
- Identify small, achievable goals the patient can meet. Provide support and encouragement. Break down tasks into small parts for the severely depressed patient. For example, rather than encouraging the patient to get dressed, have the patient focus on putting on a t-shirt.
- Encourage the patient to speak about their concerns without judgment. Use open-ended questions, such as "Tell me what concerns you today." Avoid blanket reassurance like "You are doing fine" or minimizing the patient's feelings as in "You're lucky you have a job." This might alienate a patient who is not feeling fine. Help a patient who verbalizes hopelessness to focus on describing their feelings and concerns. Then discuss one concern at a time to avoid overwhelming the patient.
- Encourage independence.
- Avoid activities that might tax memory or concentration if the patient is struggling with these.
- Monitor patient compliance with antidepressants. Include education about potential side effects and length of time until results can be expected.
- Encourage participation in activities to reduce time spent ruminating on negative thoughts.
- Promote a trusting relationship.
- Encourage the patient to challenge negative thoughts. This can be done by encouraging the patient to share a negative thought, such as "I am a bad parent," and then promoting discussion of alternative thoughts to replace that negative statement, such as "I spent quality time with my daughter yesterday."

- Promote physical activity where possible, for example, ambulating in the hall twice a day. Focusing on physical activity can promote the patient's sense of well-being.
- Promote the patient's self-esteem by identifying improvements or recent successes. The depressed patient may tend to focus only on negatives.
- If a patient gives any clues of contemplating suicide, notify other team members and the physician immediately. See Chapter 13 for more interventions for suicidal patients.

Table 11.3 provides the nursing care plan for depressed patients.

GOOD TO KNOW
Depressive disorders can contribute to confusion and social withdrawal in older adults and can lead to misdiagnosis of dementia (sometimes called **pseudodementia**). These patients need multidisciplinary assessment to obtain the correct diagnosis and treatment.

Clinical Activity
- Review effective interventions used by the nursing team to approach the depressed patient.
- Identify small goals that the depressed patient has achieved.

GOOD TO KNOW
As antidepressant drugs take effect, the patient may initially feel more energized before the mood lifts. A suicidal patient can be at increased risk during this period because they have more energy to initiate a suicide plan while still feeling hopeless. Any patient who is suicidal should be closely monitored during the first few weeks on antidepressants. All antidepressants carry a black box warning from the Food and Drug Administration (FDA) about increased risk of suicidality in children and adolescents.

Table 11.3

Nursing Care Plan for the Depressed Patient

Assessment/Data Collection	Nursing Diagnosis	Plan/Goal	Interventions	Evaluation
Withdrawn, refusing to leave their room	Impaired social interaction	To participate in conversation with nurse once a day; establish a trusting relationship.	Spend time with patient each day without pressure or demands. Ask questions that do not require demanding answers. Accept periods of silence. Encourage participation in structured activities, if possible, to reduce pressure on patient to "perform."	Track frequency of patient talking with others. Verbalizes concerns to nurse.

CONCEPT MAP

FIGURE 11.4 provides a concept map for a patient with depression. The concept map gives a clinical vignette with different interventions based on the patient's symptoms.

Patient Education

• Medication management including length of time to take effect, side effects to report to provider, mode of action, dietary restrictions if taking MAOIs, and need to continue taking medications regularly even if symptoms persist or improve
• Strategies to deal with low self-esteem and stress
• Family education on understanding the nature of depression

Clinical Activity

Review the side-effect profile of your patient's antidepressants and incorporate teaching as appropriate to promote patient compliance.

CRITICAL THINKING QUESTION

A patient is complaining of nausea and dizziness. In reviewing the medications from home, you note that the patient has been taking paroxetine for 5 years. The patient is now NPO before surgery. What do you need to know about this medication that could be a factor in the patient's postoperative recovery?

CRITICAL THINKING QUESTION

Identify some of the differences in side-effect profiles of tricyclic antidepressants and SSRIs.

Safe and Effective Nursing Care

Ensure safe administration of medications and monitor for side effects
Promote ways to increase patient's sense of self-worth
Incorporate safe practices to monitor for self-harm, especially in patients taking antidepressants
Monitor for adequate nutrition and hydration
Promote communication to enhance sense of security and self-worth

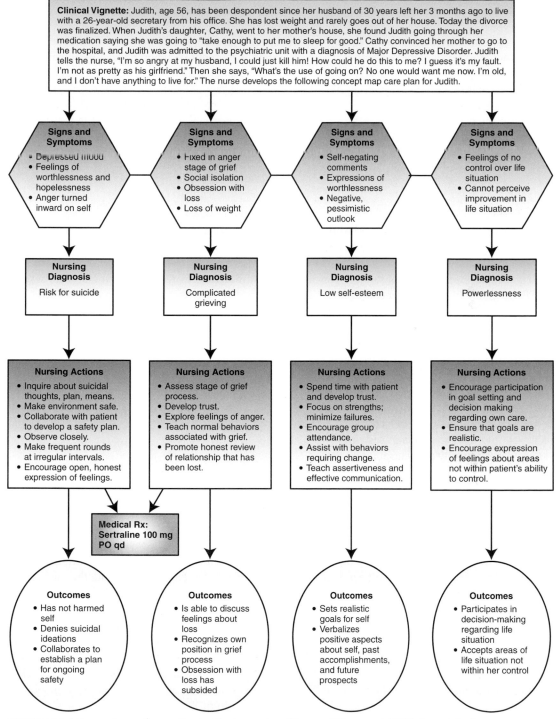

FIGURE 11.4 Concept map for a patient with depression. *(Morgan & Townsend. (2020). Essentials of Psychiatric Mental Health Nursing. Philadelphia: FA Davis.).*

Key Points

- Depressive disorders are treatable, and most people respond positively to the appropriate medications.
- Major depressive disorder is a debilitating illness that often recurs in one's lifetime.
- Depression is the most common reason for seeking out a mental health professional.
- Mood disorder due to a general medical condition is frequently seen in physically ill patients in the hospital.
- Nursing care of the depressed patient should include promotion of self-esteem and socialization.
- Antidepressants are very effective in treating depression, but side-effect profiles may require a change in drug as needed.

CASE STUDY

Marge is a 55-year-old single woman who works as a librarian. Over the past few months, she has had increasing difficulty sleeping, poor concentration, and an overwhelming sense of sadness. Her mother died 1 year earlier, and Marge attributed these changes to a grief reaction. However, as time has gone on, the symptoms have become more distressing. She has stopped exercising, has turned down social invitations, and spends most of her time alone at home. She has begun missing work because of oversleeping, and her supervisor has approached her with concern. Marge has agreed to see her health-care provider for a checkup. At the appointment, Marge appears sad, with slow speech and difficulty concentrating on the provider's questions. On specific questioning, she reports feeling that she no longer feels competent in her job despite having advanced degrees and certifications and over 20 years' experience. These feelings have increased over the past 3 months and occur daily.

The health-care provider considers major depressive disorder as a diagnosis and prescribes paroxetine.

1. What teaching would you provide to Marge about the antidepressant?
2. What other forms of treatments might be proposed?
3. What other concerns would you have for this patient?

Review Questions

1. Ms. S is admitted to your medical unit with a diagnosis of dehydration and a history of depression. She tells you, "I just can't eat. I'm not hungry." Your best therapeutic response would be:
   a. "You aren't hungry?"
   b. "If you can't eat, what is that candy bar wrapper doing in your bed?"
   c. "Why aren't you hungry?"
   d. "You really should try to eat some real food."

2. Your patient has a diagnosis of major depressive disorder and has been started on sertraline (Zoloft) 50 mg daily. After taking the medication for 3 days the patient says, "I don't think this medicine is working. I don't want to take it any longer." What would be your best response?
   a. "I'll let your doctor know, and he may order a different medication."
   b. "These medications usually take a few weeks to bring about an improvement in your symptoms."
   c. "The important thing now is getting you more involved in patient activities."
   d. "It is important to eat a more balanced diet to help this medication work."

3. Your patient appears withdrawn and depressed. Which of the following would *not* be an effective intervention?
   a. Develop trust
   b. Show acceptance
   c. Be judgmental
   d. Be honest

4. The nurse who is assessing a patient with major depression would expect to observe which of the following symptoms?
   a. Euphoria
   b. Fear
   c. Extreme sadness
   d. Compulsions

5. The nursing interventions for a patient with major depression would include all of the following *except:*
   a. Using active listening skills
   b. Maintaining a safe milieu
   c. Encouraging adequate nutrition
   d. Reassuring the patient everything will be "just fine"

6. Your new patient is taking an MAOI for severe depression. What would you tell the dietary department about her upcoming meals?
   a. No caffeine
   b. No processed lunch meat
   c. No extra salt
   d. No gluten

7. Your patient with major depressive disorder isolates herself in her room for the whole day. You find her sitting and staring out the window. What is the best therapeutic response when you walk in the room?
   a. Say to her, "Come with me. It's time for group therapy."
   b. Say to her, "I'd like to introduce you to other patients."
   c. Say to her, "What are you thinking about?"
   d. Make frequent short visits to her room and just sit there.

8. Your patient, Mr. A, had a recent myocardial infarction (MI) and open-heart surgery with an uncomplicated recovery. His wife tells you that Mr. A has changed and is now uncommunicative, sad, and discouraged about the future. How would you respond to Mrs. A?
   a. "I'll let the doctor know."
   b. "This is normal. I would just ignore it for now."
   c. "Tell me more about the changes in his behavior."
   d. "We should get a psychiatric consult."

9. Mrs. J has been diagnosed with persistent depressive disorder and has been taking paroxetine for 3 years. On arrival in your mental health clinic, she presents very differently than on her last visit. She is cheerful, energetic, and talkative. Previously, she had been fatigued and negative. What should you do?
   a. Encourage the patient to no longer take her antidepressant.
   b. Get more information from the patient about how she is feeling.
   c. Recommend that she not be seen in the clinic today.
   d. Talk with the patient's husband to confirm these behavior changes.

10. Which of the following is *not* true about depression?
    a. It is more common in men than in women.
    b. It is common after MI.
    c. Grief after a major loss can mimic depression.
    d. Children and adolescents can suffer from depression.

REVIEW QUESTIONS ANSWER KEY 1.a, 2.b, 3.c, 4.c, 5.d, 6.b, 7.d, 8.c, 9.b, 10.a

CHAPTER 12
Bipolar Disorders

KEY TERMS

Bipolar Disorder
Cyclothymic
Hypomania
Mania

CHAPTER CONCEPTS

Family
Mood and affect
Safety
Stress and coping

LEARNING OUTCOMES

1. Describe three different types of bipolar disorders.
2. Describe factors that make bipolar disorder difficult to diagnose.
3. Describe three nursing interventions for behaviors associated with mania.
4. List three medications useful in treatment of bipolar disorders and the potential side effects of each.
5. Describe two teaching points for bipolar patients on mood stabilizers.

CHARACTERISTICS OF BIPOLAR DISORDERS

Bipolar disorder (previously known as manic depression) is characterized by marked shifts in mood, energy, and ability to function, characterized by profound depression and periods of hyperactivity or **mania** interspersed with periods of normality. The common forms of bipolar disorders include bipolar I, bipolar II, and **cyclothymic**, as well as several others. These are listed in Table 12.1. Bipolar disorders are often hard to diagnose until behaviors such as grandiosity, risk-taking, and violence become exaggerated. During **hypomanic** phases (less severe hyperactivity), a person may be highly productive and not obviously symptomatic. Some highly creative people, such as the writer Ernest Hemingway and the painter Jackson Pollock, had bipolar disorder. Early onset of bipolar disorder in children and adolescents is being diagnosed more frequently (see Chapter 19). Individuals with bipolar disorder that are well managed on medication often live normal lives and are functioning members of society.

Manic episodes (also known as mania) are characterized by a distinct period of abnormality and persistently elevated, expansive, or irritable mood. Extreme mania can include psychotic behaviors such as hallucinations and delusions. Suicide risk is high in this population with 5-6% dying by suicide (American Psychiatric Association, 2022). Patients may also abuse alcohol or other substances in an effort to self-medicate to feel better. Bipolar disorder can be confused with depression, a personality disorder, schizophrenia, substance abuse, or an anxiety disorder. Clues that the illness is bipolar disorder include early onset, family history of bipolar disorder, recurrent depressions and/or manic episodes, and hyperactivity during depressive episodes (American Psychiatric Association, 2022).

See Box 12.1 for general information about bipolar disorders.

Table 12.1

Forms of Bipolar Disorders

Type	Description
Bipolar I	The classic image of bipolar disorder—a full syndrome of manic symptoms and most likely depressive episodes
Bipolar II	At least one bout of major depression with episodic occurrence of hypomania. This patient may never have experienced a full episode of mania. Mood stability can often lead to severe impairment in social and work functioning.
Cyclothymic	A chronic mood disturbance of at least 2 years' (1 year in children) duration involving numerous episodes of hypomania and depressed mood but of less intensity. The person is never without the symptoms for more than 2 months.
Bipolar disorder due to another medical condition	Prominent and persistent disturbance in mood characterized by mania that is a direct result of physiological effects of a general medical condition.
Substance/medication-induced bipolar disorder	Disturbance characterized by elevated, expansive mood with or without depression that is the direct result of the physiological effects of a substance, e.g., alcohol, amphetamines, cocaine, heavy metals

Sources: Adapted from *Diagnostic and Statistical Manual of Mental Disorders 5th ed-TR(2022), American Psychiatric Association.* (2013), American Psychiatric Association.
Morgan & Townsend. (2021). *Psychiatric Mental Health Nursing,* 10th ed. Philadelphia: F.A. Davis Company, with permission.

Box 12.1

General Facts About Bipolar Disorders

- Roughly 4.4% of the American population will have this disorder in their lifetime, with 2.8% of U.S. adults experiencing an episode in the past year.
- It affects males and females at approximately the same rate.
- Episodes may or may not be associated with periods of depression.
- Average age of onset is 25.
- After the first episode, there is a high risk of recurrence.
- Some people with the disorder have periodic episodes separated by years, and others have much more frequent cycles.
- There is strong evidence for a genetic/inherited link, but a specific genetic defect has not yet been identified.
- It occurs in children but is difficult to diagnose. Symptoms can be confused with attention deficit-hyperactivity disorder or substance abuse.

Sources: National Institute of Mental Health (2017). https://www.nimh.nih.gov/health/statistics/bipolar-disorder.shtml.
Kessler, R.C., Chiu, W.T., and Demler, O. (2005). Prevalence, severity, and comorbidity of twelve-month DSM-IV disorders in the National Comorbidity Survey Replication. *Archives of General Psychiatry,* 62(6): 617–627.
Morgan & Townsend (2021). *Psychiatric Mental Health Nursing,* 10th ed. Philadelphia: F.A. Davis Company.

Manic Phase

The manic phase may last from days to months and cause marked disruption of occupational and social functioning. It can include the following symptoms:

- being easily distracted
- little need for sleep (may feel rested after 3 hours of sleep)
- poor temper control, easily becoming agitated and irritable
- reckless behavior and lack of self-control, including:
  - drinking and/or drug use, binge eating
  - poor judgment
  - sex with many partners
  - spending sprees
- very elevated mood
- excess activity (hyperactivity)
- increased energy
- racing thoughts, flight of ideas
- talking a lot
- very high self-esteem, grandiosity (exaggerated feeling of importance, power, knowledge, ability)
- very involved in activities

In the early phase of a manic episode, an individual can become more engaging and outgoing and experience high achievement, energy, and success. As the manic phase accelerates, the individual can become frenzied and out of control, leading to impaired decision making and even altered appearance. For example, women experiencing a manic episode may apply their makeup in a distorted manner, especially lipstick. The person may be more reckless in other areas such as business decisions and physically hazardous actions. The individual in a manic phase may be prone to abusing substances such as tranquilizers and/or alcohol to sleep and control agitation. Substance abuse may also trigger bipolar disorders in susceptible individuals. The presence of substance abuse with bipolar disorder increases the negative outcomes and can confuse the illness presentation (FIG. 12.1).

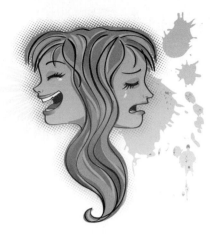

FIGURE 12.1 Depiction of bipolar disorder.

Classroom Activity

Watch films depicting people with bipolar disorder, including *Pollack, Silver Linings Playbook*, and *Lust for Life.*

Depressed Phase

The depressed phase of bipolar disorder is similar to the major depressive disorders described in Chapter 11. The following symptoms may be seen:

- low mood or sadness
- difficulty concentrating, remembering, or making decisions
- eating problems:
  - loss of appetite and weight loss
  - overeating and weight gain
- fatigue or lack of energy

GOOD TO KNOW

Patients in a manic phase can go for days without sleep and not feel tired. Reduced need for sleep is different than insomnia when the person wants to sleep.

Cultural Considerations

- Bipolar disorder is more common in higher socio-economic groups.
- As with other psychiatric disorders, misdiagnosis can occur due to misunderstood religious practices, like speaking in tongues. Language barriers can lead to misunderstanding behaviors. Bipolar disorder can be misdiagnosed as schizophrenia when culturally accepted behaviors are misunderstood.

- feelings of worthlessness, hopelessness, or guilt
- loss of pleasure in activities once enjoyed
- loss of self-esteem
- thoughts of death and suicide
- trouble getting to sleep or sleeping too much
- pulling away from friends or activities that were once enjoyed

The conversion to manic phase from the depressed phase may occur quickly. Sometimes the two phases overlap. They may occur together or quickly one after the other in what is called a *mixed* state.

Tool Box

- The general behavior inventory, which has been useful as a self-report monitoring tool in patients with bipolar disorder, is available at https://cls.unc.edu/files/2014/06/GBI_self_English_v1a.pdf (Depue, Slater, Wolfstetter-Kausch, Klein, Goplerud, & Farr).
- Mood disorder questionnaire screening tool is a well-respected tool to identify symptoms of bipolar disorder. https://www.ohsu.edu/sites/default/files/2019-06/cms-quality-bipolar_disorder_mdq_screener.pdf. Full Reference is adapted from Hirschfeld R., Williams J., Spitzer R.L., et al. Development and validation of a screening instrument for bipolar spectrum disorder: the Mood Disorder Questionnaire. Am J Psychiatry. 2000;157:1873-1875.

CRITICAL THINKING QUESTION

Your patient on the surgical unit has a diagnosis of cyclothymic disorder. Describe what behaviors you might expect postoperatively.

ETIOLOGY OF BIPOLAR DISORDERS

Biological theories predominate as the cause of bipolar disorder. Studies indicate this disorder is caused by an imbalance in neurotransmitters, particularly norepinephrine, dopamine, and serotonin. Increased levels are believed to be present in manic episodes whereas decreased levels are believed responsible for depressive ones. A genetic link has also been demonstrated through family studies. A combination of genetics and biochemical factors, along with environmental triggers such as stressful life events, may present the most comprehensive picture of the etiology of bipolar disorder. Medical conditions and medications can also trigger an episode in susceptible people. See Box 12.2 for drugs and medical conditions that can precipitate a manic state. The most common comorbid conditions include anxiety disorders, substance use disorders and attention deficit hyperactivity disorders (American Psychiatric Association, 2022).

Differential Diagnoses

- major depression
- schizophrenia
- substance abuse disorder
- borderline personality disorder
- post-traumatic stress disorder
- attention deficit/hyperactivity disorder
- dissociative disorder

GOOD TO KNOW

It can be challenging to differentiate between major depressive disorder and bipolar depression, especially when it is a new diagnosis. Often the provider must look for the presence of contributing factors such as family history of bipolar disorder, abrupt onset of symptoms, poor response to antidepressants, and/or chaotic life. The presence of any of these increases the likelihood of bipolar depression.

CRITICAL THINKING QUESTION

Your new patient on the substance abuse unit has a diagnosis of bipolar disorder I as well as alcohol use disorder. How would alcohol use contribute to symptoms in bipolar I?

TREATMENT OF BIPOLAR DISORDERS

Treatment for bipolar disorder often starts emergently when family members realize the patient is in a manic state. Patients are more likely to seek treatment for themselves during depressive phases than during manic phases. When someone is in a state of euphoria, they are less prone to accepting treatment and less likely to think there is a need for

Box 12.2

Drugs and Physical Illnesses That Can Cause Manic States

Drug Related
Steroids
Levodopa
Amphetamines
Tricyclic antidepressants
Monoamine oxidase inhibitors
Methylphenidate
Cocaine
Thyroid hormone
High doses of anticonvulsants
High doses of opioids as well as withdrawal
Anesthetics
Sulfonamides

Physical Conditions
Hyperthyroidism
Multiple sclerosis (MS)
Systemic lupus erythematosus (SLE)
Brain tumors
Traumatic brain injury (TBI)
Stroke (also called cerebrovascular accident [CVA] or
  brain attack)

Morgan & Townsend. (2021). *Psychiatric Mental Health Nursing,* 10th ed. Philadelphia: F.A. Davis Company.

it. Medications, the most common being mood stabilizers, are the primary treatment. These can be used during an exacerbation as well as for control of frequency and intensity of future episodes (see the Pharmacology Corner).

To reduce the severity of relapse and to promote medication compliance, treatment should include psychotherapy. Early diagnosis improves outcomes. After a manic phase, individual and group psychotherapy as well as family therapy may help patients and families cope with the shame and long-term effects of the manic phase. During a manic phase, the patient may have hurt loved ones emotionally with words or physically with actions. As life becomes "flatter" and less exciting without mania, the patient may need support to cope. It is common for patients to use alcohol and sedative drugs to try to sleep during manic episodes and to use stimulants during depressive phases, so substance abuse counseling may need to be part of the treatment plan.

Electroconvulsive therapy (ECT) has been used as a treatment when the individual does not tolerate or respond to traditional pharmacological treatment. ECT can also be used in emergent situations when the patient's life is threatened by dangerous behavior or exhaustion.

Pharmacology Corner

Mood stabilizers are the cornerstone treatment of bipolar disorders. See Table 12.2 for a listing of mood stabilizer medications. These include lithium and a number of anticonvulsants such as carbamazepine (Tegretol), valproic acid (Depakene), and lamotrigine (Lamictal). These medications may be used singly or in combination. These medications often are a lifelong regimen to prevent or reduce the incidence of depression as well as mania. During an acute manic phase, the patient may require antianxiety and/or antipsychotic drugs such as olanzapine (Zyprexa), aripiprazole (Abilify), or quetiapine (Seroquel). Many patients require more than one medication to remain in remission. Patients must be counseled to report side effects and not to stop medications abruptly. If side effects are too distressing, alternative medication combinations can be prescribed. See Chapter 8 for additional information on mood stabilizers. Antidepressants alone or in combination with mood stabilizers can carry a risk of triggering a manic phase in susceptible individuals. Childhood treatment of bipolar disorder often includes use of atypical antipsychotic medication. See Chapter 19 for more information on bipolar disorder in children and adolescents.

In the early phases of a manic episode, alternative treatment that includes herbs, such as chamomile and valerian, can help with mild anxiety and insomnia.

Lithium remains an important treatment in bipolar treatment. Because of its many potential adverse effects, it requires close monitoring of blood levels. Therapeutic levels are between 0.5 and 1.2mEq/L for most patients (between 1.0 and 1.5 mEq/L in acute mania), and the difference between therapeutic and toxic levels is small. Lithium blood levels can become elevated with dehydration, profuse sweating, and chronic diarrhea, leading to toxicity. Toxicity can cause tremors, confusion, seizures, coma, and even death. Early warning signs of toxicity include nausea, vomiting, and sedation. See Table 12.3 for signs of lithium toxicity. Lithium takes about 7 to 10 days to reach the desired effect and is only available orally. Because

Table 12.2
Mood Stabilizers

Drug Category	Drug Examples	Important Considerations
Lithium carbonate	Lithium (Eskalith, Lithobid)	Toxic symptoms can occur even at normal blood levels, so monitoring of adverse effects must be ongoing. May take several weeks to achieve full therapeutic effect. Use with caution in frail older persons who are at risk for dehydration. Rapid discontinuation can increase risk of relapse. Patient needs to report all other medications to avoid drug interactions. Contraindicated in presence of cardiac or renal disease. See Chapter 8 for more information.
Anticonvulsants	Carbamazepine (Tegretol) gabapentin (Neurontin), valproic acid (Depakene), lamotrigine (Lamictal), topiramate (Topamax)	Monitor CBC for possible blood dyscrasias if taking valproic acid or carbamazepine. Increased risk for suicide. Use with caution in renal, liver, or cardiac disease. See Chapter 8 for more information
Selected antipsychotics	Olanzapine(Zyprexa), aripiprazole, (Abilify) lurasidone (Latuda), quetiapine (Seroquel), risperidone (Risperdal)	May be used in acute mania Lurasidone used in depressive episodes

Source: Adapted from Morgan & Townsend. (2021). *Psychiatric Mental Health Nursing,* 10th ed. Philadelphia: F.A. Davis Company, with permission.

Table 12.3
Signs of Lithium Toxicity

Serum Levels	Symptoms
1.5–2.0 mEq/L	Blurred vision, ataxia, tinnitus, nausea, vomiting, diarrhea
2.0–3.5 mEq/L	Excessive output of dilute urine, increased tremors, muscle irritability, confusion
↑3.5 mEq/L	Seizures, coma, oliguria, arrhythmias, cardiovascular collapse

Source: Adapted from Morgan & Townsend. (2021). *Psychiatric Mental Health Nursing,* 10th ed. Philadelphia: F.A. Davis Company, with permission.

of the many contraindications to lithium, which include pregnancy, advanced age, kidney failure, and drug interactions, many people cannot take lithium. In that case, other mood stabilizers are used and are effective.

GOOD TO KNOW
Lithium has a Food and Drug Administration (FDA) black box warning that toxicity can occur at doses close to therapeutic levels. It should be prescribed only when there are resources to provide ongoing blood tests.

GOOD TO KNOW
Lithium toxicity can develop quickly, especially in dehydration. This makes it challenging to use in the older population, who are more vulnerable to dehydration.

A variety of anticonvulsants are used as mood stabilizers. Each anticonvulsant has a specific side-effect profile, so this information should be incorporated in patient teaching. Regular complete blood counts (CBCs) to monitor for anemia and blood dyscrasias may be needed.

Compliance with medication regimen is an ongoing issue with bipolar patients. If they are in a euphoric state, they may believe they do not need medications. When they are depressed, they may feel hopeless and that the medication is not helping. When they are in remission, they may be more concerned about side effects and decide to stop taking their medications. Patient teaching and follow-up counseling are part of the nursing care of these patients.

See Table 12.4 for the side effects of mood stabilizers.

GOOD TO KNOW
Bipolar women on medications should be counseled to use birth control, as many of the medications used to treat this disorder are not safe to use in pregnancy. Patients who desire to become pregnant need to be counseled to speak with their healthcare providers about their treatment options.

Cultural Considerations
Diverse populations may metabolize medications differently.

CRITICAL THINKING QUESTION
A 29-year-old patient with a history of bipolar I disorder is NPO for surgery. He is routinely taking lithium (Lithobid) and lamotrigine (Lamictal). Because he is unable to take these medications, what concerns would you have and what would you monitor?

NURSING CARE OF THE PATIENT WITH BIPOLAR DISORDERS

Common nursing diagnoses for patients with bipolar disorder include the following:

• anxiety
• coping, ineffective
• nutrition, imbalanced: less than body requirements
• self-care deficit
• sleep pattern, disturbed
• thought process, disturbed
• risk for self-directed or other-directed violence

General Nursing Interventions
• Provide clear, firm limits. Clearly define what is expected and what is not allowed. For example, if the patient needs to pace, set aside a specific area where that can be done; if they are talking too loudly, point this out and encourage them to lower their voice.
• Focus on reality, especially when the patient describes grandiose ideas. Present reality without arguing with the patient.
• Remove hazardous objects from the patient's room. Promote safety for all involved in the patient's care by identifying signs of increasing potential for violence.
• Reduce external stimulation such as extraneous noise.
• Provide an outlet for excess energy by letting the patient pace or exercise. Also promote rest periods.
• Encourage activities that do not require a lot of concentration.
• Encourage patient compliance with medication regimens and laboratory testing.
• Take the time to establish a relationship with the patient to promote a sense of safety.
• Identify ways to ensure the patient is eating and drinking adequately; for example, provide food that is easy to eat on the move.
• Encourage the patient to complete thoughts or actions rather than jumping from item to item.
• If the patient is depressed, see the nursing interventions in Chapter 11.
• Be aware that clients with bipolar disorders are at a high risk for suicide. Although clients in the manic phase are briefly agitated, energized, and elated, their underlying depression makes at risk for self-injury. See Chapter 13.
• Supervise the patient to protect them from results of poor judgment like giving away possessions or entering into risky business dealings.

Table 12.4

Side Effects of Mood Stabilizing Agents

Side Effects	Medication	Nursing Implications
Drowsiness, dizziness	Lithium, anticonvulsants	Educate patient on safety, driving. Determine whether dosing schedule allows evening dose.
Dry mouth	Lithium	Sugarless candies, saliva substitute
Gastrointestinal (GI) upset	Lithium, anticonvulsants	Administer meds with meals.
Fine hand tremors	Lithium	Report to health-care provider, dosage adjustment may be needed, avoid caffeine.
Polyuria, dehydration	Lithium	Monitor input and output (I&O) and weight. Drink adequate fluids.
Weight gain	Lithium	Need to maintain adequate sodium even if reducing calories.
Increased suicide risk	Anticonvulsants	Monitor for worsening depression, suicide risk.

Source: Adapted from Townsend. (2015). *Psychiatric Mental Health Nursing: Concepts of Care in Evidence-Based Practice,* 8th ed., pp. 520. Philadelphia: F.A. Davis Company, with permission.

GOOD TO KNOW
Patients can move quickly from social, affable, highly energetic, fun behavior to angry, violent behavior.

GOOD TO KNOW
Patients in a manic phase exhibit poor insight and judgment, and this provides a challenge to nurses to manage inappropriate behavior.

Clinical Activity
• Monitor a patient's lithium levels.
• Review potential medication side effects that can contribute to the patient's symptoms as well as affect their compliance with mood stabilizers.

CRITICAL THINKING QUESTION
A 45-year-old patient with a long history of bipolar II disorder has been in remission for 5 years. She tells you she has stopped taking her valproic acid because she feels so good and the medication prevented her from losing weight. How should you respond?

Clinical Activity
Identify the family support network for a bipolar patient and ensure that they are knowledgeable about early warning signs of manic episodes.

Table 12.5 provides the nursing care plan for patients with bipolar disorders. See Concept Map Bipolar Mania Figure 12.2.

Table 12.5

Nursing Care Plan for Patients With Bipolar Disorders

Assessment/Data Collection	Nursing Diagnosis	Plan/Goal	Interventions	Evaluation
Inappropriate behavior including loud conversation, swearing, domineering	Ineffective coping	Patient will display more socially acceptable behaviors.	Calmly point out to patient what behavior is not appropriate, e.g., "You're talking too loudly again." Avoid sounding angry or judgmental.	Patient is able to control one behavior for a set period of time.
			Set limits on swearing. Do not argue, bargain, or threaten patient. Explore how the patient can vent their frustration/energy in more socially acceptable ways. Provide alternative ways to express self.	

Classroom Activity

Review the drug categories for treatment of bipolar disorder and develop patient-teaching materials for each.

Evidence-Based Practice

Clinical Question: Can nurses effectively provide the needed education for self-management for patients with bipolar disorder?

Discussion: Teaching patients with bipolar disorder and their caregivers about their illness requires special skills to address the complex management of the disorder.

Evidence: A study conducted in the Netherlands looked at how mental health nurses gain the skills to provide this important aspect of care. The study found that five areas of expertise were needed by mental health nurses to provide this support:

1. The ability to build a trustful collaboration.
2. The ability to start a dialogue about needs and responsibilities.
3. The ability to explain bipolar disorder.
4. The ability to utilize mood monitoring instruments.
5. The ability to conceptualize self-management of bipolar disorder.

Implications for Nursing Practice: This study found that nurses utilize these five domains to provide this education. These nurses gained this knowledge through training as well as experience. The study reinforced that nurses are key to providing self-management education.

van den Heuvel, S. C. G. H., Goossens, P. J. J., Terlouw, C., Schoonhoven, L. & van Achterberg, T. (2019). Self-management education for bipolar disorders: A hermeneutic-phenomenological study on the tacit knowledge of mental health nurses. *Issues in Mental Health Nursing, 40*(11): 942-950. DOI: 10.1080/01612840.2019.1636166

Patient/Family Education

• Medication compliance is crucial even when the patient has stabilized.
• Review side-effect profiles of all medications and stress the importance of reporting these rather than stopping prescribed medications.
• If patient is on lithium, provide information on the importance of regular blood levels, drinking adequate fluids, and maintaining adequate sodium intake.
• Patients on some anticonvulsants may need follow-up CBCs.
• Educate family about the effects of bipolar disorder and signs to look for.
• Educate patients and their partners about the use of birth control if they are taking mood stabilizers.
• Lithium levels should be drawn 12 hours after the last dose for greatest accuracy.

Safe and Effective Nursing Care

• Maintain safe environment free from hazards.
• Monitor medication side effects.
• Set limits on patient behavior.
• Maintain safe environment for staff and other patients.
• Ensure proper follow-up care and monitoring are in place for patients on mood stabilizers.

Clinical Vignette: Sam and Janet had been engaged for a year. Three months ago, Sam called Janet and told her he didn't want to get married, and he was leaving to take a job in Japan. Janet became hysterical, then depressed, and then seemed to be accepting the situation. She got a new hairstyle, bought lots of new clothes, and started going to lots of parties with her roommate, Nancy. She started losing weight, exercising excessively, and sleeping very little. She became quite promiscuous. She stopped menstruating and said to Nancy, "I wonder if I'm pregnant!" Tonight she and Nancy went to a bar. Janet started buying drinks "for the house." She became quite loud and disruptive, climbing on the bar and announcing to the crowd that she had received a "message" that she would be the winner of tonight's multimillion-dollar lottery. When the bar owner eventually asked her to leave, she became violent, striking out at him and destroying bar property. He called 911, and Janet was taken to the emergency department of the hospital. She has been admitted to the psychiatric unit with Bipolar I Disorder, Manic Episode. She is agitated and restless. The nurse develops the following concept map care plan for Janet.

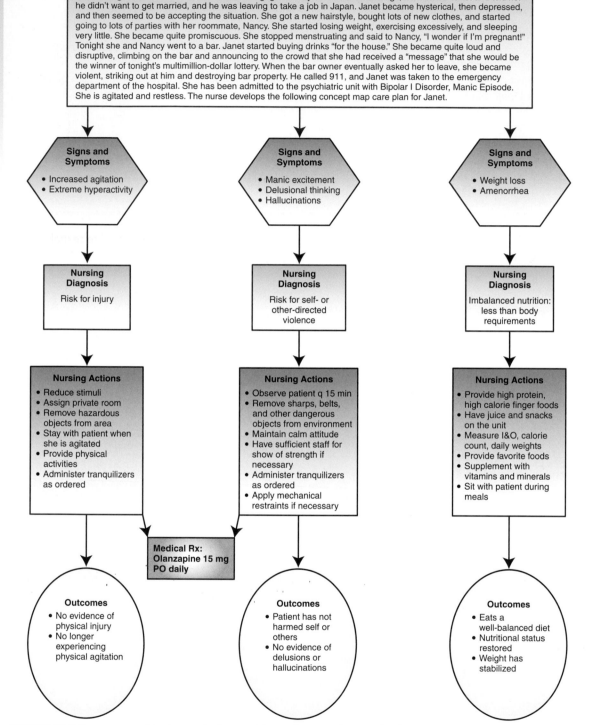

FIGURE 12.2 Concept map bipolar mania. Source: *Morgan Townsend, Essentials of Psychiatric Mental Health Nursing (2021). FA Davis.*

Key Points

- Bipolar disorders can include severe depressions with periods of extreme mania, as well as severe depressions with minor bouts of mania.
- The manic phase can last for days, weeks, or months and can cause severe disruption in all areas of functioning.
- Lithium remains a recognized treatment for bipolar disorder and requires monitoring of blood levels to ensure safety.

- A number of new medications to treat bipolar disorder are now used as well, including many anticonvulsants.
- Ongoing medication management is challenging, as the euphoric patient will often deny the need for these medications.
- Primary nursing interventions for a patient in mania include maintenance of safety, promotion of health, and medication compliance.

CASE STUDY

Jonathan is a 30-year-old single attorney living in New York City. He recently joined a prestigious law firm and is anxious to make a good impression on the partners. He has a long history of success in life, including graduating from a top law school with excellent scores, making a large income, and having many friends and associates. He is gregarious and always seems to be the center of attention wherever he is. His new position is more stressful than his previous jobs were. He has been sleeping only 2 to 3 hours a night and then coming in to the office at 4:00 a.m. to keep up with the workload. He drinks heavily at night to try to sleep and uses stimulants in the morning to keep going. He has received a lot of attention in the office for a recent successful litigation. However, his assistant notes that Jonathan is increasingly irritable and demanding, often changing from charming to angry at the slightest frustration. A woman in the office reports him to the superiors for inappropriate sexual advances. When he is brought into the office to discuss the allegations, he explodes and storms out of the office. Later that night, he is arrested in a bar for fighting with a patron and tells the police he is friends with the chief of police and will get the officer fired.

Jonathan is brought to the emergency department (ED) by the police, where he acknowledges he was diagnosed with bipolar disorder in college but stopped taking his lithium 1 year ago.

1. What other information would you need to know regarding what type of bipolar disorder Jonathan has?
2. What were the early signs that Jonathan was escalating into a manic phase?
3. What questions would you ask him regarding his history?

Review Questions

1. Mrs. A is admitted to the medical-surgical unit with a diagnosis of dehydration and pneumonia. She has a history of bipolar disorder and is controlled on lithium. As her nurse, you know you must:
   a. Treat her carefully because she may become catatonic.
   b. Observe for signs of lithium toxicity from dehydration.
   c. Alert the other staff of the "psych" patient on the unit.
   d. Treat the medical illness only.

2. Mrs. D has an appointment with the doctor. She began taking lithium 1 month ago as prescribed. She now states that her mouth and lips are constantly dry and she sometimes feels confused. She says, "I stagger like I'm drunk sometimes when I walk." You suspect:
   a. She is drinking to combat her depression.
   b. She is making it up to get different medications.
   c. She took too much lithium.
   d. She is dehydrated.

3. Marge is a 68-year-old woman with a long history of bipolar disorder I. She is brought to the ED by her sister, who reports that Marge has been increasingly agitated, is unable to sleep, and told her daughter that the mayor was calling her for advice on running the city. The behavior is an example of:
   a. Delusions of grandeur
   b. Delusions of persecution
   c. Auditory hallucinations
   d. Schizophrenia

4. The health-care provider orders lithium carbonate 600 mg tid for a patient newly diagnosed with bipolar disorder. The therapeutic blood level of lithium for acute mania is:
   a. 1.0–1.5 mEq/L
   b. 10–15 mEq/L
   c. 0.6–1.2 mEq/L
   d. 6–10 mEq/L

5. Which of the following drugs is NOT classified as a mood stabilizer?
   a. Carbamazepine
   b. Olanzapine
   c. Valproic acid
   d. Gabapentin

6. Your patient, who is manic, says, "Everything I do is great." How should you respond?
   a. "Yes, I am happy for you."
   b. "Tell me about a time in your life when things didn't go as planned."
   c. "No one can be great at everything."
   d. "Keep it up."

7. Your patient, who is manic, has lost 5 pounds and is underweight. Which meal is most appropriate?
   a. Grilled chicken and baked potato
   b. Spaghetti and meatballs
   c. Chili and crackers
   d. Chicken fingers and French fries

8. A newly admitted patient in an acute manic state has a nursing diagnosis of risk for injury related to hyperactivity. Which nursing intervention is most appropriate?
   a. Place the patient in a room with another hyperactive patient.
   b. Have the patient sit in his room while you review all the rules of the unit.
   c. Administer antipsychotic medication as ordered prn by the physician.
   d. Reinforce previously learned coping mechanisms to calm the patient down.

9. Which statement is most true about bipolar disorder?
   a. Bipolar disorders all follow the same pattern of behavior.
   b. Bipolar disorders always include periods of major depression.
   c. Manic depression is the same as hypomanic disorder.
   d. Patients with bipolar II have major depression with hypomanic symptoms.

10. Which category of medication would *not* be given to a patient with bipolar disorder?
    a. Stimulant
    b. Antipsychotic
    c. Antianxiety
    d. 2 and 3

11. What is cyclothymic disorder?
    a. A chronic mood disorder of at least 2 years
    b. A one-time event of hypomania
    c. A continuous state of hypomania for 2 years
    d. A chronic depression for 2 years

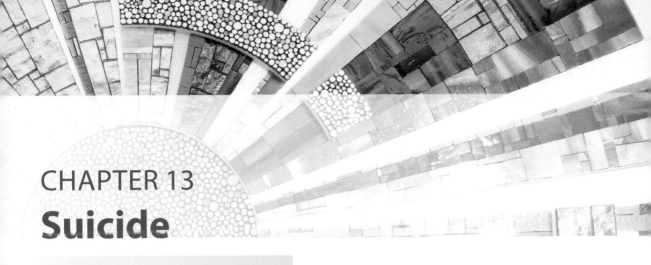

CHAPTER 13
Suicide

KEY TERMS

Ambivalence
Lethality
Suicidal ideation
Suicide
Suicide attempt
Suicide pact
Survivor of suicide

CHAPTER CONCEPTS

Grief and loss
Mood and affect
Safety
Stress and coping

LEARNING OUTCOMES

1. Identify populations at risk for suicide.
2. Identify myths and truths about suicide.
3. Identify warning signs of suicide.
4. Identify nursing care for people who are suicidal.
5. Describe the management of a suicidal patient in the acute hospital.

 THE REALITY OF SUICIDE

Suicide is defined as self-inflicted death, with evidence that the person intended to die. Many people experience momentary self-destructive thoughts during a bout of depression or a setback in life, but they do not take action on these thoughts. Suicidal thoughts are not always an indicator of a psychiatric diagnosis. Thinking about suicide does not mean the individual will act on those thoughts; however, anyone who talks about or threatens suicide or who makes a **suicide attempt** (any act with the intention of taking one's own life that the individual survived) must be taken seriously. A suicide attempt might or might not lead to injury or serious medical consequences. Factors that influence the medical consequences of a suicide attempt include type of planning, knowledge about the lethality of the chosen method, amount of ambivalence, and chance intervention by others (American Psychiatric Association, 2013). Because suicide is viewed as unacceptable in Western culture, it generates anxiety that has led to a number of myths. See Table 13.1 for a list of common myths.

Here are some important facts about suicide in the United States:

• Suicide is the 12th leading cause of death in the United States, accounting for more than 1% of all deaths.
• Suicide is the second-leading cause of death in the age group 15 to 34.
• Since 1999, the total suicide rate has increased by 35% in the United States, with much of the increase driven by suicides during midlife.
• More years of life are lost to suicide than to any other single cause except heart disease and cancer.

Table 13.1

Clearing Up the Myths About Suicide

Myth	Truth
Asking people about their suicidal thoughts will make them more likely to act on them.	Most people are not afraid to talk about their thoughts of committing suicide and are usually grateful that someone is available and cares. Talking can reduce the sense of isolation.
All people who attempt suicide have a psychiatric disorder.	People can become overwhelmed with life circumstances without having a psychiatric disorder.
A person who talks about suicide will not do it.	Approximately 80% of individuals who attempt or complete suicide give some definite verbal or indirect clues. As many as 50% have seen their health-care provider within the previous month, often with vague somatic complaints.
A person who attempts suicide will not try again.	Almost 50% to 80% of those individuals who complete suicide have attempted it at least once before.
People who attempt suicide are always determined to die.	Many individuals are ambivalent and are using the suicide as a cry for help. Suicide is often an attempt to end one's suffering rather than a wish to die.
People who attempt suicide just want attention.	Even if the suicide attempt is manipulative, the individual may go on to complete the suicide.
As the person becomes less depressed, the risk of suicide decreases.	As the depression begins to lift, the individual's energy level can increase before feelings of hopelessness are relieved. Once the individual makes the decision that suicide is an effective solution, their mood may even elevate.

Source: From Gorman and Sultan (2008). *Psychosocial Nursing for General Patient Care,* 3rd ed. Philadelphia: F.A. Davis Company, with permission.
  National Alliance on Mental Illness (2020). 6 Common Misconceptions about suicide debunked. https://www.nami.org/Blogs/NAMI-Blog/September-2020/5-Common-Myths-About-Suicide-Debunked

- Females attempt suicide three times more often than males.
- Suicide crosses all cultural, age, gender, racial, and socioeconomic groups. Native Americans have the highest suicide rate of any racial group in the United States.
- Other high-risk groups include members of the Lesbian, Gay, Bisexual, Transgender, Queer (LGBTQ+) community, military veterans, people who are incarcerated, and young people in child-welfare settings.
- Rates of suicide in older adults continue to be greater than the general population. Suicides in older adults may be less obvious as in intentional over-doses, self-starvation, and "accidents" that may not be immediately recognized as suicide (Fig. 13.1).
- The ratio of attempts to completed suicides is at least 12 to 1.
- A high percentage of people who complete suicide have made a previous attempt.
- Over 90% of people who kill themselves have a diagnosable mental illness, with the most common being mood disorders (depression or bipolar) and substance use disorders.
- About 46,000 Americans died by suicide in 2018. There are 2.5 times more suicides than there are homicides in the United States.
- **Suicide pacts,** or "copycat" suicides, among some adolescent groups have been seen in some communities.
- Single-vehicle auto crashes are generally investigated as possible suicides.

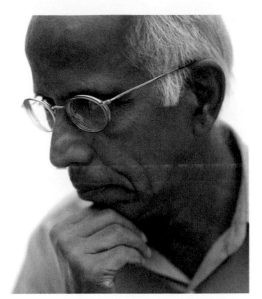

FIGURE 13.1 Older adults often have difficulty coping with loss, loneliness, and depression, and they have very high rates of suicide.

- Around 4.8% of adults have had thoughts about suicide during the past year, with those in the 18 to 25 age group being more likely to have these thoughts than those in other age groups.
- The most common methods of suicide include firearms, hanging, and overdose. The **lethality,** also known as *level of risk*, of suicide methods is a factor in the assessment of the patient. Men more commonly use highly lethal methods such as firearms or hanging, accounting for their higher death rate. Those who overdose have a greater chance of surviving because the medications take a longer time to produce death. They can receive treatment if found in time.
- For every person who commits suicide, six persons on average are left behind as **survivors of suicide** (family or friends of those who commit suicide).

(References include Suicide and Self-Harm [CDC, 2020] Suicide [National Institute of Mental Health, 2020]; Key Substance Use and Mental Health Indicators in the United States: Results from the 2019 National Survey on Drug Use and Health [SAMSHA, 2019]; CDC National Center Health Statistics, Suicide Mortality in the US, 1999-2019 [2021]; National Center for Health Statistics, Provisional Numbers for Suicide 2020 [2021]).

Classroom Activity
- Discuss factors that contribute to suicide in today's society.
- Discuss the impact of suicide of a well-known person.

Suicide remains a major public health problem, and all nurses must be familiar with risk factors, warning signs, and interventions to provide support to individuals at risk. Suicide can be a long-planned action or an impulsive act when the person is overwhelmed. People with a variety of psychiatric disorders, including depression, bipolar disorder, anxiety disorders, personality disorders, post-traumatic stress disorder (PTSD), and substance abuse, may consider suicide. Drugs or alcohol can contribute to accidental overdoses when the individual's judgment is impaired or they can be part of the self-destructive cycle. The *Diagnostic and Statistical Manual of Mental Disorders,* 5th edition (DSM-5), created a new category, suicidal behavior disorder, for an individual who initiates a behavior with the expectation that it will lead to the individual's own death within the next 24 months. Psychotic individuals can also experience hallucinations in which they believe they are being told to kill themselves by voices or powers outside themselves. Being alert to signals that the patient is at risk for suicide requires good observation skills and communication with the patient and the health-care team.

Cultural Considerations
In the United States, white males constitute the largest group of suicides. Native American males are also at high risk. African Americans, Asian Americans, and Hispanic Americans tend to have lower rates than the population as a whole (American Foundation of Suicide Prevention, n.d.). Some groups are less prone to suicide based on religion, for example, Roman Catholics. Some cultures, however, are more tolerant of suicide. Socioeconomic factors, including unemployment, add to an individual's risk.

CRITICAL THINKING QUESTION
Your teenager tells you her friend plans to kill herself because her boyfriend rejected her. Your teen says her friend swore her to secrecy and asks you not to tell anyone. What action should you take?

ETIOLOGY OF SUICIDE

The risk for suicide is associated with changes in brain chemicals called neurotransmitters, including serotonin. Decreased levels of serotonin have been found in people with depression, impulsivity disorders, and a history of suicide attempts, as well as in suicide victims.

Psychological factors including anger turned on oneself and an overwhelming sense of hopelessness, shame, guilt, and/or humiliation have been linked to **suicidal ideation**, that is, suicidal thoughts. Suicide may be viewed by some as a relief from overwhelming suffering (physical or emotional); some see it as a way to reunite with a loved one who has died. A psychotic individual may view suicide as a way to stop hallucinations, or the hallucinations may be telling the patient to commit suicide.

See Box 13.1 for a list of common risk factors for suicide.

Suicide occurs in all age groups. See Chapter 19 for more information on suicidal behavior in children and adolescents. Older adults, especially those facing health issues and multiple losses, may be at risk for

Box 13.1

Risk Factors for Suicide

- prior suicide attempt
- family history of mental disorder, substance abuse, family violence, sexual abuse, or suicide
- history of alcohol or substance use
- exposure to the suicidal behavior of others, such as peers or media figures
- poor support system, isolation
- easy access to lethal methods
- impulsive and/or aggressive tendencies
- grief from recent loss
- physical illness
- barriers to accessing mental health treatment

Source: From Centers for Disease Control and Prevention (2019), Risk for Suicide. Available at https://www.cdc.gov/violenceprevention/suicide/riskprotectivefactors.html

suicide. It is common for suicidal older adults to have seen a health-care provider in the prior year, so identifying any risk factors in older patients is an important part of the care plan.

The Warning Signs of Suicide

Having one of these signs does not necessarily mean the person is considering suicide, but having several of them may signal a call for help. Because the majority of suicidal individuals give some sign of their intention, these warning signs can save lives if recognized in time. Suicidal people often reach out for help and generally retain some **ambivalence** or contradictory feelings experienced at the same time. Consequently, getting help to someone who is considering suicide can save a life.

Suicide warning signs include the following:

- verbal suicide threats, such as, "You'd be better off without me," "Maybe I won't be around," or "I won't be here when you come back to work"
- expressions of hopelessness and helplessness and the inability to see alternatives
- previous suicide attempts
- talking about suicide methods to which the person has access
- saving pills
- asking questions about/researching different methods of committing suicide
- daring or risk-taking behavior
- personality changes
- depression
- lack of interest in future plans

Other warning signs may include the following:

1. *Noticeable improvement in mood occurs:* When this happens in a suicidal person, it is often a sign that the person has made the decision to go through with suicide. The pain will soon be over for that person. The feelings of those who will be left behind may or may not be a consideration. It has been said that suicide is the ultimate controller. For some people, this may be the only situation they feel they can control in their lives. Some people are not concerned about the survivors because their own pain overrides that of others. Some people, especially younger ones, may view death in a more romanticized way. Television, movies, and video games that show death often do so in a way that is glamorous or humorous. Young people may not make the connection

between the fantasy of the media and the reality of life, or they become so caught up in seeking revenge or making others suffer that they do not consider the finality of what they are attempting.

2. *Person starts giving away personal items:* When someone has made the decision to terminate their own life, it is no longer necessary to keep certain things. Some people will even attempt to give away a beloved pet. These individuals do want those items cared for. In an attempt to "tie up loose ends," they decide who will get certain items. The items will be given away for reasons other than "because I am going to kill myself," although people sometimes use that honest approach and are not taken seriously. Usually, these people will simply say that it is time to clean out a certain room or that they no longer need a certain item and they would like it to go to a special friend. Individuals may also write or change a will when contemplating suicide.

3. *Person starts talking about death and suicide or becomes preoccupied with learning about these things:* Curiosity about death is not unusual. People tend to be curious about what they do not know. When this curiosity becomes a preoccupation and a single thought for the patient, it signals that the patient has ideas of attempting suicide. Reporting this to the charge nurse and documenting the concerns are required.

Tool Box

A number of screening tools are available for health-care professionals as well as family/friends of individuals who are potentially suicidal. These tools are all available in multiple languages:

- The Columbia suicide severity rating scale has been used in many settings as a screening tool when suicidal ideation is suspected. Available at https://www.cms.gov/files/document/cssrs-screen-version-instrument.pdf
- The National Institute of Mental Health has developed a validated tool called the *ask suicide-screening questions* (known as *ASQ*), four questions used to assess if an individual is contemplating suicide. These questions can take less than a minute to ask and can identify youth and adults who are at risk for suicide. See Box 13.2.

Available at https://www.nimh.nih.gov/research/research-conducted-at-nimh/asq-toolkit-materials/

Classroom Activity

Movies and streaming programs with suicide themes that can promote discussion include *The Hours; Girl, Interrupted; Dead Poets Society; 13 Reasons Why;* and *Whose Life Is It Anyway?*

Differential Diagnosis

- borderline personality disorder
- major depression
- substance use disorder
- anxiety disorder
- PTSD
- bipolar disorder
- prolonged grief disorder
- psychotic disorder such as schizophrenia

 TREATMENT OF INDIVIDUALS AT RISK FOR SUICIDE

Suicide is a major public health concern. Prevention is focused on identifying people who display the warning signs and risk factors and providing them with support and interventions. Anyone who talks about suicide must be taken seriously, and interventions must be instituted immediately to address that person's concerns and problems. Individual and group psychotherapy; emergency psychiatric care; access to hotlines and on-call mental health professionals; pharmacological treatment for depression, psychosis, and anxiety; and inpatient hospitalization if the person is at high risk for suicide are some of the approaches that can be used. Patients who make multiple suicide attempts need ongoing psychotherapy to address their issues and impulses. Patients at low-to-moderate risk for suicide can be followed as outpatients with a treatment plan that includes adequate support, such as family and friends, medications, and regular mental health appointments.

Family and friends, as well as health-care providers, of anyone who commits suicide need special support. These survivors of suicide are at risk for long-term emotional distress, especially related to guilt and anger and their elusive search to understand why. The stigma of suicide adds to the complexity of a lifetime of trying to recover. Grieving for survivors of suicide is complicated and often prolonged. Support groups are available in many communities for survivors of suicide.

Tool Box

- Suicidology.org has many resources for suicidal patients, their families, and professionals, including support programs for survivors: www. suicidology.org/suicide-survivors
- National Suicide Prevention Lifeline offers a 24/7 free and confidential nationwide network of crisis centers: 1-800-273-TALK (8255) or 988 or text HOME to 741741
- For deaf or hard of hearing use the preferred relay service or dial 711 then 1-800-273-8255.

NURSING CARE OF THE SUICIDAL PATIENT

Common nursing diagnoses in those at risk for suicide include the following:

- hopelessness
- violence to self, risk for
- anxiety
- coping, ineffective
- self-concept, disturbed
- spiritual distress
- thought processes, altered

Nursing responsibilities for patients who are suicidal are many. The goal, of course, is always

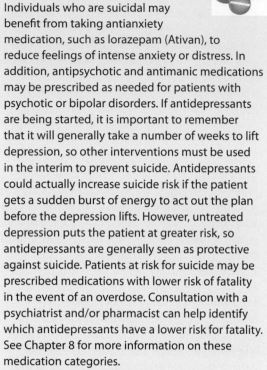

Pharmacology Corner

Individuals who are suicidal may benefit from taking antianxiety medication, such as lorazepam (Ativan), to reduce feelings of intense anxiety or distress. In addition, antipsychotic and antimanic medications may be prescribed as needed for patients with psychotic or bipolar disorders. If antidepressants are being started, it is important to remember that it will generally take a number of weeks to lift depression, so other interventions must be used in the interim to prevent suicide. Antidepressants could actually increase suicide risk if the patient gets a sudden burst of energy to act out the plan before the depression lifts. However, untreated depression puts the patient at greater risk, so antidepressants are generally seen as protective against suicide. Patients at risk for suicide may be prescribed medications with lower risk of fatality in the event of an overdose. Consultation with a psychiatrist and/or pharmacist can help identify which antidepressants have a lower risk for fatality. See Chapter 8 for more information on these medication categories.

Patients at high risk for suicide may need to have medications administered in liquid or parenteral form to avoid "cheeking" and hoarding pills that could be collected to use for an overdose. Outpatients should be given only a few days' supply of any medication that could potentially be used in a suicide attempt.

Adequate symptom management for pain and other distressing symptoms must be provided to the patient with a serious or terminal illness. A patient's belief that their symptoms cannot be controlled could be a contributing factor in hopelessness and suicide.

to prevent the suicide. Because the nurse may not know when suicide potential exists, especially for a first attempt, using excellent observational and communication skills is mandatory. Nurses are bound (under the *Meier v. Ross General Hospital* case) to report any reasons they have to suspect the patient may be suicidal. Nurses must report their observations to their team and document preventive actions in the health-care record. Once a nurse suspects suicidal ideation, informing all members of the health-care team is essential so that appropriate treatment can be initiated and patient safety can be ensured. Never keep information about a patient's suicide plan to yourself as part of maintaining a relationship with a patient. If a patient is considered suicidal, the following interventions can be helpful.

General Nursing Interventions

1. *Frequent monitoring:* In the in-patient setting, check on the suicidal patient frequently but avoid a predictable routine and ensure that the patient is checked during extra busy times like shift change. If the patient is actively suicidal, a psychiatric consultation will be required, and the patient may be placed on 1:1 precautions until the patient can be moved to an appropriate treatment setting. On 1:1 precautions, a staff member will be required to accompany the patient to and remain with the patient in the bathroom. Nurses must follow their agency policies on providing safety for the suicidal patient.
2. *Safety:* Keep any potentially harmful items away from the patient, such as knives, scissors, glass, razor blades, belts, nail files, electrical cords, and even linens. Inform visitors of any restrictions so that they do not bring items the patient may request. Ensure that windows cannot be opened. The room may need to be searched periodically, and the patient may need a body search and close monitoring in the bathroom. It is common for patients who are at very high risk for suicide to wear paper gowns and to have paper bedding. Large objects that can be used to break a window also need to be removed. Plastic trash bags that the patient could use to suffocate themself should not be used in the patient's room.

Tool Box

Use this reference to establish a safe environment for your patient who is suicidal in the inpatient setting:
Revisiting "Suicide Proofing" an Inpatient Unit Through Environmental Safeguards: A Review by Cardell, Bratcher, and Quinnet (2009) available at https://www.researchgate.net/publication/23802104_Revisiting_Suicide_Proofing_an_Inpatient_Unit_Through_Environmental_Safeguards_A_Review

Clinical Activity

• If your patient has been identified as suicidal, review the care plan for all the safety measures in place for this patient.
• Review policies from assigned hospitals on how to manage suicidal patients.

3. *Communication:* Ask outright if the patient is considering suicide and, if so, how and when. A patient is at higher risk if they have a specific plan with a highly lethal method that is available to them. **Asking a patient to talk about suicidal thoughts does not increase the chance of their completing a suicide.** Rather, it demonstrates caring and acknowledges their value as a person. Ask if the patient has attempted suicide in the past. In addition, be prepared to talk to the patient about their feelings, work to reframe hopelessness, and assist in problem-solving to identify alternative solutions to problems the patient views as insurmountable. When talking to someone who is suicidal, avoid platitudes like, "Think what this would do to your children." Often the suicidal person is so immersed in feelings of hopelessness and isolation that they are unable to identify with how others are feeling. In addition, the patient may believe that the family will be better off without them. When working on problem-solving, break down one problem into manageable steps rather than looking at the whole picture, which can be overwhelming. Most people who are suicidal have ambivalent, or mixed, feelings about taking action. Supporting the reasons the person does not want to commit suicide can help the person to reevaluate the situation.

GOOD TO KNOW

• If you suspect someone is suicidal, be direct in asking about their plans.
• Suicide is an emotional subject, and great care must be taken with anyone who expresses suicidal ideation. Report any suicidal ideation or behavior immediately.
• The hopelessness experienced by a suicidal patient can be draining and overwhelming for the nurse. Recognize that team members need extra support when working with anyone who is suicidal.

Clinical Activity

If your patient has a history of suicide attempts, discuss any concerns with your instructor.

See Box 13.3 for suggestions on talking with a suicidal patient to evaluate lethality.

CRITICAL THINKING QUESTION

Your 85-year-old patient is a recent widower. He is in the hospital to recover from a recent fall. He tells you he wants to go home so that he can be with his wife. How would you respond to that statement?

CRITICAL THINKING QUESTION

Your patient with multiple chronic health problems has been diagnosed by the psychiatrist as actively suicidal. She is too ill to be transferred to the psychiatric unit. Describe what actions the team should take to prevent a suicide attempt on your medical surgical unit.

Table 13.2 provides a nursing care plan for suicidal patients.

Box 13.3

Talking With a Suicidal Patient to Evaluate Lethality

1. Do you think about hurting or killing yourself? If yes, ↓
2. Do you have a plan? How have you considered doing it? If yes, ↓
3. Do you think you may or will do something to act on your thoughts? If yes, where and when? Do you feel you have control over your own behavior?
4. Do you have the means available (such as rope, rolled-up sheet, gun, saved-up pills [note lethality of plan])?
5. Have you ever tried to harm yourself in the past? If yes, how? Did you expect to survive?
6. Are you willing to notify staff/therapist whenever you feel you may act on these thoughts?

   *If the patient denies having a suicide plan, ask about other plans for the future and support systems.

1. What do you see yourself doing in a week, in a month, and in a year from now?
2. Do you feel optimistic or pessimistic about the future?
3. Do you have family members or friends with whom you can freely discuss your problems?

Source: From Gorman and Sultan (2008). *Psychosocial Nursing for General Patient Care,* 3rd ed. Philadelphia: F.A. Davis Company, with permission.

Table 13.2

Nursing Care Plan for Suicidal Patients

Assessment/ Data Collection	Nursing Diagnosis	Plan/Goal	Interventions/Nursing Actions	Evaluation
Patient describes hopelessness; unable to view the future in a positive manner; denies options to resolve dilemmas; verbalizes suicide as only alternative	Hopelessness	Verbalize possible solutions to current problems	Listen to patient's concerns and worries. Avoid minimizing them. Help patient identify one problem and discuss alternative ways to view it. Provide a different perspective on the problems. Appeal to the patient's ambivalence by stressing reasons they do not want to do this. Describe a recent situation where you observed the patient being successful.	Patient agrees to try one alternative solution to recent problem.

Classroom Activity

Obtain information about local suicide prevention programs, such as counseling centers and hotlines. Then, share this information with other students and with nursing staff caring for patients.

GOOD TO KNOW

Patients who are terminally ill may verbalize vague suicidal thoughts such as, "I will kill myself if my pain gets too bad." Encourage your patient to talk about fears and discomforts. Patients with good symptom management are much less likely to think about suicide. If you are practicing in a state that has "right-to-die" (also known as *assisted death*) legislation, patients with terminal illnesses may want to discuss their thoughts if they are considering this option. Nurses in these states need to be aware of agency policies concerning the nurse's role with these patients.

Patient/Family Education

- Ensure that family/friends are available for support and supervision.
- Educate family/friends on what to look for regarding suicidal behavior.
- Provide hotline numbers to patient and family.
- Recognize that the vast majority of suicidal individuals are ambivalent and are searching for a way not to act on suicidal thoughts.
- Ensure that any prescriptions that could be used in a suicide attempt are dispensed in small amounts (1–3 day supply) to reduce risk of overdose.
- Ensure that appointments for mental health follow-up are in place.
- Family members and friends can participate in developing a safety plan with the patient. This plan can help identify early symptoms of suicidality, who to call for help, and how to create a safe environment without access to lethal methods such as firearms.

Evidence-Based Practice

Clinical Question: "No-suicide contracts" have been an approach used by mental health clinicians in preventing suicide in the past. Are they effective in reducing the risk of suicide?

Discussion: These contracts are verbal or written agreements in which the patient agrees to contact the professional before acting on a suicide plan.

Evidence: There are little data that this practice has been effective. Its use is not based on research. In fact, use of these agreements can give a false sense of security to the clinician that the patient will uphold the contract. These contracts are particularly risky in short-term encounters with the patient, like in an emergency department where there is no long-term relationship. Emphasis should rather be on establishing a safety plan, also known as a *crisis response plan*, of what to do in case of increased suicidality rather than a contract.

Implications for Nursing Practice: Interventions must be individualized rather than relying on a standardized contract.

Hoffman, R. (2013). Contracting for safety: A misused tool. *Pennsylvania Patient Safety Advisory*, 10(2):82-4. Available at http://patientsafety.pa.gov/ADVISORIES/Pages/201306_82.aspx
Puskar, K., Urda, B. (2011). Examining the efficacy of no-suicide contracts in inpatient psychiatric settings: Implications for psychiatric nursing. *Issues Ment Health Nurs.* 32(12):785-8. doi: 10.3109/01612840.2011.599476. PMID: 22077751

Clinical Activity

When administering medications to suicidal patients, consider having a colleague with you to double-check that the patient has swallowed the pills.

Key Points

- Suicide is the 12th leading cause of death in this country and remains a serious public health problem. All nurses must be aware of risk factors and warning signs for suicide in their patients and take action as needed.
- Caring for a suicidal patient requires excellent observation and communication skills, including working collaboratively with team members to keep the patient safe.

- Open communication with the person who expresses suicidal ideation is essential.
- The most common psychiatric diagnoses for suicidal patients include depression and substance abuse.
- Most people considering suicide have some ambivalence, so they will often leave clues as to their plans.
- Family, friends, and health-care providers of someone who commits suicide need special support.

Safe and Effective Nursing Care

Provide a safe environment, free from potential hazards for self-injury.

Maintain adequate supervision.

Support open communication for the patient to express fears and feelings.

Ensure adequate support is available for the suicidal patient and for staff caring for a potentially suicidal patient.

CASE STUDY

Jeff is a 54-year-old man who is recently divorced with four grown children. He is living alone in a furnished apartment and was recently laid off from his accounting job. He spends most days alone and has started drinking in the morning. He recently got a DUI and had to give up his driver's license. He has been a hunter all his life and has a variety of guns in a local storage unit. He has several close friends who report that Jeff is depressed, irritable, and much less sociable than he used to be. They call him to go out, but he repeatedly declines. One friend calls Jeff's ex-wife to tell her that Jeff called him and was quite emotional, saying he feels guilty for the way he treated her and his children over the years. Jeff told the friend he feels like a failure in life and wonders if his kids would be better off if he were not around. The friend tells Jeff's ex-wife that he believes Jeff is thinking of moving away. Jeff's friend and ex-wife decide to work together to get help for Jeff.

1. With the information presented, what signs suggest that Jeff may be suicidal?
2. What suggestions would you give Jeff's ex-wife and his friend to address potential suicidal ideation?
3. If Jeff's friend brought him to your mental health clinic, what information would you want to know initially?
4. What should be considered for a safety plan for Jeff?

Review Questions

1. A nursing intervention that is appropriate for a patient who is suicidal is:
   a. Report the patient to the police.
   b. Ignore the patient's suicidal comments, considering them "attention getting."
   c. Tell the patient that they "have so much to live for!"
   d. Listen to the patient's concerns and worries.

2. A person is more likely to commit suicide when they:
   a. Are in deepest depression
   b. Have a sudden lift from previous depressed mood
   c. Are confused
   d. Are feeling loved and appreciated

3. Your patient tells you, "I am just a burden. Everyone would be better off if I was dead." Nurses are aware that:
   a. Suicide talk is just an attention-getting device.
   b. Suicide is an impulsive act; it is not thought out.
   c. Suicidal talk or ideation can lead to suicidal behavior.
   d. Suicidal people seldom really attempt suicide.

4. Mr. P is brought to the hospital by his wife. She states that he has been treated for depression recently, but that tonight he said, "You and the kids don't need me messing up your lives." Mr. P tells you he has been thinking about suicide for some time now. A nursing diagnosis for Mr. P would be:
   a. Knowledge deficit related to family needs
   b. Ineffective individual coping as evidenced by manipulation of wife's feelings
   c. Anxiety related to hospitalization
   d. Potential for violence, self-directed, as evidenced by stating suicidal thoughts

5. Your charge nurse tells you that Mr. P must be placed on suicide precautions. The first intervention you begin is:
   a. Place Mr. P in a locked unit.
   b. Begin one-on-one observation at least every 15 minutes.
   c. Call the security code over the public address system.
   d. Allow Mr. P to shave and carry out his bedtime care.

6. Further discussion with Mr. P reveals that he believes there is honor in dying for one's religion. He does not understand why everyone is so afraid to die in this country. As his nurse, you:
   a. Document the discussion and remove the suicide precautions, citing religious freedom.
   b. Encourage him to present his beliefs at group tomorrow.
   c. Document the discussion but tell him that the suicide precautions remain in effect.
   d. Thank him for his explanation and bring him his next dose of medication.

7. Statistically, which of the following people is at highest risk for suicide based on the information provided?
   a. Nancy is a 33-year-old mother of two who just lost her mother in a motor vehicle accident.
   b. Jim is a 68-year-old recent widower with a long history of alcohol abuse.
   c. Carol, age 18, has a long history of sickle cell disease and is depressed over chronic pain and the inability to attend her prom.
   d. Hans is a 55-year-old man with end-stage pancreatic cancer who is entering a hospice program.

8. Susan is 27 years old and has been admitted from the emergency department (ED) with an overdose of an antidepressant. She tells you, "My boyfriend broke up with me, and I can't live without him." What is your best response?
   a. "You are young. You will find someone else."
   b. "Forget him. You can do better than him. He isn't worth losing your life for."
   c. "Why did he break up with you?"
   d. "You must have been feeling very sad."

9. The next day, Susan tells you that she has another plan to "finish the job when I get out of here. Please don't tell anyone." What would be your best response?
   a. "You are safe here."
   b. "What are you planning to do?"
   c. "I won't tell anyone if you promise not to do anything to yourself."
   d. "I was hoping you were feeling better."

10. The fact that Susan is telling you she has another plan indicates what?
    a. She is reaching out for help and is ambivalent about wanting to die.
    b. She is committed to her suicide plan.
    c. She is psychotic.
    d. She needs antidepressants started right away.

REVIEW QUESTIONS ANSWER KEY 1.d, 2.b, 3.c, 4.d, 5.b, 6.c, 7.b, 8.d, 9.b, 10.a

CHAPTER 14
Personality Disorders

KEY TERMS

Anhedonia
Antisocial personality disorder
Avoidant personality disorder
Borderline personality disorder
Dependent personality disorder
Histrionic personality disorder
Magical thinking
Narcissistic personality disorder
Obsessive-compulsive disorder (OCD)
Obsessive-compulsive personality disorder
Paranoid personality disorder
Personality
Personality disorder
Schizoid personality disorder
Schizotypal personality disorder
Self-mutilating behavior
Splitting

CHAPTER CONCEPTS

Communication
Family
Mood and affect
Self
Stress and coping

LEARNING OUTCOMES

1. Define and differentiate between personality and personality disorder.
2. Describe three personality disorders designated by the *Diagnostic and Statistical Manual of Mental Disorders,* 5th edition, Text Revision (DSM-5-TR).
3. Describe two behavioral symptoms of each of these three personality disorders.
4. Identify nursing interventions for these three disorders.
5. Discuss some of the challenges in caring for a patient with borderline personality disorder.

Personality is defined as the complex characteristics that distinguish an individual. It includes that person's thoughts, feelings, and attitudes. Personality traits are enduring patterns of perceiving, relating to, and thinking about the environment and oneself that are exhibited in a wide range of social and personal contexts. Personality development occurs in response to a number of biological and psychological influences.

Theorists of personality development include Erik Erikson, Harry Stack Sullivan, and Margaret Mahler.

Personality disorders occur when these traits become inflexible and contribute to maladaptive patterns of behavior or impairments in functioning. Most people display some traits of these disorders from time to time, but only when these traits contribute to some dysfunction in different areas of life do they become personality disorders. Personality disorders are frequently seen and are estimated at 9.1% of the general population (Lenzenweger, Lane, Loranger, & Kessler, 2007). They may coexist with other psychiatric disorders. They are most commonly diagnosed in adulthood after one's personality is fully developed. The most common characteristic of personality disorders is dysfunction in interpersonal relationships (Bornstein, Bianucci, Fishman, & Biars, 2014). It is common that more than one personality disorder exists in these patients. Patients with these disorders as their primary diagnosis are often not treated in psychiatric settings. However, nurses will encounter these patients in all areas of health care. Patients with these disorders can present challenges for the nurse, as maladaptive mechanisms including manipulation are used to cope with the stresses of their illnesses.

Cultural Considerations

Personality development is influenced by culture. Thoughts, feelings, and attitudes are shaped by the cultural values surrounding people.

The DSM-5-TR describes 10 personality disorders and groups them in three clusters based on their similarities (see Table 14.1).

Generally, personality disorders include one or more of the following traits:

- negative affect: frequently experiences negative emotions
- detachment: withdraws from others
- antagonism: is difficult to get along with
- disinhibition: is impulsive
- inflexibility: clings to rigid or fixed ideas

Personality disorders often have their roots in difficult relationships with parental figures. Although each disorder has its own dynamics, this relationship is the thread that runs through all of them. Genetics may be a factor in some of these disorders as well.

TYPES OF PERSONALITY DISORDERS

Cluster A
Paranoid Personality Disorder

Individuals with **paranoid personality disorder** present with behaviors of suspiciousness and mistrust of other people. The person displays consistent mistrust of others' motives. These individuals may seem "normal" in their speech and activity, except for the fact that they consistently feel people treat them unfairly. People with paranoid personality disorder are prone to filing lawsuits when they feel wronged in some way. They tend to be guarded and secretive because they cannot trust others. They may have difficulty maintaining focused eye contact, for example, because they are so alert to other activity around them. People with paranoid personality disorder are not easily able to laugh at themselves; they take themselves very seriously. They may not show tender emotions and may seem cold and calculating in their relationships. They are reluctant to confide in others and tend to take comments, events, and situations very personally, perhaps thinking that others are going to take advantage of them. Sometimes these individuals are said to "have a chip on their shoulder." They have an excessive need to be self-sufficient, which can create challenges if they become ill. As a general rule, a person with paranoid personality disorder avoids the health-care system, if possible.

Patients with paranoid personality disorder are not psychotic and do not have hallucinations and

Table 14.1
The Personality Disorder Clusters

Cluster A (Behaviors Described as Odd)	Cluster B (Behaviors Described as Dramatic)	Cluster C (Behaviors Described as Anxious or Fearful)
• Paranoid personality disorder • Schizoid personality disorder • Schizotypal personality disorder	• Antisocial personality disorder • Borderline personality disorder • Histrionic personality disorder • Narcissistic personality disorder	• Avoidant personality disorder • Dependent personality disorder • Obsessive-compulsive personality disorder

delusions as in schizophrenia; they are, however, suspicious of other people and situations. The suspiciousness may cross into other areas of the person's life. For instance, it may be very challenging to enlist the cooperation of a person with this disorder when it comes to taking medications if the patient suspects ulterior motives.

Paranoid personality disorder seems to have a high incidence of occurrence within families with a history of schizophrenia, which supports the theory of a genetic component to this disorder. Difficult parental relationships in which the child is used as a scapegoat for parents' aggression and childhood neglect can be contributors as well.

DIFFERENTIAL DIAGNOSES
- schizophrenia spectrum
- substance use disorder
- schizoid or schizotypal personality disorders

Cultural Considerations

Recent immigrants to the United States may exhibit some traits that can be viewed as paranoid by others due to their unfamiliarity with society's rules and expectations. This would not be considered a paranoid personality disorder unless it became pervasive and created more problems for the person.

Schizoid Personality Disorder

People with **schizoid personality disorder** have a pattern of detachment from social relationships and a restricted range of expression of emotions in interpersonal settings. They may appear shy, awkward, and introverted. They have trouble developing friendships. They tend to respond in a very serious, factual manner that is pleasant, but not warm or inviting. They may be described by others as "cold."

It is unusual to see patients hospitalized in a psychiatric facility for this disorder because they are so quiet that the disorder often goes unnoticed. They often are described by others as "loners." It is common to see people with this type of personality become very engrossed in books. The books may be a substitute for human companionship. Partly because of this aversion to social interaction, people with schizoid personalities tend to be very intellectual and can be very successful in life, if they choose a career that fits their personality. They may

appear indifferent to the approval or criticism of others.

It is believed that ineffective and unemotional parenting may contribute to this disorder. A family history of schizophrenia or schizotypal personality disorder supports a genetic link. Parental relationships are often lacking in empathy and nurturance.

DIFFERENTIAL DIAGNOSIS
- schizophrenia spectrum
- autism spectrum disorders
- obsessive compulsive personality disorder
- substance use disorder

Schizotypal Personality Disorder

Behaviors in **schizotypal personality disorder** are often odd and eccentric, but not to the level of schizophrenia (see Chapter 15). However, under stress, this person may decompensate with psychotic symptoms such as delusions and hallucinations. Individuals with this disorder are more similar to people with schizophrenia than to people with schizoid personality disorder. Because they can seem to be living in their own world, individuals with schizotypal personalities can experience unusual reactions such as **magical thinking**, a primitive form of thinking in which an individual believes that thinking about a possible occurrence can make it happen. They can exhibit belief in clairvoyance or superstitions. These individuals are aloof and isolated and may use language and gestures that only they understand. They have reduced capacity for close relationships. Often appearing blank and apathetic, their emotional responses may seem inappropriate. They also may display paranoia and social anxiety. Diagnosis is made by a mental health professional who looks at symptoms and life history.

Origins of this disorder may include poor relationships with parental figures characterized by discomfort with affection and closeness, leading to distrust in personal relationships. This disorder is more common among first-degree relatives of people with schizophrenia, suggesting genetic and biological links. Schizotypal personality disorder is now considered part of the genetic spectrum of schizophrenia (American Psychiatric Association, 2013).

DIFFERENTIAL DIAGNOSIS
- schizophrenia spectrum
- paranoid or schizoid personality disorders
- substance use disorders
- neurodevelopmental disorders in children

Cluster B
Antisocial Personality Disorder

Sometimes referred to as *sociopaths*, people with **antisocial personality disorder** disregard the rights of others with a pattern of irresponsibility and exploitation. This often leads them to a path of violating rules, lying, stealing, participating in a variety of illegal activities, and other infringements of the law. The disorder seems to affect males more frequently than females and affects about 3% of the total U.S. population versus 50% of the prison population (Hatchett, 2015). The serial killer Ted Bundy is one of the best-known sociopaths. When these individuals end up in the court system, they may become part of the healthcare system to avoid legal consequences or due to court order. These individuals have difficulty handling frustration and anger. They seldom feel affection, loyalty, or guilt, and show very little concern for the rights or feelings of anyone else. It is rare that they display true remorse for their acts. People who have this disorder are also at high risk for substance abuse. In addition, impulsiveness and irresponsibility are major features of the disorder, with actions poorly planned. This type of person has difficulty with close relationships and may change jobs and relationships frequently. Abusive relationships can occur.

In spite of their inability to feel or show affection, patients with antisocial personality disorder are usually gregarious, intelligent, charismatic, and likable but can quickly move to aggression if frustrated. They may take risks with little regard for the safety of others.

Because people with antisocial personality disorder are frequently highly intelligent, they learn the jargon of psychology and know how to manipulate it. Those with antisocial personality disorder are difficult to treat as they often have little motivation to change. Healthcare professionals need to approach these patients with consistency and set clear limits and boundaries.

It is widely believed that the roots of this disorder stem from dysfunctional parenting and family life. This may be from a permissive or authoritarian parenting style that does not include guidelines for appropriate social behavior and includes abuse.

A chaotic family life is often found. This personality disorder may be displayed in childhood with signs of callousness and lack of empathy. Childhood bullying and cruelty, animal abuse, as well as manipulative behaviors are seen at an early age. Individuals may have been diagnosed with conduct disorder before age 15 (see Chapter 19). These behaviors can run in families, so a genetic link is also suspected. Some evidence also exists that there may be brain abnormalities in how the individual processes emotions.

DIFFERENTIAL DIAGNOSES
- substance use disorder
- bipolar disorder
- narcissistic, borderline, or histrionic personality disorders

GOOD TO KNOW

Patients with an antisocial personality can be challenging as they can use unscrupulous means to accomplish their goals without the staff realizing it.

CRITICAL THINKING QUESTION

You are working on a substance abuse unit. When you walk on the unit, you see a patient named **Brad** chatting with a number of nursing staff. He is telling funny stories about celebrities, and many of the nurses seem to be enjoying themselves. Brad is quite handsome and charming. After this occurrence, Brad asks one of the nurses for a special privilege to take a walk off the unit. How would you advise this nurse to handle this request?

When the nurse denies the patient's request, he quickly changes from charming to cruel as he insults the nurse and then knocks over a lamp. How should the staff respond?

Borderline Personality Disorder

Borderline personality disorder (sometimes known as BPD) is the most frequent personality disorder seen in the clinical setting, affecting 1.4% of the general population and 20% of psychiatric inpatients (Lenzenweger, Lane, Loranger, & Kessler, 2007; National Educational Alliance for Borderline Personality Disorders, 2021). *Instability* is often the first word associated with BPD. Individuals with this disorder often exhibit both clinging and distancing behavior as they struggle with fears of separation and abandonment. They are known for intense and chaotic relationships as well as self-destructive, impulsive, and dramatic coping. A chronic sense of emptiness, poor self-image, and excessive self-criticism are part of this disorder. These individuals operate using ingrained behavior patterns that involve manipulating others to achieve their goals to reduce anxiety. These patients may also utilize **self-mutilating behaviors**, including self-inflicted superficial cuts (known as *cutting*), which usually are not performed with suicidal intent (FIG. 14.1). Cutting can be a way to reduce tension, to inflict pain to validate one's feelings, to challenge a pervasive sense of emptiness, or to seek attention. However, suicide attempts can be part of the self-destructive pattern. Substance abuse is also often a factor as the person tries to control the anxiety.

BPD is much more common in females than in males. It usually begins in adolescence and early adulthood. BPD is a relatively new classification as it was not recognized by psychiatry until 1980. It was given the name *borderline* originally as a way to categorize individuals who did not classically conform to the standard categories of neuroses or psychoses, although this really does not describe the condition very well. Current ideas about BPD focus on ongoing patterns of difficulty with self-regulation (the ability to soothe oneself in times of stress) and trouble with emotions, thinking, behaviors, relationships, and self-image. Some people refer to BPD as *emotional dysregulation*.

The origins of BPD can include coming from an abusive background where one was dismissed by authority figures. Poor relationships with parental figures involving issues of abandonment and dependency are often seen. Traumatic childhood experiences that cause the individual to feel unsafe may be another factor. Defense mechanisms of denial, projection, and **splitting** (the inability to integrate positive and negative feelings at the same time) are known to be commonly used. Splitting is manifested by a patient who needs to see others as all good or all bad. For example, a nurse who is caring during one shift may be viewed by a borderline patient as the idealized "perfect" nurse, and then the nurse who sets limits on another shift is called "a poor excuse for a nurse."

Because of the high incidence of major depression and substance use disorders in first-degree relatives of people with BPD along with the challenges to self-regulation, genetic and biological factors are believed to contribute to this diagnosis. See FIGURE 14.2 for a concept map for a patient with BPD.

DIFFERENTIAL DIAGNOSES
- depressive disorders
- anxiety disorders
- post-traumatic stress disorder
- eating disorders
- substance use disorders

GOOD TO KNOW

Recognizing staff splitting is essential for good care of the patient with BPD. If a patient complains about other staff members, never encourage them. Rather, point out that the patient needs to address their concerns with the individual and not complain about staff members to others. Avoid taking sides or acting as an intermediary.

Tool Box

Psych Central has a 12-question screening test for BPD: https://psychcentral.com/quizzes/borderline-test/

Clinical Activity

When you are informed that your patient has a borderline personality, get specific information on interventions that the team has been using to avoid getting in the middle of conflict between the patient and staff.

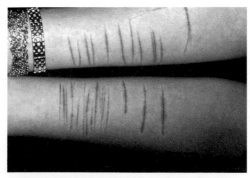

FIGURE 14.1 Self-inflicted lacerations on a teenage girl's arms.

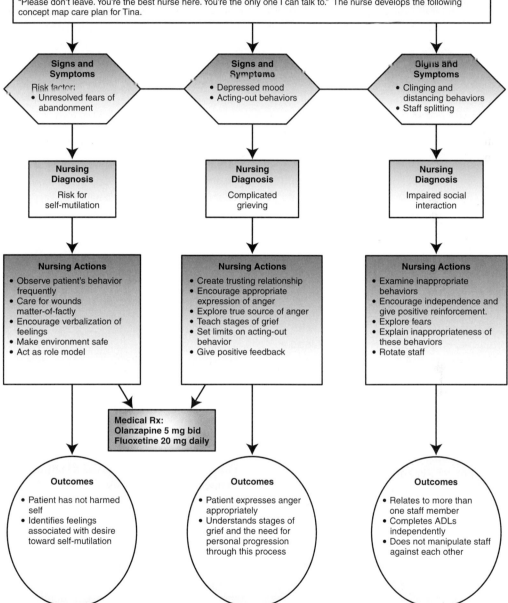

Clinical Vignette: Tina, age 37, was diagnosed with Borderline Personality Disorder when she was 22 years old. She has had counseling with the same therapist since the initial diagnosis. She suffers from chronic depression and unstable personality. Two days ago, at her regular counseling session, the therapist told Tina that in 1 month she was getting married and would be moving across the country with her new husband. She told Tina that she would help her find a new therapist. Tina became hysterical and shouted, "You can't leave me! I don't want another therapist!" That evening, Tina's husband, Bill, found her sitting in a pool of blood in the bathroom, having sliced the back of both calves with a razor blade. Bill took Tina to the hospital where she is well known by the staff. Her wounds were treated in the emergency department, and she was transferred to the psychiatric unit. She clings to the admitting nurse saying, "Please don't leave. You're the best nurse here. You're the only one I can talk to." The nurse develops the following concept map care plan for Tina.

Signs and Symptoms

Risk factor:
- Unresolved fears of abandonment

Signs and Symptoms
- Depressed mood
- Acting-out behaviors

Signs and Symptoms
- Clinging and distancing behaviors
- Staff splitting

Nursing Diagnosis

Risk for self-mutilation

Nursing Diagnosis

Complicated grieving

Nursing Diagnosis

Impaired social interaction

Nursing Actions
- Observe patient's behavior frequently
- Care for wounds matter-of-factly
- Encourage verbalization of feelings
- Make environment safe
- Act as role model

Nursing Actions
- Create trusting relationship
- Encourage appropriate expression of anger
- Explore true source of anger
- Teach stages of grief
- Set limits on acting-out behavior
- Give positive feedback

Nursing Actions
- Examine inappropriate behaviors
- Encourage independence and give positive reinforcement.
- Explore fears
- Explain inappropriateness of these behaviors
- Rotate staff

Medical Rx:
Olanzapine 5 mg bid
Fluoxetine 20 mg daily

Outcomes
- Patient has not harmed self
- Identifies feelings associated with desire toward self-mutilation

Outcomes
- Patient expresses anger appropriately
- Understands stages of grief and the need for personal progression through this process

Outcomes
- Relates to more than one staff member
- Completes ADLs independently
- Does not manipulate staff against each other

FIGURE 14.2 Concept map: borderline personality disorder. (From Morgan & Townsend [2021]. Psychiatric Mental Health Nursing, 10th ed. Philadelphia: F.A. Davis Company, with permission.)

GOOD TO KNOW
Although cutting behaviors are more common in adolescents, they can occur in adults.

Tool Box

Borderline Personality Disorder information for patients and families:
https://www.nimh.nih.gov/health/topics/borderline-personality-disorder/index.shtml
BPD Central with information for patients and families:
www.bpdcentral.com/
Useful books for family members include *The Essential Family Guide to Borderline Personality* (2008) by Randi Kreger and *The Stop Walking on Eggshells Workbook* by Paul T. Mason and Randi Kreger.

CRITICAL THINKING QUESTION

A 25-year-old woman is admitted from the emergency department (ED) to your unit with superficial cuts on both arms and a high blood-alcohol level. She states that she was attacked by her boyfriend. She is emotional and angry. As you sit with her to complete the admission, she shares with you that she cut her arms to get her boyfriend to "love" her. You are called out of the room. When you return, the patient yells at you and says she wants another nurse. She does not trust you.

This patient was diagnosed with borderline personality. Describe why she may have reacted so negatively to you when you returned to the room.

Histrionic Personality Disorder

Histrionic personality disorder is characterized by dramatic, excessive, extroverted behaviors in someone who has a pattern of strong emotions. Excessive attention-seeking, seductive, and provocative behaviors are additionally seen. Some may describe the person as theatrical. They are known to be highly distractible and even flighty. Delaying gratification is challenging for them as is maintaining close, intimate relationships, despite their gregarious and flirtatious behaviors. Their constant need for approval and affection can lead to disappointment, dejection, and anxiety.

This disorder is more common in women. Childhood experiences of needing to be dramatic to get recognition or needs met and lack of feedback from parents about appropriate behavior contribute to the development of this disorder. Genetics also are believed to play a role, as histrionic personality is common among first-degree relatives of people with this disorder.

DIFFERENTIAL DIAGNOSES
- other personality disorders including borderline, antisocial, and narcissistic
- substance use disorder

GOOD TO KNOW
Having histrionic traits does not mean the person has histrionic personality disorder. To have the disorder, the person would have consistent problems functioning in life as a result of these traits.

Cultural Considerations

Cultural background can dictate social behavior. It is important to consider the patient's whole picture, including their cultural norms, before making assumptions about a potential diagnosis.

Narcissistic Personality Disorder

Those who have **narcissistic personality disorder** tend to display an exaggerated impression of self with an inflated sense of self-importance. They are preoccupied with fantasies of unlimited success. Another characteristic is limited ability to empathize with others' problems because they see everything through their own eyes. They have a tendency to overestimate their abilities, are attention seeking, and are surprised if they do not receive admiration from others. While projecting an image of invulnerability, their deep sense of emptiness is hidden from others. These individuals have difficulty maintaining close relationships. Narcissistic personality disorder is more common in men.

People with this disorder will seem to take criticism lightly. In reality, deep feelings of anger, resentment, and poor self-esteem are being repressed. Friends will be chosen according to how good they make the person with the narcissistic personality feel.

Often, these people are children of narcissistic parental figures who were perfectionistic as well as very critical and demanding of their children. The children then model their parent's behaviors. Another environmental factor can be parents who live vicariously through their child and do not subject the child to restrictions and limitations. Narcissistic traits are particularly common in adolescents even though they do not necessarily have the disorder.

DIFFERENTIAL DIAGNOSES
• bipolar disorder (tendency toward grandiosity)
• other personality disorders including borderline, antisocial, and histrionic

CRITICAL THINKING QUESTION
You are working on a psychiatric unit, and your patient with narcissistic personality disorder tells you that she plans to get the lead in a play once she leaves the hospital. She tells you she has always been successful in every audition she has had. What concerns would you have for this patient? How would you respond to her statements?

Cluster C
Avoidant Personality Disorder
Individuals with **avoidant personality disorder** are extremely sensitive and may avoid social situations to protect themselves from possible rejection. They appear awkward and uncomfortable in social settings. They may be considered shy, but the pattern of avoiding close relationships goes beyond shyness and leads to a restricted life. These people have a strong need to be accepted, but they often view others as critical of them. They want a close relationship but avoid it because of fear of being rejected. Characteristics include low self-esteem, avoidance of close relationships, anxiety, and **anhedonia**, or lack of pleasure in life. They are very hesitant to engage in new activities due to fear of failure. Highly critical parental figures are believed to be the origin. A history of early trauma or neglect may lead to fears of abandonment. There also may be a hereditary link.

DIFFERENTIAL DIAGNOSES
• depressive disorders
• anxiety disorder
• dependent personality disorder

Dependent Personality Disorder
Dependent personality disorder is characterized by a pervasive and excessive need to be taken care of that leads to submissive and clinging behaviors along with fears of separation. These behaviors tend to elicit caregiving responses in others, including nurses. People with dependent personality disorder want others to make decisions for them; they tend to feel inferior, to be suggestible, and to have a tendency toward self-doubt. These individuals often appear helpless and avoid responsibility. They often have an intense fear of being alone. They may go out of their way to be generous and giving to others as a way to find acceptance, but internally they lack confidence and anticipate rejection. Individuals with this disorder tend to take everything to heart and go out of their way to satisfy people they feel close to and try to change those personality traits that people criticize.

An inordinate amount of fear exists among people who experience dependent personality disorder. It may be the fear of criticism that brings about their inability to make decisions. Inability to make decisions can be severe enough as to limit a person's meaningful social interactions. In the health-care setting, these dependency behaviors can lead to a disturbed nurse-patient relationship. The need to accept some dependency is often part of facing a serious illness. Those with dependent personality exhibit more maladaptive and extreme behavior than would be seen in more adaptive forms of dependency.

Cultural Considerations
The behaviors described here as symptomatic of dependent personality disorder are typical behaviors expected of women in certain cultures.

Seriously overprotective parents who discourage independence and promote dependence in the child can be a contributing factor for this disorder. These parents may "protect" the child from unfamiliar experiences. The child can fear a loss of parental love when seeking out autonomous experiences. Chronic physical illness in childhood can also predispose a person to this disorder.

DIFFERENTIAL DIAGNOSES
• other personality disorders, including histrionic and borderline

• depressive disorders
• panic disorder

Obsessive-Compulsive Personality Disorder

Individuals with **obsessive-compulsive personality disorder** are disciplined and rigid to an extreme. They are meticulous and demand accuracy and discipline in others. They exhibit rigid perfectionism that is polar opposite to disinhibition (American Psychiatric Association, 2017). They are preoccupied with details, rules, and order. They display a stubborn streak in order to maintain control so that things are done their way, and they have trouble expressing emotions. A calm exterior may hide the anger, ambivalence, and conflict the person is experiencing. They may appear polite and formal but can be autocratic and critical with others. They demonstrate persistence at tasks long after the behavior has ceased to be functional or effective and continue the same behaviors despite repeated failures or obvious annoyance by others. The fear of making mistakes can lead to an inability to make any decisions. The origins of obsessive-compulsive personality include overcontrolling parents. The disorder does run in families, so a genetic component is also suspected. This personality disorder differs from what is known as **obsessive compulsive disorder (OCD)**.

OCD is characterized by recurrent obsessions (repetitive thoughts, urges, or emotions) and compulsions (repetitive acts that may appear purposeful) that interfere with daily functioning and are an effort to maintain control. This disorder is now believed to be a neurological "short circuit" that causes repetitive behaviors. A genetic link among families who display OCD has also been suggested. Previously thought to be an anxiety disorder, OCD is now in its own category, obsessive-compulsive and related disorders, in the DSM-5. An example of compulsive behaviors is repeatedly checking that doors are locked before being able to leave the house. This can escalate to the person being unable to leave the house because they are unable to stop thinking about or acting on locking the doors. Another example is a person who has a strict, ritualistic way of doing something and who, if interrupted, has to start over at the beginning. When these thoughts and behaviors negatively affect the person's life, the diagnosis of OCD can be made.

DIFFERENTIAL DIAGNOSES
• OCD
• hoarding disorder
• schizoid personality disorder
• anxiety disorder

GOOD TO KNOW

It is possible for an individual to have more than one personality disorder. Often, the additional diagnosis is in the same cluster group.

Classroom Activity

Watch films that portray characters with personality disorders and discuss their characteristics: *One Flew Over the Cuckoo's Nest* (antisocial), *Fatal Attraction* (borderline), *Wall Street* (narcissistic), *Taxi Driver* (schizoid), *Nightcrawler* (antisocial), *Welcome to Me* (borderline), *The Squid and the Whale* (narcissistic), *Girl, Interrupted* (borderline)

PSYCHIATRIC TREATMENT OF PERSONALITY DISORDERS

Because personality disorders become ingrained early in life, treatment is often difficult. People with personality disorders may not seek treatment for their disorder at all, or they may wait until it drains their coping reserves. At times, these patients will demonstrate resistance to treatment. Treatment may be involuntary after a crisis or due to entrance into the legal system. Psychotherapy, cognitive behavioral therapy (CBT), and group therapy may be useful in some situations. Maintaining a long-standing trusting relationship with a therapist can be advantageous. Medications to treat anxiety, depression, and delusions are often used. Family members of people with personality disorders often benefit from family therapy and psycho-education around coping with them.

GOOD TO KNOW

Although people with personality disorders may not seek mental health treatment, they often enter the health-care system for other problems. Patients with personality disorders present many challenges to nurses. These patients may display rigid behavior patterns and be socially inappropriate.

Pharmacology Corner

Many patients with these disorders experience anxiety, so antianxiety medications are often prescribed. Borderline personality patients may be treated with SSRIs (selective serotonin reuptake inhibitors) to manage impulsivity. SSRIs have been used to treat obsessive compulsive personality disorder as well as OCD. Antipsychotics may be used with patients with psychotic features such as schizotypal disorders. For patients prone to violence, antipsychotics may also be needed. Because many of these patients are susceptible to substance abuse to self-medicate, close monitoring of drug abuse should be included in the treatment plan.

GOOD TO KNOW

Compliance with a prescribed medication regimen can be challenging. Some patients may have a tendency to avoid following instructions or may act impulsively.

GOOD TO KNOW

Nurses need to display much patience and acceptance as part of the care plan for an individual with a personality disorder.

CRITICAL THINKING QUESTION

Your patient with a diagnosis of avoidant personality requests alprazolam (Xanax) before a group therapy session. Describe what this medication accomplishes for the patient and suggest alternative approaches in place of medication.

NURSING CARE OF PATIENTS WITH PERSONALITY DISORDERS

Common nursing diagnoses used with personality disorders include the following:

- coping, defensive
- personal identity, disturbed
- self-esteem, disturbed
- self-mutilation, risk for
- social interactions, impaired
- violence, self-directed, risk for

General Nursing Interventions for Personality Disorders

See Table 14.2 for a summary of nursing interventions for each personality disorder and Table 14.3, which details the nursing care plan for patients with borderline personality.

Table 14.2
Nursing Interventions for Personality Disorders

Type	Symptoms	Nursing Interventions
Antisocial	• Requires immediate self-gratification • Often in trouble with the law • Has difficulty handling frustration and anger • Seldom feels affection, loyalty, guilt, or remorse • Shows very little concern for the rights or feelings of others • Good at manipulating others for personal gain • High risk for substance abuse • Usually gregarious, charming, intelligent, and likable	• Promote positive, healthy interpersonal relationships • Monitor for violent behaviors • Provide feedback on negative behaviors • Encourage appropriate expression of anger • Support analysis of feelings • Point out effect of manipulative behavior • Avoid negotiating rewards • Set limits. Establish clear expectations

Continued

Table 14.2

Nursing Interventions for Personality Disorders—cont'd

Type	Symptoms	Nursing Interventions
Avoidant	• Avoids social situations • Preoccupied with thoughts of being rejected or criticized • Low self-esteem • Avoids new activities for fear of being embarrassed • Anhedonia	• Promote self-esteem by acknowledging any success • Encourage participation in supportive social situations • Provide emotional support • Teach calming techniques to deal with anxiety • Reinforce strengths
Borderline	• Moods unstable and changeable • Uncertainty regarding self-concept • Substance abuse • Suicide attempts • Difficulty handling strong emotion • Bored and empty feelings • Fear of being alone • Self-destructive behaviors • Self-mutilation (including cutting) • Manipulative • Feels most comfortable by creating chaos around them	• Remain calm in presence of patient's drama • Build trusting relationship • Set limits and establish clear ground rules that are followed by everyone • Establish therapeutic communication • Demonstrate positive role modeling • Monitor for self-destructive behaviors • Provide safety/security • Communicate a consistent plan of care among all staff • Encourage patient to verbalize feelings rather than act them out • Avoid power struggles • Involve family and friends in treatment plan • Recognize patient's need to create instability, see others in extremes (e.g., all good or all bad)
Dependent	• Dependent and submissive • Wants others to make decisions for them • Tends to feel inferior, is suggestible, and doubts self • Tends to appear helpless and to avoid responsibility • Tends to take everything to heart—eager to satisfy people they feel close to and to change personality traits that people criticize • Inordinate amount of fear	• Allow patient to make some decisions for their treatment • Reinforce the patient's decisions • Encourage patient to make truthful, positive self-statements each shift • Recognize patient's insecurities and anxieties

Table 14.2

Nursing Interventions for Personality Disorders—cont'd

Type	Symptoms	Nursing Interventions
Histrionic	• Demonstrates dramatic behaviors, especially in situations where this would not be expected • Exaggerated, theatrical, and demonstrative emotions • Easily influenced by others • Rapidly shifting emotions • Provocative behaviors to draw attention to self	• Support healthy coping • Offer reassurance • Support consistent healthy relationships • Give appropriate feedback • Maintain calm demeanor
Narcissistic	• Exaggerated self-image • Appears self-centered • Lacks empathy for others' problems • Expresses need for self-importance • Appears to take criticism lightly but in reality represses feelings of anger and resentment • Expresses sense of entitlement • Cheerful, carefree mood can quickly change to distress if criticized	• Encourage patient to learn to accept limitations in self and others • Give patient feedback on how others are responding to patient • Prepare patient for possible setbacks • Recognize the patient is very sensitive to hurt feelings • Encourage the patient to talk about their vulnerabilities
Obsessive-compulsive	• Rigid behavior • Preoccupied with rules • Formal • Perfectionistic • Intense fear of making mistakes • Appears calm on outside, deals with intense conflict and hostility internally	• Acknowledge patient's fears and be flexible to their needs • Allow patient to make simple decisions with limited choices • Establish trusting, supportive relationship • Discuss alternative strategies for dealing with new situations • Support healthy coping mechanisms to deal with stress
Paranoid	• Suspicious and mistrustful of other people • May seem "normal" in speech and activity • Believes that people treat them unfairly • Hypersensitive to activity in the environment • Finds it difficult to maintain focused eye contact • Not easily able to laugh at themselves • Takes themself very seriously • May not show tender emotions • May seem cold and calculating in their relationships • Tends to take comments, events, situations personally • Few social interactions • Loners • Appears to be shy and introverted	• Avoid situations that the patient may perceive as demeaning • Encourage trusting relationship and behaviors • Encourage verbalizing their perceptions of the situations • Acknowledge alternate explanations for others' motives

Continued

Table 14.2

Nursing Interventions for Personality Disorders—cont'd

Type	Symptoms	Nursing Interventions
Schizoid	• Detached • Chooses solitary activities • Avoids social situations • Loner • Often excels in fields where limited social interaction needed	• Accept behavior • Encourage appropriate, brief social interactions • Meet patient on their own terms • Help patient understand how behaviors may contribute to satisfactory relationships
Schizotypal	• Eccentric behavior • Inappropriate affect • Aloof • Psychotic symptoms under stress	• Brief, concrete conversations that are focused on reality • Accept behavior • Encourage appropriate social behaviors • Recognize need for personal space • Reinforce reality gently

Table 14.3

Nursing Care Plan for Patients With Borderline Personality Disorder

Assessment/Data Collection	Nursing Diagnosis	Plan/Goal	Interventions/Nursing Actions	Evaluation Criteria
After drinking heavily, got in physical fight with acquaintance, then made attempt at cutting wrists	Risk for self-directed violence	Verbalize alternative coping mechanisms when under stress	Provide safe, secure environment Convey acceptance of patient as a person Discuss alternative ways to express anxiety, irritation Identify alternative actions to reduce destructive impulses	Able to describe alternative coping mechanisms Able to utilize these coping mechanisms next time in a stressful situation

Clinical Activity

• Be alert to possible manipulation or staff splitting; patients may view nursing students as being more vulnerable and try to take advantage of them.

• At the same time, make efforts to avoid stereotyping or judging such patients based on information that they have a personality disorder.

Evidence-Based Practice

Clinical Question: How can nurses be helped to challenge the negative attitudes they commonly have about patients with personality disorders?

Evidence: Working with people with personality disorders is very challenging. Previous studies found nurses to have a generally negative attitude about this population, due to some of the difficult and at times unpredictable behaviors these patients exhibit. Stacey et al. (2018) used a focus-group study to explore student nurses' experiences of an educational intervention designed for nurses working with people with a diagnosis of personality disorder. By examining the challenges presented by these patients and using a model with a knowledge-and-understanding framework, student nurses gained information on the behaviors often seen. After the focus group, students exhibited positive attitudes toward people with a diagnosis of personality disorder and expressed confidence to influence negative attitudes in practice. Student nurses reported shifts in focus from identifying patient behaviors as problematic to understanding that their difficulties with patient behaviors arose from the students' own emotional responses.

Implications for Nursing Practice: By gaining knowledge about personality disorders and understanding the challenges presented by patients with these disorders, nurses can achieve more positive approaches to working with these patients.

Stacey, G., Baldwin, V., Thompson, B.J., Aubeeluck, A. J. (2018). A focus group study exploring student nurse's experiences of an educational intervention focused on working with people with a diagnosis of personality disorder. *Psychiatr Ment Health Nurs.* Sep;25(7):390-399. doi: 10.1111/jpm.12473. Epub 2018 Jul 16. PMID: 29782073.

Patient/Family Education

- Ensure that patient and family receive education on the diagnosis to better understand the patient's behaviors and their effect on family relationships.
- Ensure that referrals for counseling appointments are made.
- Address concerns with taking medications to control uncomfortable symptoms, especially with any patient at risk for substance use disorder.

Key Points

- Personality disorders are maladaptive responses to personality development.
- People with personality disorders are seldom hospitalized for their diagnosis. Many of these people do not see a need for obtaining help, and those who do are not always taken seriously by the medical community.
- BPD is the most common personality disorder seen in the mental health setting.

- People with personality disorders often present challenges to nursing staff when receiving care for physical ailments due to their challenging behaviors, which can include poor interpersonal skills, negative emotions, and inflexibility.
- Common traits of people with personality disorders include socially inappropriate behavior, negative emotions, and difficulty with close relationships.

Safe and Effective Nursing Care

Maintain a safe environment.

Establish ongoing communication between all staff caring for those patients to ensure a consistent treatment plan.

Establish appropriate limits for acceptable behavior.

CASE STUDY

Marsha, a 25-year-old woman, is brought to the emergency department by her friend after threatening to take sleeping pills because her boyfriend broke off their relationship. On questioning, Marsha acknowledges a long history of problems. She has made multiple suicide attempts, which include cutting her arms and taking handfuls of sleeping pills. Each attempt occurred after a rejection by a boyfriend or, in earlier years, by her parents. Marsha describes falling in love easily and a history of intense relationships that often are discontinued by the man after Marsha becomes increasingly clingy and demanding.

She describes a chaotic childhood in which her mother was away a lot, and Marsha moved around to live with a variety of relatives. She barely finished high school and has struggled to find unskilled jobs.

On interviewing her, you find her cheerful and charming. She does not appear depressed. When you leave the room to attend to another patient, she cries out that she is being ignored. She calls multiple friends to visit her in the ED so that she will not be alone, thus creating a chaotic environment that must be monitored by security.

Her long-term psychiatrist comes to see her and tells you she is treating Marsha for BPD.

1. Which behaviors in this case study are indicative of this diagnosis?
2. What treatment options are used to treat this disorder?
3. What medications would you expect Marsha to have prescribed?

Review Questions

1. When setting limits with patients with personality disorders, the consequences of violating those limits should be set:
   a. When the behavior is done
   b. Just before the nurse anticipates the behavior
   c. When the staff or family complains about the behavior
   d. When the limit is set

2. David, 30 years old, comes to your unit for treatment of multiple broken bones following a car accident. He is friendly and flirtatious but very demanding. As you gather data from him, you learn that the police have been looking for him for petty theft. He laughs and says, "Like they don't have better things to do!" He states he has changed jobs three times in the past year and has just broken off his second engagement. His former fiancée is visiting and privately tells you that you need to be careful because "He doesn't always tell the truth." You suspect which of the following personality disorders?
   a. Paranoid
   b. Dependent
   c. Antisocial
   d. Schizoid

3. A primary mechanism used by people with personality disorders is:
   a. Manipulation
   b. Depression
   c. Projection
   d. Euphoria

4. For the patient with antisocial personality disorder, which of the following behaviors would be the most difficult for the patient to comply with?
   a. Listening to music
   b. Abiding by the rules in the hospital
   c. Playing volleyball
   d. Organizing a patient committee

5. A patient who has committed multiple crimes would be more likely to have which of the following personality disorders?
   a. Narcissistic
   b. Schizoid
   c. Antisocial
   d. Borderline

6. Patients who display very bizarre behavior but who are still functional in society are most likely to have which of the following types of personality disorder?
   a. Narcissistic
   b. Schizotypal
   c. Antisocial
   d. Borderline

7. Which intervention describes an important component in treatment of personality disorders?
   a. Antidepressants are most effective with most personality disorders.
   b. Inpatient psychiatric hospitalization is particularly effective.
   c. Self-awareness by the nurse is necessary to ensure a therapeutic relationship.
   d. Long-term psychoanalysis is the treatment of choice.

8. Your patient has been admitted with a diagnosis of bilateral pneumonia. You have trouble communicating with this patient, who is pouty and is demanding your constant attention. She talks for long periods about the smallest details of her life. Besides the pneumonia, you ask the physician if the patient has a history of which of the following personality disorders?
   a. Schizoid
   b. Antisocial
   c. Narcissistic
   d. Borderline

9. Nursing care for people with personality disorders includes all of the following *except:*
   a. Nurse self-awareness
   b. Trust
   c. Limit setting
   d. Vague communication (to decrease feelings of inferiority)

10. You are caring for a 25-year-old man who has been admitted for infections that resulted from self-inflicted burns. He denies suicidal ideation. You are told he has been admitted before with self-inflicted injuries. You suspect he has a history of which one of the following personality disorders?
    a. Narcissistic
    b. Borderline
    c. Schizoid
    d. Passive-aggressive

REVIEW QUESTIONS ANSWER KEY 1.d, 2.c, 3.a, 4.b, 5.c, 6.b, 7.c, 8.c, 9.d, 10.b

CHAPTER 15
Schizophrenia Spectrum and Other Psychotic Disorders

KEY TERMS

Catatonia
Delusions
Echolalia
Echopraxia
Extrapyramidal symptoms (EPS)
Hallucinations
Illusions
Psychosis
Schizoaffective disorder
Schizophrenia
Schizophrenia spectrum disorder
Schizophreniform disorder

CHAPTER CONCEPTS

Cognition
Family
Mood and affect
Self
Stress and coping

LEARNING OUTCOMES

1. Define schizophrenia.
2. Differentiate between positive and negative symptoms seen in schizophrenia.
3. Identify two other psychotic disorders.
4. Identify treatment modalities for people with schizophrenia.
5. Describe catatonic features in schizophrenia.
6. Identify nursing care for people with schizophrenia.

The term schizophrenia, which literally means "split mind," was first used by Swiss psychiatrist Eugen Bleuler (FIG. 15.1). **Schizophrenia** is a serious, chronic psychiatric disorder characterized by impaired reality testing, **hallucinations** (false sensory perceptions), **delusions** (fixed, false beliefs), and limited socialization. It is a psychotic thought disorder in which hallucinations and delusions dominate the patient's thinking. People with schizophrenia have a "split" between their thoughts and their feelings and between their reality and society's reality, which can lead to unusual, confusing, bizarre, and/or frightening behaviors.

Schizophrenia is a frequent cause of psychiatric hospitalizations and long-term disability. The suffering for a patient with schizophrenia and their family can last a lifetime. As a chronic illness, schizophrenia is characterized by remissions and exacerbations throughout one's life. The first psychotic break often responds well to treatment; but the relapse rate is high, and over time, the person may become increasingly disabled.

Individuals with schizophrenia are vulnerable to substance abuse as they self-medicate to control their symptoms, contributing to co-occurring disorders (see Chapter 17). These patients can also be at risk for

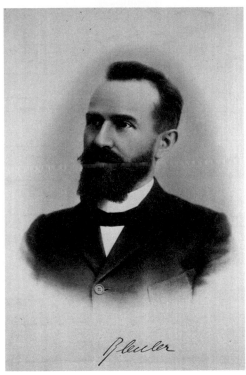

FIGURE 15.1 Eugen Bleuler (1857–1940) was a Swiss psychiatrist who coined the term *schizophrenia* and contributed to the understanding of the disorder.

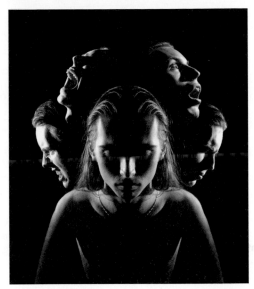

FIGURE 15.2 Schizophrenia can create extreme distress.

suicide, either because of voices telling the patients to kill themselves or because patients perceive suicide as a means to end their suffering. These individuals also have a high rate of unemployment, poverty, and homelessness. Frequently, schizophrenia is initially diagnosed in adolescents and younger adults, with the first psychotic break often occurring between the ages of 16 and 35, although later onset does occur. A common scenario is that a young person leaves home for college or the military and suddenly exhibits psychotic behavior (FIG. 15.2); however, analysis of earlier behaviors may indicate this individual was withdrawn, had problems with social relationships, and exhibited possible antisocial behavior. Schizophrenia is rare in young children. It is estimated that 0.3% to 0.7% of the U.S. population has schizophrenia (American Psychiatric Association, 2022).

The *Diagnostic and Statistical Manual of Mental Disorders,* 5th edition, Text Revision (DSM-5-TR) categorizes schizophrenia under the global title of **schizophrenia spectrum disorders** (2022). The schizophrenia spectrum is a gradient of psychopathology that a patient can experience from least to most severe, with schizophrenia being the most severe. Other disorders on this spectrum include **schizoaffective** and **schizophreniform** disorders, which are generally less severe than schizophrenia. See Table 15.1 for definitions of these and other disorders with schizophrenic features.

Individuals with disorders on the schizophrenia spectrum are considered to have a **psychosis**, a disorganization of the personality and loss of contact with or distortion of reality. Psychoses can also occur in bipolar disorder and major depression. Another psychotic disorder is brief psychotic disorder, which includes postpartum-onset psychosis (see Chapter 20). Medical conditions that can contribute to psychoses include brain tumors, central nervous system (CNS) infections, delirium, endocrine disorders, exposure to toxins, and substance abuse. All of these conditions may exhibit some of the same symptoms as schizophrenia, including hallucinations, delusions, abnormal sensations, and bizarre behaviors, but they have different etiologies and durations of disability.

GOOD TO KNOW

Sudden onset of hallucinations and delusions requires quick action to identify the cause. Causes can include a variety of medical conditions, metabolic changes, as well as drug reactions.

Table 15.1

Other Disorders With Schizophrenic Features

Type	Characteristics
Brief psychotic disorder	Sudden onset of psychotic symptoms that may or may not be preceded by severe psychosocial stress. These last at least 1 day and not more than a month.
Delusional disorder	Delusions without the other symptoms or disabilities of schizophrenia
Schizoaffective	Symptoms of schizophrenia along with symptoms of major depression or manic episodes that require treatment of both disorders
Schizophreniform	Schizophrenia symptoms without the level of impairment of functioning usually seen in schizophrenia and lasting more than 1 month and fewer than 6 months
Schizotypal	A personality disorder characterized by odd and eccentric behavior that does not decompensate to the level of schizophrenia (see Chapter 14)
Substance/medication-induced psychotic disorder	Hallucinations and delusions directly linked to substance intoxication or withdrawal from or exposure to a medication or toxin

Source: Adapted from *Diagnostic and Statistical Manual of Mental Disorders, 5th edition, Text Revisions (2022)* and Morgan &Townsend (2021).

Classroom Activity

View and discuss movies that feature schizophrenic characters, including *A Beautiful Mind, The Soloist,* and *I Never Promised You a Rose Garden.*

CRITICAL THINKING QUESTION

Your patient has a diagnosis of schizophreniform disorder. How is this different from a diagnosis of schizophrenia?

Classroom Activity

Contact a local NAMI (National Alliance on Mental Illness) support group and ask permission to attend a meeting, if possible.

GOOD TO KNOW

The coronavirus disease 2019 (COVID-19) pandemic had a devastating effect on those with serious mental illness such as schizophrenia. Prolonged isolation and reduced availability of mental health treatment affected everyone, but especially those with serious mental illness. Precautions taken during the pandemic such as mask wearing and staying home may even have contributed to their relapses and deterioration (Sukut & Balik, 2020).

 PRESENTING SYMPTOMS

Symptoms of schizophrenia are divided into two types: positive and negative.

Positive Symptoms

Positive symptoms are those that are found among people with schizophrenia but not present among those who do not have the disorder. They reflect an excess or distortion of normal functions and can include:

- delusions, including delusions of grandeur and persecution
- hallucinations, including auditory, visual, tactile, gustatory, olfactory
- speech disturbances, such as loose associations, neologisms (making up words), perseveration (repeating the same words or ideas in response to different questions), **echolalia** (repeating words or phrases), disorganized speech
- **illusions** (misperceiving real external stimuli)
- **echopraxia** (imitating movements made by others)
- magical thinking (believing that one's thoughts can control others)

Negative Symptoms

Negative symptoms are those found among people who do not have the disorder but are missing or lacking among individuals with schizophrenia. Negative symptoms reflect a lessening or loss of normal functions. These symptoms make holding a job, forming relationships, and other day-to-day functions especially difficult for people with schizophrenia and may include:

- avolition (lack of desire or motivation to accomplish goals)
- lack of self-care
- lack of desire to form social relationships
- inappropriate social behavior, such as pacing, rocking, or posturing (assuming bizarre or inappropriate postures)
- blunted affect and emotion

- anhedonia, apathy
- lack of insight
- concrete thinking (literally interpreting the environment)
- difficulty concentrating
- difficulty processing information to make a decision

Symptoms also include impairment in one or more areas of functioning, such as work, school, personal relationships, or self-care. Some disturbance needs to be evident for at least 6 months. Schizophrenia can also have features of **catatonia**, which include any of the following: motor immobility to stupor, excessive motor activity, and peculiar voluntary movements. Making a diagnosis requires looking at patterns of behavior and thought over time. See Tables 15.2 and 15.3 for lists of common delusions and hallucinations.

Cultural Considerations

Schizophrenia occurs in people of all races and cultures.

Cultural Considerations

A person's culture often influences the content of hallucinations and delusions. Familiarity with the patient's culture can provide insight into the origin of some of these thought disorders.

Table 15.2
Common Delusions

Delusion	Example
Grandeur (belief of exaggerated importance)	"I am Napoleon Bonaparte."
Paranoia (belief of deliberate harassment and persecution)	"The FBI is following me and wants to kill me."
Reference (belief that the thoughts and behavior of others are directed toward self)	"Those people on the TV show are talking to me."
Physical sensations (belief that parts of one's body are diseased, distorted, or missing)	"I have no blood in me."
Thought insertion	"The devil made me say that."

Source: Adapted from Gorman and Sultan (2008). *Psychosocial Nursing for General Patient Care,* 3rd ed. Philadelphia: F.A. Davis Company, with permission.

Table 15.3
Recognizing Hallucinations

Affected Sense	Example
Visual	"I watch angels bring different babies to my apartment each night."
Auditory (most common)	"The voices are calling me a prostitute."
Tactile	"When I touched my arm, I could tell my arm is made of stone."
Olfactory	"I don't want to stay in that room. I can smell the odors of the people who died there."
Gustatory	"I taste milk in my mouth all the time."
Kinesthetic (bodily movement or sense)	"It feels as if the rats in my head are eating up my brain."

Source: Adapted from Gorman and Sultan (2008). *Psychosocial Nursing for General Patient Care,* 3rd ed. Philadelphia: F.A. Davis Company, with permission.

GOOD TO KNOW

Schizophrenia is a debilitating and painful lifelong disease for the patient and family requiring long-term management and compassion.

DIFFERENTIAL DIAGNOSES

- substance use disorder
- psychotic disorder due to medical condition
- autism spectrum disorder (ASD)
- major depressive or bipolar disorder with psychotic or catatonic features
- post-traumatic stress disorder (PTSD)

CRITICAL THINKING QUESTION

Your patient with a schizophrenia diagnosis tells you that his mother has communicated with him. She has told the patient that he needs to leave the hospital right now to help save the mayor from peril. What type of delusions and hallucinations is this patient experiencing?

ETIOLOGY OF SCHIZOPHRENIA

No single cause has been identified for schizophrenia; rather, it is a brain disorder that can have many different origins. Disruption of neurotransmitters, including

dopamine, has been identified as one cause. Some dysfunction in neuron functioning is another. Cerebral changes in the limbic system and prefrontal cortex are still others. These factors may contribute to problems with attention and information processing. The person is unable to filter stimuli, leading to disorganization of mental functioning. Although family dysfunction may contribute to schizophrenia, it appears that psychological factors by themselves do not cause this condition. There is also evidence of genetic predisposition; the most significant risk factor for schizophrenia is having a close relative with this disorder.

Cultural Considerations

Behaviors that may be normal in some cultures can be confused with psychotic behavior in others. For example, in some cultures, speaking "in tongues" and talking to spirits is considered normal behavior in certain situations. If psychotic behavior is suspected, it is important to obtain information on what is normal behavior for the culture of your patient.

PSYCHIATRIC TREATMENT OF SCHIZOPHRENIA

A comprehensive, multidisciplinary treatment plan including pharmacotherapy, social support, social/life skills training, self-help groups, group therapy, and family therapy can be helpful to maintain the patient effectively. Gaining life skills to deal with everyday challenges, occupational training, and family education have also proven helpful. Intensive individual psychotherapy is generally not effective, but reality-based therapy that focuses on changing behaviors can be incorporated into the treatment plan. Ongoing support can promote compliance with anti-psychotic medications; this is probably one of the most important treatment approaches because man agement of antipsychotic medications is generally the primary treatment (see Pharmacology Corner). Early diagnosis is also associated with a better prognosis. Educating family caregivers about the disorder has been shown to reduce the stress and sense of burden on loved ones caring for someone with schizophrenia (Bulut, Arslantas, & Ferhan Dereboy, 2016).

Tool Box

Brief Psychiatric Rating Scale (BPRS): This is a standardized tool used to track changes in schizophrenia symptoms over time: https://www.webmd.com/schizophrenia/what-is-bprs#1

Classroom Activity

Invite a local mental health professional to class to discuss the treatment approaches available to schizophrenic patients in your community.

Antipsychotic medications are of two types: typical and atypical. Most people respond to one of the typical or atypical antipsychotic agents to a degree during the first psychotic episode. Typical antipsychotics have been around since the 1950s and work by blocking postsynaptic dopamine receptors. These agents are generally used to treat the positive symptoms of schizophrenia. Atypical antipsychotics (sometimes referred to as novel or second generation agents) have been available since the 1990s and are weaker dopamine-receptor antagonists but more potent antagonists of serotonin receptors. New atypicals are added to the market regularly. These drugs treat both positive and negative symptoms and generally have fewer side

Pharmacology Corner

Antipsychotic medications are key to returning a patient with schizophrenia to a stable state. Once the patient is stabilized, maintenance therapy is established to prevent exacerbations. Most patients will relapse off their medications, so incorporating a plan for medication compliance is essential. Once established on appropriate medications, the patient is usually more open to counseling and supportive interventions. It can take time to establish the appropriate medication and dosages, so the patient and family must be monitored closely. Some patients may require months or even years to find the best available medication, the right dosage, and the most manageable side-effect profile. New drugs are entering the market regularly, so providers may add one to help address symptoms not responding to the current regimen. A trial of any one medication should last for a substantial period, usually 6 to 8 weeks, unless intolerable side effects occur earlier. In the future, medication choices will be based more on biological markers that identify the antipsychotic that would be most effective for an individual (Janicak, 2014).

effects than the typical antipsychotics do. Even though the atypical agents have a better side-effect profile for long-term treatment, the typical, or older, agents may be chosen for short-term management of psychosis or long-term management of symptoms that do not respond to the atypical agents. See Table 15.4 for a list of the common typical and atypical antipsychotics with their side-effect profiles. A few are available as a long-acting injection that is given every 2 to 12 weeks. These include haloperidol (Haldol), fluphenazine (Prolixin), paliperidone palmitate (Invega), aripiprazole (Abilify Maintena), and risperidone (Risperdal). These can be effective if a patient is unable to take oral medications. This option can be helpful to caregivers to avoid the daily struggle of getting the patient to take the pills. Some medications come in liquid forms or quick dissolving tablets, which can be given orally and can be useful if the patient is not cooperative with swallowing pills.

Table 15.4

Comparison of Side Effects Among Typical and Atypical Antipsychotic Agents

Class	Generic Name	EPS	Sedation	Anticholinergic	Orthostatic Hypotension	Weight Gain
Typicals	Chlorpromazine (Thorazine)	3	4	3	4	*
	Fluphenazine (Prolixin)	5	2	2	2	
	Haloperidol (Haldol)	5	2	2	2	
	Loxapine (Loxitane)	3	2	2	2	*
	Perphenazine (Trilafon)	4	2	2	2	*
	Pimozide (Orap)	4	2	3	2	*
	Thioridazine (Mellaril)	2	4	4	4	*
	Thiothixene (Navane)	4	2	2	2	*
	Trifluoperazine (Stelazine)	4	2	2	2	*
Atypicals	Aripiprazole (Abilify)	1	2	1	3	2
	Asenapine (Saphris)	1	3	1	3	4
	Clozapine (Clozaril)	1	5	5	4	5
	Iloperidone (Fanapt)	1	3	2	3	3
	Lurasidone (Latuda)	1	3	1	3	3
	Olanzapine (Zyprexa)	1	3	2	2	5
	Paliperidone (Invega)	1	2	1	3	2
	Quetiapine (Seroquel)	1	3	1	3	4
	Risperidone (Risperdal)	1	2	1	3	4
	Ziprasidone (Geodon)	1	3	1	2	2
	Brexpiprazole (Rexulti)	1	1	1	1	5
	Cariprazine (Vraylar)	3	2	1	1	1

1

Key: 1 = very low, 2 = low, 3 = moderate, 4 = high, 5 = very high
*Weight gain occurs, but incidence is unknown.
Source: Adapted from Townsend & Morgan (2018): *Essentials of Psychiatric Mental Health Nursing,* 9th ed. Philadelphia: F.A. Davis, with permission. Page 74.

CRITICAL THINKING QUESTION

You realize your patient has been "cheeking" his risperidone (hiding the pill in his cheek). What might be some of the reasons the patient is doing this? Identify two pharmacological alternatives for this medication.

Managing the side effects of antipsychotics is a major component of the treatment plan as this can determine compliance with the regimen. Typical antipsychotics can be particularly effective in controlling psychotic symptoms; however, they are more prone to **extrapyramidal symptoms (EPS)** as well as anticholinergic effects. See

Chapter 8 for more information on the categories of EPS. See Box 15.1 for a list of extrapyramidal side effects and Table 15.5 for a list of anticholinergic side effects. EPSs are generally managed with anticholinergic drugs such as benztropine (Cogentin), trihexyphenidyl (Artane), dopaminergic agonists such as amantadine (Symmetrel), or antihistamines such as diphenhydramine (Benadryl). Anticholinergic effects can often be managed with education (see Table 15.5). Newer medications to treat specific forms of EPS are being developed, including deutetrabenazine (Austedo) for tardive dyskinesia.

Another side effect that is common with antipsychotics is weight gain, which can be a factor in patient noncompliance with taking these medications.

Box 15.1

Extrapyramidal Side Effects

- Dystonia: muscle rigidity, torticollis (neck turned in awkward angle)
- Pseudoparkinsonism or dyskinesia: stiffness, tremors, shuffling gait
- Akathisia: restlessness, inability to sit still
- Oculogyric crisis: uncontrolled rolling back of the eyes
- Tardive dyskinesia: late onset movement disorder that includes lip smacking, grimacing, tongue protrusion

Table 15.5

Anticholinergic Effects and Interventions

Symptom	*Nursing Action*
Dry mouth	Offer sugarless candy, good oral hygiene, saliva substitute
Orthostatic hypotension	Instruct patient to get out of bed slowly, monitor blood pressure
Constipation	Promote high-fiber diet, fluids, stool softeners, laxatives as needed
Urinary retention	Instruct patient to report symptoms promptly
Dry eye	Lubricant eye drops

Antipsychotics can also be associated with sedation, diabetes, and elevated prolactin levels. Elevated prolactin is associated with sexual dysfunction, amenorrhea, and osteoporosis.

The atypicals are generally less associated with EPS than the typical agents, but there is a wide range of other side effects, so close monitoring of the prescribed drug is essential. Some atypicals are prone to anticholinergic effects. Serious side effects in specific atypicals can include reduced seizure threshold, blood dyscrasias, and cardiac arrhythmias. One of the most serious blood dyscrasias is agranulocytosis, which is a rare blood complication of clozapine (Clozaril), requiring close monitoring of the white blood cell count. The specific side effects of the atypicals must be reviewed and monitored whenever these drugs are ordered.

GOOD TO KNOW

Tracking the patient's weight is generally part of each health-care visit to monitor for weight gain with antipsychotic medications.

GOOD TO KNOW

EPSs can be devastating to a patient's quality of life. Close monitoring to treat these and prevent long-term consequences must be part of the treatment plan. They also contribute to patients discontinuing these medications on their own, which contributes to relapse.

GOOD TO KNOW

Compliance with antipsychotic medication therapy is a lifelong challenge for the patient and their family. It is important to regularly monitor medication compliance and the current side-effect profile. Reinforce education each time the patient is seen in any health-care setting.

Tool Box

Abnormal Involuntary Movement Scale (AIMS): This tool is a rating scale developed by the National Institute of Mental Health to measure involuntary movements associated with tardive dyskinesia.

https://www.psychiatrictimes.com/view/aims-abnormal-involuntary-movement-scale

Clinical Activity

As you read patient charts during your clinical experience

- Review a chart for complete white blood cell counts (CBC) if the patient is on clozapine.
- Review the chart for evidence of side effects of antipsychotic medications.
- Discuss management of side effects with the patient and their family.

CRITICAL THINKING QUESTION

Your patient with schizophrenia has been taking clozapine for 2 years. He is now in the hospital and is NPO awaiting an appendectomy. What concerns would you have that the patient has been without his medications for 2 days? Why is the health-care provider monitoring the patient's white blood cell counts closely?

NURSING CARE OF THE PATIENT WITH SCHIZOPHRENIA

Nursing care of the patient with schizophrenia requires knowledge and compassion. Common nursing diagnoses for these patients include:

- self-care deficit
- sensory perception, disturbed
- social isolation
- thought processes, disturbed
- verbal communication, impaired
- violence, risk for

General Nursing Interventions

- Watch for clues that the patient is hallucinating, for example, darting eyes, mumbling to self, staring at a vacant wall for long periods. You can also ask if the patient is hearing voices.
- If the patient is hallucinating, acknowledge what the patient is experiencing without reinforcing it as your reality. For example, your response could be, "I don't see the devil standing there, but I understand how upsetting this is for you."
- If your patient is delusional, reinforce reality with calm statements of fact. For example, you might say, "That man works for the hospital, not the FBI"

or "Yes, there was a man at the nurse's station, but I did not hear him talk about you." Remind the patient that there are alternative ways to view reality.
- Work to slowly build trust in small ways. Avoid over-reacting to patient's bizarre behavior or appearance.
- Maintain a calm, consistent environment with a regular routine.
- Even though the patient appears to be in another world, continue to include the patient in conversations and activities. Acknowledge their presence and importance.
- Focus on reality. For example, rather than listening to a long monologue about a delusion, talk to the patient about the schedule for the day.
- Never argue with the patient about what they are experiencing.
- Incorporate Quality and Safety Education for Nurses (QSEN) competencies to maintain a safe environment for the psychotic patient (www. qsen.org). For example, remove sharp objects and provide adequate supervision.
- Take action to provide medications before agitation escalates. Make sure there are orders for prn medications for agitation.
- **Never** reinforce hallucinations, delusions, or illusions. An example of an inappropriate response from the nurse is, "Jesus wants you to take these pills." That response reinforces the patient's delusion about Jesus.
- Avoid whispering or laughing when the patient cannot hear the whole conversation; such behavior can promote paranoia.
- Avoid putting the patient into situations that are competitive or embarrassing.
- Build trust by using therapeutic communication skills.
- Attempt to decode incomprehensible communication by restating what you think the patient is talking about. If not sure, then seek clarification as in "I don't understand what you mean by that."
- If the patient is catatonic, provide for basic physical needs and safety, and make brief supportive contact with the patient without pressuring the patient to communicate.

Table 15.6 provides a sample nursing care plan for patients with schizophrenia. See Table 15.7 for interventions for patients with schizophrenia who are hallucinating. See Figure 15.3 Concept Map for the patient with Schizophrenia.

Table 15.6

Nursing Care Plan of the Patient With Schizophrenia

Assessment/Data Collection	Nursing Diagnosis	Plan/Goal	Interventions/Nursing Actions	Evaluation Criteria
Patient is mumbling to himself, looks suspiciously at staff, avoids contact with staff, other people avoid patient.	Social isolation	Patient will spend time in a social activity.	• Approach patient for brief periods in a nonthreatening manner. • Avoid touching patient without asking permission. • Talk about concrete unit activities. • Demonstrate acceptance of patient's behavior and appearance by avoiding reacting to bizarre behavior. Point out possible alternative behaviors once relationship established.	Patient will participate in unit activity once a day.

Table 15.7

Suggested Interventions for Patients With Schizophrenia Who Are Hallucinating

Suggested Nursing Action	Rationale
1. "Mr. R, I don't see any bugs. It is time for lunch. I will walk to the dining room with you."	1. This lets the patient know you heard him but brings him immediately into the reality of time of day and the need to go to the dining room.
2. "I see a crack in the wall, Mr. R. It is harmless; you are safe. Susan is here to take you down to occupational therapy now."	2. This is in response to a probable illusion. It lets the patient know that you see something. It validates his fear but tells him what you see and then moves him into the here and now.
3. "I know that your thoughts seem very real to you, Ms. C, but they do not seem logical to me. I would like you to come to your room and get dressed now, please."	3. Again, you are validating the patient's concern without exploring and focusing on the delusion.
4. "Ms. C, it appears to me that you are listening to someone. Are you hearing voices other than mine?"	4. This is a method of validating your impression of what you see. This is as far as you will go into exploring what she may be hearing.
5. "Thank you, Ms. C. I want to help you focus away from the other voices. I am real; they are not. Please come with me to the reading room."	5. In this statement, you respond to her in the present and reinforce her response to you. This response attempts to redirect her thinking.

Source: Adapted from Gorman and Sultan (2008). *Psychosocial Nursing for General Patient Care,* 3rd ed. Philadelphia: F.A. Davis Company, with permission.

Evidence-Based Practice

Clinical Question: What do family caregivers need to provide support for the patient with schizophrenia?

Discussion: The trend to have people with schizophrenia living outside the psychiatric hospital setting means family members often become primary caregivers and must manage medication regimens. Medication compliance is essential for the best outcomes.

Evidence: A study of family caregivers of patients with schizophrenia found that medication management is a major concern. Five main themes for family members emerged from the study: insight into illness (poor understanding of illness), treatment factor (thinking about medication, poor guidance for medication compliance), resources and support (availability of medication and cost of medication), health-care provider factors (communication gap and poor assessment with follow-up), and social dysfunction (social isolation, disruption in life routine) of the primary caregivers. Knowing the concerns of family members can help direct education to better meet their needs.

Implications for Nursing Practice: Including family caregivers in the treatment plan and education will lead to improved treatment outcomes when the patient is in the community.

Alasmee, N. & Hasan, A. A. (2020). Primary caregivers' experience of antipsychotic medication: A qualitative study. *Archives of Psychiatric Nursing.* 34(6): p520-8 September 09, 2020 DOI: https://doi.org/10.1016/j.apnu.2020.06.002

Patient/Family Education

- Explain medication regimen with side-effect profile.
- Provide resources for life-skills training and socialization.
- Provide referrals for ongoing counseling, including psychiatric follow-up for medication management, group therapy, and family therapy.
- Arrange for scheduled blood tests for patients on clozapine.
- Provide family education on what to expect with the patient's behavior and tools for managing behaviors.
- Monitor weight gain.

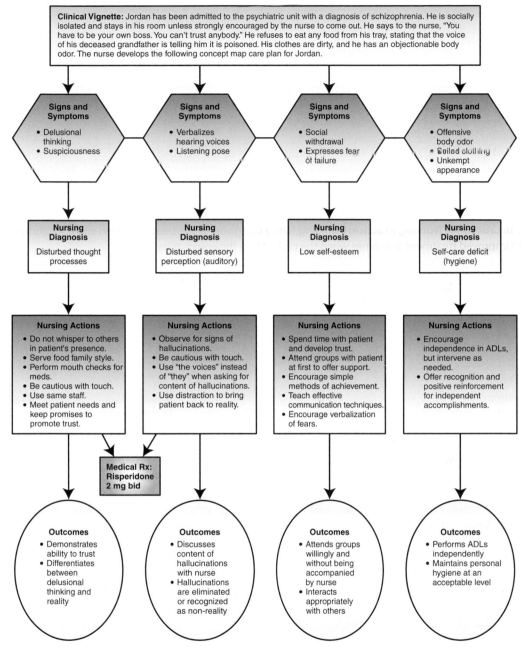

FIGURE 15.3 Concept map for the patient with schizophrenia. (From Morgan & Townsend [2021]. Essentials of Psychiatric Mental health Nursing. FA Davis.)

GOOD TO KNOW

It is important for you to avoid reinforcing patients' psychotic thinking. For example, avoid asking the patient what "they" are telling him or her. Rather, let the patient know you are concerned but do not hear these voices.

GOOD TO KNOW

Remember that patients with schizophrenia are often very concrete thinkers, so it is important to speak clearly and plainly. Make only one request at a time. Avoid joking as it can easily be misinterpreted.

Classroom Activity

Have a mental health counselor from a local clinic present information on managing schizophrenia to your class.

Tool Box

National Institute of Mental Health information on schizophrenia for patients and their families: http://www.nimh.nih.gov/health/topics/schizophrenia/index.shtml

CRITICAL THINKING QUESTION

Your 19-year-old patient with a new diagnosis of schizophrenia begins yelling, "Stay away! Don't touch me!" as you walk into his room. His mother is in the room and is trying to comfort the patient. What approaches might be helpful for the patient and his mother?

Key Points

- Schizophrenia is a chronic, serious, often debilitating psychiatric disorder that affects all aspects of the patient's life and their loved ones.
- Schizophrenia is a brain disorder.
- Not all psychoses are schizophrenia. Other psychotic disorders can include brief psychotic disorder, psychosis in bipolar disorder, substance abuse, and major depression.
- Schizophrenia is a spectrum disorder, which means there is a gradient of less to more severe

conditions. Schizophrenia is usually diagnosed in a person's late teens and young adulthood, but often continues for the rest of the patient's life.
- Hallucinations and delusions are examples of positive patient symptoms that present challenges to all health-care professionals.
- The main treatment for schizophrenia remains antipsychotic medications. Because of the side-effect profile of these medications, close monitoring is needed to achieve the best outcomes and patient compliance.

Safe and Effective Nursing Care

Prevention of falls
Maintenance of safe environment free from hazards for self-harm
Safe medication administration including appropriate route
Structured environment to promote feeling of safety for patient
Effective communication to reduce patient misinterpretation of reality

CASE STUDY

Ralph, a 20-year-old college student, is admitted to your psychiatric facility by his parents. Ralph is in his second year at an out-of-state college. Over the past 6 months, he has been exhibiting increasingly bizarre behavior, such as walking the halls of his dorm at night knocking on doors, asking strange questions, mumbling to himself, and sleeping on the floor during the day. He has also been exhibiting disruptive behaviors in class. Students report being afraid of him, and he has become increasingly isolated. Most recently, he became violent in the college cafeteria. Then, the school's mental health counselor reported to Ralph's parents that he needed immediate hospitalization.

The parents report that Ralph had a normal childhood and never displayed any unusual behavior until the last year. The parents tell you they feel guilty that they did not monitor his behavior more closely in the last few months.

On meeting Ralph, you note that he avoids eye contact and appears to be talking to someone he sees in the corner of the room. When his parents walk into the room, he begins hitting his head repeatedly against the wall.

1. How should you respond to Ralph when first meeting him?
2. How would you address the parents' fears?
3. What medications might be useful for this patient?

Review Questions

1. Brian, an 18-year-old with schizophrenia, is delusional, hears voices, and is withdrawing from others. A nursing intervention that is appropriate for promoting activity for Brian is:
   a. Tell him "the voices" told you he should participate in the weekly party.
   b. Remind him that he does not want to get worse by sitting alone.
   c. Tell him he must join the party; it is part of his care plan.
   d. Invite him to join in the party.

2. Shawna is a 22-year-old woman who has episodes of extreme muscle rigidity. She sometimes repeats a word or a phrase over and over. Attempts to move her are met with even more muscle resistance. What is she exhibiting?
   a. Catatonia
   b. Disorganized schizophrenia
   c. Brief psychotic disorder
   d. Schizotypal personality

3. Mr. G is calling out, "Nurse!" When you arrive in his room, he tells you to be careful of the snake in the corner. You do not see anything in the corner. Mr. G is experiencing a/an:
   a. Hallucination
   b. Attention-getting behavior
   c. Illusion
   d. Delusion

4. Of the following responses, which would be your *best* response to Mr. G regarding the snake that he sees?
   a. "Don't worry; I'll get rid of it." (You pretend to remove the snake.)
   b. "I don't see a snake; what else do you see that isn't there?"
   c. "I don't see a snake. It is time for your group meeting. I'll walk with you to the meeting room."
   d. "Where is it? I hate snakes. Let's get out of here."

5. Which of the following is *not* a sign of untreated schizophrenia?
   a. Experiencing loss of reality
   b. Living in one's own world
   c. Maintaining satisfactory performance on the job
   d. Experiencing delusions, hallucinations

6. A nursing intervention for a person with schizophrenia is to:
   a. Reinforce the hallucinations.
   b. Keep the person oriented to reality and to the present.
   c. Encourage the patient to begin psychoanalysis.
   d. Encourage competitive activities.

7. Mr. S states, "Look at the snakes on the ceiling." You see some cracks in the plaster. Mr. S is experiencing a/an:
   a. Hallucination
   b. Illusion
   c. Delusion
   d. Flashback

8. Your best response to Mr. S might be:
   a. "How many snakes do you see, Mr. S?"
   b. "Yes, I see them, too. Let's go to the dayroom."
   c. "I see some cracks in the plaster, but I do not see snakes. Let's go to the day room."
   d. "I don't think your medication is working. I'll call the doctor."

9. A patient who repeats a word or part of a word over and over might be said to have which of the following symptoms?
   a. Echolalia
   b. Echopraxia
   c. Illusion
   d. Word salad

10. An individual stands on the train track with the train coming nearer. The person exclaims, "I am invincible! The train will not hurt me." This is an example of:
    a. Delusions of grandeur
    b. Echolalia
    c. Sensory hallucinations
    d. Extrapyramidal symptoms

11. Which of the following pairs of symptoms are closely associated with EPS?
    a. Muscle rigidity and protruding tongue
    b. Overly emotional and depressed
    c. Shuffling gait and depression
    d. Fatigue and painful joints

12. The primary goal in working with an actively psychotic, suspicious patient is to:
    a. Improve her relationship with her parents
    b. Encourage participation in individual psychotherapy
    c. Decrease her anxiety and increase trust
    d. Promote healthy living habits

13. The most current thinking on the cause of schizophrenia is that it is:
    a. A brain disorder
    b. Primarily related to a disturbed mother/child relationship
    c. Brain damage caused by the mother's use of tranquilizers during pregnancy
    d. An alteration in opioid receptors

REVIEW QUESTIONS ANSWER KEY 1.d, 2.a, 3.a, 4.c, 5.c, 6.b, 7.b, 8.c, 9.a, 10.a, 11.a, 12.c, 13.a

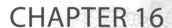

CHAPTER 16
Neurocognitive Disorders: Delirium and Dementia

KEY TERMS

Agnosia
Agraphia
Alzheimer's disease
Apraxia
Chemical restraint
Delirium
Dementia
Lewy body disease
Major neurocognitive disorder
Mild neurocognitive disorder
Neurocognitive disorder
Nocturnal delirium
Physical restraint
Pseudodementia
Vascular dementia

CHAPTER CONCEPTS

Cognition
Comfort
Family
Safety

LEARNING OUTCOMES

1. Describe the differences between delirium and dementia.
2. Define neurocognitive disorders.
3. List the most common forms of dementia.
4. List common causes of delirium.
5. Describe effective treatments for each.

Neurocognitive disorders (NCDs) are clinically significant deficits in cognition or memory representing a major change from a previous level of functioning. In the past, these conditions were referred to as organic mental syndromes and disorders by the American Psychiatric Association. NCDs include delirium and dementias.

 DELIRIUM

Delirium is a neurocognitive disorder that is an acute reaction to underlying physiological (e.g., toxins, drugs, illness) or psychological (e.g., sensory overload) stress. Delirium is a temporary condition characterized by a disturbance in attention (i.e., reduced ability to direct, focus, sustain, and shift attention) and orientation to the environment. For example, the patient may need questions repeated due to inattention, be easily distracted, or need repeated orientation to the situation. Delirium can also include memory deficit, language disturbance, and/or perceptual disturbance. Those with delirium may exhibit alterations in sleep-wake cycle. These alterations can include a wide gamut of responses, including being overly vigilant to any stimuli all the way to stuporous in others. The patient may exhibit **nocturnal delirium**, known as *sundowning*, when confusion and agitation increase at dusk. See Table 16.1 for types of delirium with common symptoms.

Delirium usually develops quickly and often fluctuates throughout the day. The condition often resolves once the

Table 16.1
Types of Delirium

Assessments	Hypoactive Hypoalert	Hyperactive Hyperalert	Mixed
Level of alertness	Lethargic, falls asleep between questions, difficult to arouse	Overly attentive to cues	Alternates between hyperalert and lethargic states within hours or days
Motor activity	Decreased activity	Moves quickly	Alternates within one episode of delirium
Ability to follow commands	Follows a simple command, for example, lift your foot Is passively cooperative	May be combative, pulls at tubes, tries to climb out of bed	Alternates between hypoactive and hyperactive states, may be unpredictable
Thinking ability	Difficulty in focusing attention, disorganized	Easily distracted, rambles May mumble, swear, or yell	Alternates between hypoactive and hyperactive states in an unpredictable manner

Source: Adapted from Forrest et al. (2007) and Gorman & Sultan (2008).

underlying cause is identified and treated. Delirium should be considered when the person exhibits sudden onset of confusion, memory impairment, incoherence, fluctuating levels of consciousness, sleep-wake cycle disruption, hallucinations, and/or delusions. Emotional instability such as anger, irritability, and fear can also be seen.

Delirium is an extremely common condition seen in the acute hospital, nursing home, and home settings, particularly in older patients. It is estimated that 29% to 64% of the general hospital population has delirium and it is especially common in the older population. It is also common post operatively (American Psychiatric Association, 2022). The condition also contributes to mortality and morbidity. The DSM-IV-TR (2000) reports that 15% of older people die within 1 month of an episode of delirium. Delirium prevalence surpasses all other psychiatric syndromes in the general medical setting (Maldonado, 2016). Common causes of delirium include electrolyte imbalance, poor oxygenation, medication side effects or misuse, urinary tract infections, and dehydration. See Table 16.2 for a more comprehensive list of causes. Identifying the cause can be challenging in people with complex medical conditions, as multiple factors may contribute to the delirium. Substance-induced delirium is a separate category. It is defined as delirium developing during or within 1 month after severe intoxication or withdrawal from a substance capable of producing delirium.

Treatment of Delirium

Treatment of delirium must focus on finding and treating the cause. Often, symptoms of delirium can resolve quickly once the appropriate treatment for its underlying cause is begun. Supportive interventions to maintain patient safety, control agitation, prevent further complications, and reorient the patient can be very helpful.

Clinical Activity

If your patient has a delirium diagnosis or exhibits a sudden change in consciousness and/or behavior, review their medical record for possible causes, including medication side effects, recent laboratory results, and recent infections.

DIFFERENTIAL DIAGNOSES

- psychotic disorders, for example, bipolar or depressive disorders, schizophrenia spectrum
- other neurocognitive disorders, for example, Alzheimer's disease
- substance use disorder
- acute stress disorder

Table 16.2
Causes of Delirium

Biological Factors	Other Factors
Hypoxia	Medication side effect
Nutritional deficiencies, for example, iron, B12	Anesthesia reaction
Electrolyte imbalances, for example, ↑calcium	Overdose of medication
Hypoglycemia/hyperglycemia	Substance abuse/withdrawal, for example, alcohol, cannabis, opioids, anxiolytics, sedatives
Kidney failure, hepatic encephalopathy	Sensory overload and deprivation
Sepsis and other infections including urinary tract infection (UTI)	Head trauma
Hypothyroidism	Emotional stress
Cardiac insufficiency	
Febrile illness	
Primary brain disorders, for example, brain tumors, Parkinson's disease, head trauma	
Pain	

Source: Adapted from Gorman & Sultan (2008) and Morgan & Townsend (2021).

Pharmacology Corner

Prescribing medications to control delirium symptoms is risky because these medications can mask or compound the confusion and agitation. However, at times, low-dose antipsychotic medications such as haloperidol (Haldol), risperidone (Risperdal), quetiapine (Seroquel), and olanzapine (Zyprexa) may be needed to address agitation. The benefits of the medications must be weighed against the possible side effects. Generally, benzodiazepines like lorazepam (Ativan) should be avoided as they further confuse the picture of alterations in consciousness and can contribute to delirium on their own.

GOOD TO KNOW

Your patient with delirium needs to be monitored closely. They can appear normal at times and then suddenly become agitated and try to get out of bed unsupervised.

CRITICAL THINKING QUESTION

An 81-year-old woman is admitted from the emergency department (ED) with a diagnosis of delirium manifested by acute confusion, rambling speech, and new onset of incontinence. Her husband reports this all started 24 hours ago after several episodes of diarrhea. She had recently been in the hospital for complications from diabetes. List the possible causes of delirium that should be evaluated.

DEMENTIA

Dementia is defined as a gradual loss of previous levels of cognitive functioning, which can include memory, language, executive functions (includes organizing), and attention in a state of being fully alert. In the DSM-5, the term dementia has been replaced with neurocognitive disorder, which can be classified as mild or major. These are further classified by the cause, such as Alzheimer's disease or Lewy body disease. A **mild neurocognitive disorder** is characterized by modest cognitive decline in one or more of six areas (see below) and does not interfere with the capacity for independence. A **major neurocognitive disorder** is characterized by significant decline from the previous level of performance in one or more of the six cognitive domains and does interfere with independence in everyday activities. The six cognitive domains are complex attention; executive function such as planning and organizing; learning and memory; language; perceptual motor; and social cognition (how people process, store, and apply information about other people and social situations).

Dementia remains a commonly used term in clinical practice, so it will be used in this chapter. In contrast with delirium, dementia is a slowly progressive condition that eventually affects all aspects of mental and social functioning. Primary dementias, including Alzheimer's disease, are those in which the dementia itself is the major cause. Secondary dementia, including vascular and HIV-related dementias, is caused by another disease or condition.

Depression is a common disorder in older patients. Sometimes depression can mimic dementia; in that case, it is referred to as pseudodementia. At times, the symptoms of depression can be misdiagnosed as dementia without a thorough work-up. See Table 16.3 for a comparison of neurocognitive disorder (dementia) and pseudodementia (depression).

Alzheimer's Disease

This most common form of neurocognitive disorder was initially recognized by Dr. Alois Alzheimer (FIG. 16.1) in 1906 as a form of impairment of brain function. **Alzheimer's disease** currently accounts for 60% to 80% of dementias. However, these numbers can be misleading because misdiagnosis is common (see below). It is estimated that 11.3% of Americans more than 65 years old have this diagnosis, and incidence increases with age. The effect of this disease on society is a profound one, as people are living longer. Alzheimer's disease is not reversible. It is the fifth leading cause of death in the over-65 population, and this number will only increase as other major causes (e.g., heart disease, cancer) decline. The official causes of death for people with Alzheimer's disease are often

Table 16.3

A Comparison of Neurocognitive Disorder and Pseudodementia (Depression)

Symptom Element	Neurocognitive Disorder (NCD)	Pseudodementia (Depression)
Progression of symptoms	Slow	Rapid
Memory	Progressive deficits; recent memory loss greater than remote; may confabulate for memory "gaps"; no complaints of loss	More like forgetfulness; no evidence of progressive deficit; recent and remote loss equal; complaints of deficits; no confabulation (will more likely answer "I don't know")
Orientation	Disoriented to time and place; may wander in search of the familiar	Oriented to time and place; no wandering
Task performance	Consistently poor performance but struggles to perform	Performance is variable; little effort is put forth
Symptom severity	Worse as the day progresses	Better as the day progresses
Affective distress	Appears unconcerned	Communicates severe distress
Appetite	Unchanged	Diminished
Attention and concentration	Impaired	Intact

Source: Morgan and Townsend (2021). *Psychiatric Mental Health Nursing,* 10th ed. Philadelphia: F.A. Davis Company, with permission.

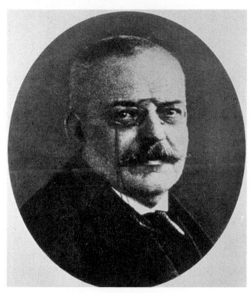

FIGURE 16.1 Alois Alzheimer (1864–1915) was a German neurologist who first identified Alzheimer's disease in 1906.

aspiration pneumonias, infections, and complications from falls, which are all outcomes of immobility, swallowing disorders, and malnutrition, which can be present in late stages of the disease (Alzheimer's Association, Alzheimer's Disease 2021 Facts and Figures). See Box 16.1 for the symptoms of Alzheimer's disease and Box 16.2 for warning signs.

There are three broad phases of Alzheimer's disease: preclinical Alzheimer's disease, mild neurocognitive impairment (see the following sections) due to Alzheimer's disease, and dementia due to Alzheimer's disease. The Alzheimer's dementia phase is further broken down into the stages of mild, moderate, and severe, which reflect the degree to which symptoms interfere with one's ability to carry out everyday activities. See Box 16.3 for the Stages of Alzheimer's Disease. How long individuals spend in each part of the continuum varies. The length of each phase of the continuum is influenced by age, genetics, gender, and other factors.

Box 16.1

Symptoms of Alzheimer's Disease

- memory loss that disrupts daily life
- challenges in planning or solving problems (executive functions)
- difficulty completing familiar tasks at home, at work, or at leisure
- confusion with time or place
- trouble understanding visual images and spatial relationships
- new problems with words in speaking or writing
- misplacing things and losing the ability to retrace steps
- decreased or poor judgment
- withdrawal from work or social activities
- changes in mood and personality
- **agnosia:** loss of ability to recognize objects
- **agraphia:** difficulty writing and drawing
- **apraxia:** inability to carry out motor activities despite intact motor function

Source: Adapted from Alzheimer's Association (2021) and Townsend & Morgan (2017).

Box 16.2

Warning Signs of Alzheimer's Disease

1. asking the same question over and over again
2. repeating the same story, word for word, again and again
3. losing one's ability to pay bills or balance one's checkbook
4. getting lost in familiar surroundings or misplacing household objects
5. relying on someone else, such as a spouse, to make decisions or answer questions they previously would have handled themselves
6. finding it hard to remember things
7. losing things or putting them in odd places

Source: Adapted from National Institute on Aging (2019). Alzheimer's Disease Fact Sheet; Alzheimer's Association 2021 Facts and Figures.

Tool Box

Review the government's national plan to address Alzheimer's disease (2013) along with a 2017 update:

https://aspe.hhs.gov/system/files/pdf/102526/NatlPlan2012%20with%20Note.pdf

https://aspe.hhs.gov/report/national-plan-address-alzheimers-disease-2017-update

Realizing the National Plan to Address Alzheimer's Disease: available at https://www.alz.org/aaic/downloads2021/2021_Milestones_Brochure.pdf

The Alzheimer's Association publishes facts and figures about Alzheimer's disease that review the most current treatment. Available at https://www.alz.org/media/Documents/alzheimers-facts-and-figures.pdf.

In addition to symptom assessment, including cognitive testing and brain imagery to rule out other causes, the diagnosis of Alzheimer's disease can be made by a positron emission tomography (PET) scan, which can detect physical and chemical changes in the brain. The changes seen in the brain include development of plaque (chemical deposits made of degenerating nerve cells and proteins called *beta amyloid*) and tangles (malformed nerve cells). Both plaques and tangles are greatly increased in someone with this form of dementia. As they increase, they create a toxic environment for normal brain cells. Spinal taps are now being used for early detection of plaque. An enzyme used to produce the neurochemical acetylcholine is reduced as well. Some of the medications that slow the progression of this disease increase the level of acetylcholine in the brain.

Biomarkers identify inflammation processes in the brain that can also be an indicator of Alzheimer's disease. There are genetic markers for some forms of this disease. Research is ongoing as to the causes of these brain changes (FIG. 16.2). Genetics plays a role in early onset Alzheimer's (onset before age 65) and research is being conducted to understand its role in later age onset. Other specific causes are still unclear.

GOOD TO KNOW

The reported number of people with Alzheimer's disease may be misleading because patients are often diagnosed based on clinical symptoms alone, which could be confused with other forms of dementia. When use of biomarkers becomes more common, the statistics will be more accurate.

GOOD TO KNOW

Since 2011, the annual Medicare wellness visit has included a required cognitive evaluation. The Alzheimer's Association (2021) found that only one in three older adults was aware that these visits should include a cognitive assessment.

A diagnosis of mild neurocognitive disorder (also called mild cognitive impairment [MCI]) is a risk factor for Alzheimer's disease. Mild neurocognitive disorder is a condition in which a person has mild deficits with memory, language, or another essential cognitive ability. The person begins making changes in their life to compensate for these, and it begins to affect daily living. Mild neurocognitive disorder is *not* normal aging.

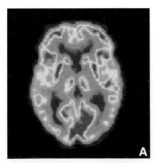
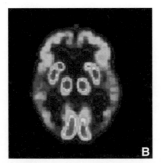
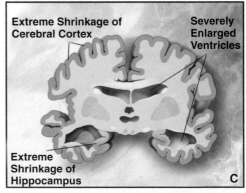

FIGURE 16.2 Changes in the Alzheimer's brain. A, Metabolic activity in a normal brain. B, Diminished metabolic activity in Alzheimer's diseased brain. C, Late-stage Alzheimer's disease with generalized atrophy and enlargement of the ventricles. (*Source: Alzheimer's Disease Education & Referral Center, A Service of the National Institute on Aging.*)

Many people fear that forgetfulness is a sign of developing Alzheimer's disease. See Table 16.4 for the differences between Alzheimer's disease and normal aging.

GOOD TO KNOW

Alzheimer's disease is a progressive, eventually terminal, illness. Nurses should be aware of signs of late-stage Alzheimer's disease, when hospice care may be an appropriate referral. Signs such as being bedbound or incontinent as well as having multiple infections or aspirations can indicate the patient is an appropriate candidate for hospice care.

Classroom Activity

View and discuss movies that address dementia, including *Iron Lady, The Savages, Still Alice, The Father,* and *The Notebook,* or read and discuss the novel *Elizabeth Is Missing* by Emma Healey.

Tool Box

The mini-mental state examination (MMSE) is a widely used test of cognitive function. It is a 30-point questionnaire used extensively with patients with dementia to track changes over time. The MMSE is available online at https://www.dementiacarecentral.com/mini-mental-state-exam.pdf.

Other Forms of Dementia

Neurocognitive disorder with Lewy bodies (or **Lewy body disease)** is the second-most common form of dementia. This has a similar presentation to Alzheimer's disease, with the addition of visual hallucinations and parkinsonian features (e.g., shuffling gait, rigid muscles). These symptoms may occur in the absence of major memory deficits. Lewy body disease is characterized by the presence of abnormal proteins in the cerebral cortex and brainstem called *Lewy bodies*. The cause is unknown.

Vascular dementia, also known as NCD due to vascular disease, is caused by small strokes, which over time result in interruption of blood flow to the brain. Vascular dementia is also sometimes referred to as multi-infarct dementia or vascular neurocognitive disease. Progression of this form of dementia can vary from Alzheimer's disease depending on the occurrence of vascular events; dementia progresses with each new stroke. Sudden onset of vascular dementia can occur if the vascular damage is severe, but the disease can follow a slower progression with periods of stability if the patient has no new strokes. Other forms of major neurocognitive disorders include dementia associated with Parkinson's disease, substance abuse, HIV, and traumatic brain injury, among others. Each of these forms of dementia has its own unique components in addition to core diagnostic features of dementia.

Differential Diagnosis of Delirium and Dementia

A new patient presenting with confusion and agitation can sometimes be misdiagnosed. Symptoms of delirium and dementia can seem similar, especially on first meeting a patient. See Table 16.5 and Box 16.4 to

Table 16.4

Differentiating Alzheimer's Disease From Normal Aging

Alzheimer's Disease	*Normal Aging*
Making poor judgments and decisions a lot of the time	Making a bad decision once in a while
Having problems taking care of monthly bills	Missing a monthly payment
Losing track of the date or time of year	Forgetting which day it is and remembering it later
Experiencing difficulty holding a conversation	Sometimes forgetting which word to use
Misplacing things often and being unable to find them	Losing things from time to time

Source: Adapted from The National Institute on Aging (2015).

Box 16.3

The Stages of Alzheimer's Disease

Mild Alzheimer's disease (early stage)

In the early stage of Alzheimer's, a person may function independently. They may still drive, work, and be part of social activities. Despite this, the person may feel as if they are having memory lapses, such as forgetting familiar words or the location of everyday objects.

Friends, family, or others close to the individual begin to notice difficulties. During a detailed medical interview, health-care providers may be able to detect problems in memory or concentration. Common difficulties include:

- recalling the right word or name
- remembering names when introduced to new people
- having difficulty performing tasks in social or work settings
- forgetting material that one has just read
- losing or misplacing a valuable object
- experiencing increased trouble with planning or organizing

Moderate Alzheimer's disease (middle stage)

Moderate Alzheimer's is typically the longest stage and can last for many years. As the disease progresses, the person with Alzheimer's will require a greater level of care.

You may notice the person with Alzheimer's confusing words, getting frustrated or angry, or acting in unexpected ways, such as refusing to bathe. Symptoms that vary from person to person may include:

- being forgetful of events or about one's own personal history
- feeling moody or withdrawn, especially in socially or mentally challenging situations
- being unable to recall information about themselves such as their own address or telephone number or the high school or college they attended

- experiencing confusion about where they are or what day it is
- requiring help choosing proper clothing for the season or the occasion
- having trouble controlling bladder and bowels
- experiencing changes in sleep patterns, such as sleeping during the day and becoming restless at night
- showing an increased risk of wandering and becoming lost
- demonstrating personality and behavioral changes, including suspiciousness and delusions or compulsive, repetitive behavior like hand-wringing or tissue shredding

Severe Alzheimer's disease (late stage)

In the final stage of this disease, individuals lose the ability to respond to their environment, to carry on a conversation and, eventually, to control movement. They may still say words or phrases, but communicating pain becomes difficult. As memory and cognitive skills continue to worsen, significant personality changes may take place, and individuals need extensive help with daily activities.

At this stage, individuals may:

- require round-the-clock assistance with daily activities and personal care
- lose awareness of recent experiences as well as of their surroundings
- experience changes in physical abilities, including walking, sitting and, eventually, swallowing
- have difficulty communicating
- become vulnerable to infections, especially pneumonia

Reprinted with permission from the Alzheimer's Association (2021). https://www.alz.org/alzheimers-dementia/stages

differentiate between delirium and dementia and learn common factors leading to misdiagnosis. A work-up to determine possible etiologies for different forms of dementia should also be done before giving the diagnosis of Alzheimer's disease.

DIFFERENTIAL DIAGNOSES FOR DEMENTIA

- major depressive disorder
- alternate neurocognitive disorders
- other neurological conditions
- delirium

Treatment of Dementias

No treatment is available to stop the deterioration of brain cells in Alzheimer's disease. Currently, pharmacological treatment is available to temporarily slow the worsening of symptoms for some patients (see Pharmacology Corner). Some other forms of dementia can be treated to slow progression if an etiology can be identified and addressed.

In addition to medications, supportive care, maintaining safety, prevention of infections, and caregiver support are the major interventions. Once diagnosed, the patient and their family need to develop a plan to provide care as the disease

Table 16.5

Characteristics of Delirium and Dementia

Delirium	*Dementia*
• Fluctuating levels of awareness and symptoms • Sudden onset • Clouding of consciousness • Perceptual disturbances (hallucinations, illusions) • Memory disturbance, more often for recent events • Highly distractible • Reversibility possible with treatment	• Slow, insidious onset with less fluctuation of symptoms • Deterioration of cognitive abilities • Impaired long- and short-term memory (memory impairment always present) • Personality changes • May focus on one thing for a long time • Usually irreversible

Source: Adapted from Gorman and Sultan (2008). *Psychosocial Nursing for General Patient Care,* 3rd ed. Philadelphia: F.A. Davis Company, with permission.

Box 16.4

Factors That Contribute to Misdiagnosis in Dementia and Delirium

• Some symptoms of dementia and delirium are similar.
• Several causes may occur simultaneously to bring about dementia.
• Delirium occurring in a patient with a dementia can exacerbate already existing symptoms.
• Health-care personnel may harbor unfounded beliefs that serious memory deficits, confusion, and other progressive intellectual deficits are a normal part of the aging process.
• Health-care personnel may harbor unfounded beliefs that confusion always indicates Alzheimer's disease in an older patient.
• Confusion and behavioral changes may be the first signs of medical illness in older patients.
• Head injuries and other conditions causing brain tissue trauma may present with symptoms similar to those of dementia.
• Confusion is an adverse reaction to many medications.

Source: Linda Gorman (author).

progresses. This is important in the early stages so that the patient can participate in decisions about future care while they still can. For example, identifying options for home care or facilities in the area based on the patient's wishes can be documented early on, and financial arrangements can be established to ensure future support. Family members of

these patients need to be prepared for what to expect as the disease progresses (FIG. 16.3).

Clinical Activity

If your patient has dementia, talk with the family about how they are coping.

GOOD TO KNOW

People with early stage Alzheimer's disease should be encouraged to complete an advance directive so that they can document their wishes for care and treatment as the disease progresses.

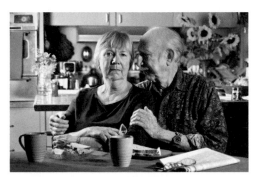

FIGURE 16.3 Alzheimer's disease has a tremendous effect on the family.

Pharmacology Corner

The U.S. Food and Drug Administration (FDA) has approved two types of medications—cholinesterase inhibitors (donepezil, rivastigmine, galantamine) and memantine (Namenda)—to treat the cognitive symptoms (memory loss, confusion, and problems with thinking and reasoning) of Alzheimer's disease (Alzheimer's Association, 2021). Cholinesterase inhibitors work by inhibiting acetylcholinesterase, which increases concentrations of acetylcholine in the brain. Memantine works as a receptor antagonist of N-methyl-d-aspartate (NMDA) and has been shown to slow the decline in cognitive and daily functioning in some patients with more advanced disease. One medication, Namzaric, combines one of the cholinesterase inhibitors (donepezil) with memantine. Patients with NCD due to Lewy bodies have also been found to benefit from cholinesterase inhibitors.

In 2021, the FDA approved aducanumab (Aduhelm) for early stage Alzheimer's disease. The medication is administered as an intravenous infusion. This is the first drug that treats the actual cause of the disease by removing beta-amyloids, which are the cause of Alzheimer's disease.

As Alzheimer's progresses, brain cells die, and connections among cells are lost, causing cognitive symptoms to worsen. Often, cholinesterase inhibitors have decreasing effectiveness as the disease progresses. Although current medications cannot stop the damage Alzheimer's causes to brain cells, they may help lessen or stabilize symptoms for a limited time by affecting certain chemicals involved in carrying messages among the brain's nerve cells. See Table 16.6 for the medications used to treat Alzheimer's dementia. Early treatment with these medications in patients with mild neurocognitive disorder may be helpful.

In some cases, extreme agitation requires the use of antipsychotic medications in patients with dementia. The FDA has ordered black box warnings on atypical antipsychotics due to increased risk of death in older patients with psychotic behaviors associated with dementia. These deaths were cardiovascular related. In 2008, all typical antipsychotics were added to this warning (see Chapter 15, Schizophrenia Spectrum and Other Psychotic Disorders, for a discussion of typical and atypical antipsychotics). Therefore, close monitoring is required when any of these medications is used. These medications present a dilemma to the health-care provider. They can control undesirable behavior and promote safety, but there is a risk of untoward effects. The adage "start low and go slow" when using any medications in the older population is particularly true for typical antipsychotics.

Medications to treat depression, anxiety, and insomnia may also be utilized; however, benzodiazepines like lorazepam can contribute to more confusion. Buspirone (Buspar) is a nonbenzodiazepine that is an alternative. Certain antidepressants like mirtazapine (Remeron) and trazodone (Desyrel) are also useful for insomnia. Because depression and anxiety are especially common if the person is aware of their cognitive decline, these medications can be very helpful. Be aware that paradoxical reactions (when a drug has the opposite of its intended effect) sometimes occur with antianxiety medications used in older patients. Managing anxiety with these medications can be useful to reduce the patient's suffering and disruptive behaviors.

GOOD TO KNOW

It can be challenging to give oral medications to patients with dementia. An effective strategy is to crush the pills and put them in sweet foods like pudding or applesauce. Some medications come in transdermal form as well as extended-release oral formulations to ease administration.

GOOD TO KNOW

Close monitoring of side effects of all medications can be challenging, as the patient may not be able to tell you what they are experiencing, for example, dry mouth, itching, or constipation. When monitoring side effects, it is important to remember that patients at home may miss doses or take extra doses of prescribed medications due to poor memory.

Table 16.6
Alzheimer's Medications

Cholinesterase Inhibitor	Side Effects
Donepezil (Aricept)	Insomnia, dizziness, headache, gastrointestinal (GI) upset, weight loss
Rivastigmine (Excelon)	Dizziness, headache, fatigue
Galantamine (Razadyne)	Dizziness, headache, GI upset
Memantine (Namenda	Dizziness, headache, constipation

Source: Morgan & Townsend (2021).

CRITICAL THINKING QUESTION

Your 72-year-old patient with advanced dementia has been screaming all night, calling for her mother. All attempts to console her are ineffective. Every time someone walks by her room, her screaming increases. You have orders for several medications to control agitation, including haloperidol (Haldol) and lorazepam (Ativan). Before administering one of these, what should you consider?

Clinical Activity

Monitor side effects of any medications your patient is taking. Your observations are important, as your patient may not be able to verbalize about symptoms.

NURSING CARE OF PATIENTS WITH DELIRIUM AND DEMENTIA

Common nursing diagnoses in patients with delirium and dementia include the following:

- anxiety
- injury, risk for
- memory, impaired
- self-care deficit
- sensory perception, disturbed
- sleep pattern, disturbed
- thought processes, disturbed

General Nursing Interventions

The nursing interventions for patients with either or both of these diagnoses are based on the patient's symptoms.

1. *Collect data:* Collect information on vital signs, medications used by the patient, circumstances immediately preceding symptom onset, and any other information the patient or person who may be accompanying the individual can provide. Note anything that is considered to be a change in the patient's condition. Question family or caregivers on interventions that have been useful in the past.

2. *Stay calm:* Be ready for anything. Patients with symptoms of delirium and/or dementia can be very changeable. No matter what the situation, you must diffuse it calmly and maintain safety. It is very important to make every attempt to also maintain the patient's dignity during periods of excitability. Due to memory deficits, these patients can exhibit impulsive behaviors and labile emotions as they forget the context of the situation. By remaining calm, you will reinforce maintaining a calm environment.

GOOD TO KNOW

A patient with early to moderate dementia may suffer intense anxiety due to confusion and awareness of losing their memory. This can be the cause of agitation and paranoia.

GOOD TO KNOW

For sleep problems, offering chamomile tea at bedtime or using aroma therapy, such as spraying pajamas with a lavender fragrance, can be helpful to avoid use of sleeping pills.

3. *Do not argue with the patient:* Patients with dementia and/or delirium have cognitive impairment. They do not have the capacity to make rational decisions during an agitated episode. Attempting to model desired behavior or simply waiting a few minutes and repeating verbal instructions may prove successful. These patients may no longer have the filters to control

their behavior or act in a socially acceptable manner. Distraction can be helpful in some cases. Be aware that patients may use disruptive behaviors such as swearing or insulting others as a way to express frustration.

4. *Use clear, simple verbal communication:* Sensory overload is a common experience for patients experiencing delirium and dementia. To avoid a behavioral "short circuit," it is a good idea to use simple communication and calm activity in the room. Keep the area quiet. Keep curtains drawn or partially open; keep televisions and radios off or at a very low volume. The stimulation can be adjusted according to the patient's tolerance. Focus on one task at a time. Do not give the patient two to three instructions at the same time.

5. *Allow time for the patient to respond:* The ability to function cognitively and physically is diminished when a person is in delirium or dementia. Nurses and other health-care workers must remember to allow more time for performing care. Patience is an important intervention. This can be frustrating for caregivers, but by following this plan, the patient will have more opportunities to remain independent and reduce their anxiety. This will ultimately make your job easier with better outcomes.

6. *Use touch when appropriate:* Although it is impossible not to touch patients while providing care, recognize that in this population there can be a danger for misinterpretation of that touch. People who have challenges in their ability to process and understand information may not remember the situation as it actually happened. They may have forgotten the episode of incontinence and not understand why "that nurse had to touch me there!" Having a second person—another nurse or a family member—in the room can be a helpful protection for both you and the patient. Documenting all nursing actions and patient responses very carefully is also necessary.

7. *Prevent wandering:* Patients in a state of delirium or dementia may wander. This can occur if the patient becomes stressed as they attempt to search for something that is familiar. It can also be related to sensations of hunger, thirst, or the need to eliminate that the person is not able to verbalize. Wandering is a major safety risk that frequently encourages nurses

to request restraint orders from the physician. **Restraints should be used only as a last resort, when alternative interventions are unsuccessful.** Interventions to use before requesting restraints include:

- providing a safe environment where the patient can walk or pace
- maintaining a structured schedule when providing care
- distracting the patient with other activities
- putting up large signs in the area reminding patients of their rooms or of areas that are off-limits
- using alarms either on the patient or on doors to off-limit areas (e.g., exit door to a stairwell); GPS tracking devices that patients can wear are available as well
- engaging family and volunteers to closely watch the patient's movements

When the health-care provider has ordered restraints, your responsibilities include careful observation and documentation of alternative interventions that have been tried. **Physical restraints** are defined as any physical method of restricting an individual's freedom of movement, activity, or normal access to their body; these restraints cannot be easily removed. For physical restraints, each state has guidelines for how often to check, release, and reposition or exercise the patient. Assessing for signs of pressure injuries and stiffness of muscles helps to maintain skin integrity and full range of motion. Physical restraints can cause more problems than they solve. So every effort must be made to use them only as a last resort (American Academy of Nursing, 2014). **Chemical restraints** are defined as the use of a medication as a restriction to manage the patient's behavior or restrict the patient's freedom of movement. These medications are not a standard treatment or dosage for the patient's condition. Again, each state may have guidelines on the use of chemical restraints. For chemical restraints, you must document the effect of the medication and any possible side effects. Many medications have side effects, such as confusion, restlessness, and forgetfulness, which are counterproductive for people with delirium and dementia. **Medications should not be used as a substitute for appropriate activities, programming, and personal interaction.**

8. *Assist with activities of daily living (ADLS) as appropriate to the situation:* You will be doing as much for the patient physically as the individual's condition requires. For temporary delirium and early stages of dementia, you may only have to give the patient some verbal cues as to what they need to do. For deeper delirium and later stages of dementia, performing total care for the patient may be necessary. Always maintain the patient's dignity and allow them to do as much independently as they are able.

9. *Provide adequate stimulation:* It is as detrimental to under-stimulate people with cognitive disorders as it is to overload them. The brain needs some encouragement to activate. This will be a "trial-and-error" situation between you and the patient, and it will be different for every patient. Some success has been had with music, pets, art, and physical therapies.

10. *Maintain appropriate milieu:* People living with irreversible, progressive dementia require special attention to the environment. Caregivers and family must come to accept that the disease is progressive and will not improve. With patients with dementia, do not emphasize "reality orientation" by asking or reminding the patient of their name, the year, and current location—especially in later stages of the disease. Changes in the brain will not allow the memory to function successfully and may, in fact, cause the patient to experience frustration, feel agitation, and increase acting-out behaviors if reality orientation is emphasized. Reality orientation may be helpful in delirium and in early stages of dementia, where the patient gains a sense of comfort from being reoriented; however, with short-term memory gaps, this approach may be helpful only for a brief time.

Having old photos of the patient or familiar smells such as a favorite perfume or food in the environment can have a reassuring effect. Many memory-care facilities ask families to bring in special personal items, such as photos or mementos that are meaningful to the patient that can be housed in a "memory box" in the patient's room to provide a calming influence.

11. *Provide emotional support:* The patient will often experience anxiety as they realize loss of mental abilities. The person can become panicky when disoriented. A consistent, calm environment is important. Patients can also suffer from depression, especially in early stages when the full effect of the progressive disease is understood. Family caregivers also need much support, as caring for this patient is exhausting. Family members often need assistance in identifying support groups and resources for additional caregivers and facilities.

See Table 16.7 for the nursing care plan of confused patients. See Concept Map for Dementia Figure 16.4.

Table 16.7

Nursing Care Plan of the Confused Patient

Assessment/Data Collection	Nursing Diagnosis	Goal	Interventions	Evaluation
Confused as to time, place Becomes agitated when efforts made to reorient patient	Disturbance in sensory perception	Reduced episodes of agitation	• Encourage family to provide familiar items in patient's room, for example, old photos, mementos. • Place a large sign on door to identify patient's room, bathroom. • Spend time with patient to reminisce about an important event in the past. • Play music or TV shows that are meaningful from patient's past. • Judge whether reorienting patient regularly is effective. If it increases agitation, then avoid this.	Patient will have periods of calmness.

GOOD TO KNOW

Review agency policies on the use of restraints. Be aware of which alternatives to restraints are useful with different patients.

GOOD TO KNOW

Music therapy has been found to be helpful for some patients with Alzheimer's disease. Playing music that has special meaning in the patient's life can be a calming influence for some.

Evidence-Based Practice

Research Question: To what extent are nurses in nursing homes affected by the sleep disturbances in patients with dementia?

Evidence: A multicenter cross-sectional study assessed nurses' burden associated with sleep disturbances in residents with dementia. This burden was assessed using the sleep disorder inventory (SDI). Seventy-eight percent of nurses in the study reported being regularly confronted with patients with sleep disturbances on the night shift.

Implications for Nursing Practice: The frequency of sleep disturbances in patients with dementia means that nurses need to have skills to deal with this common symptom in patients with neurocognitive disorders. Education programs on managing sleep disturbance need to be part of the education for all nursing staff in skilled nursing facilities.

Wilfling D, Dichter MN, Trutschel D, Köpke S. (2020). Nurses' burden caused by sleep disturbances of nursing home residents with dementia: Multicenter cross-sectional study. *BMC Nurs.* 19:83. doi: 10.1186/s12912-020-00478-y. PMID: 32943980; PMCID: PMC7487724.

Patient/Family Education

- Explain effective safety measures for the family to incorporate when arranging for home care.
- Provide information on support programs for caregivers, such as the Alzheimer's Association.
- Provide information on factors that may contribute to the development of delirium.
- Provide family information on strategies that have been effective to reassure the patient, such as presence of family photos and familiar objects.
- Review medications that can be useful or hazardous to patient care.
- For a patient in early dementia, ensure that the patient and family are addressing the need to complete an advance directive while the patient still has the capacity to participate.
- Review strategies to help family address difficult behaviors such as agitation and wandering.
- If the patient is still driving, provide information to the family on addressing when and how to take away the car keys.

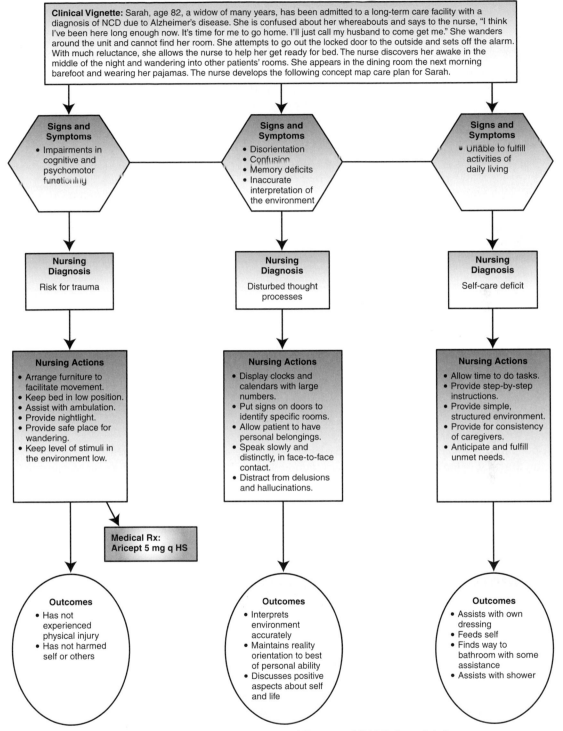

Clinical Vignette: Sarah, age 82, a widow of many years, has been admitted to a long-term care facility with a diagnosis of NCD due to Alzheimer's disease. She is confused about her whereabouts and says to the nurse, "I think I've been here long enough now. It's time for me to go home. I'll just call my husband to come get me." She wanders around the unit and cannot find her room. She attempts to go out the locked door to the outside and sets off the alarm. With much reluctance, she allows the nurse to help her get ready for bed. The nurse discovers her awake in the middle of the night and wandering into other patients' rooms. She appears in the dining room the next morning barefoot and wearing her pajamas. The nurse develops the following concept map care plan for Sarah.

Signs and Symptoms
• Impairments in cognitive and psychomotor functioning

Signs and Symptoms
• Disorientation
• Confusion
• Memory deficits
• Inaccurate interpretation of the environment

Signs and Symptoms
• Unable to fulfill activities of daily living

Nursing Diagnosis
Risk for trauma

Nursing Diagnosis
Disturbed thought processes

Nursing Diagnosis
Self-care deficit

Nursing Actions
• Arrange furniture to facilitate movement.
• Keep bed in low position.
• Assist with ambulation.
• Provide nightlight.
• Provide safe place for wandering.
• Keep level of stimuli in the environment low.

Nursing Actions
• Display clocks and calendars with large numbers.
• Put signs on doors to identify specific rooms.
• Allow patient to have personal belongings.
• Speak slowly and distinctly, in face-to-face contact.
• Distract from delusions and hallucinations.

Nursing Actions
• Allow time to do tasks.
• Provide step-by-step instructions.
• Provide simple, structured environment.
• Provide for consistency of caregivers.
• Anticipate and fulfill unmet needs.

Medical Rx:
Aricept 5 mg q HS

Outcomes
• Has not experienced physical injury
• Has not harmed self or others

Outcomes
• Interprets environment accurately
• Maintains reality orientation to best of personal ability
• Discusses positive aspects about self and life

Outcomes
• Assists with own dressing
• Feeds self
• Finds way to bathroom with some assistance
• Assists with shower

FIGURE 16.4 Concept Map for Dementia. (From Morgan & Townsend [2021]. Essentials for Psychiatric Mental Health Nursing. FA Davis.)

Cultural Considerations

The type of care the family wants for the patient with dementia will be influenced by their culture. In some cultures, the family will maintain the patient in the home, no matter how difficult the care. Home care needs to incorporate cultural values to help the family provide the needed care.

Language barriers can also add to complications in understanding the patient's needs, especially for those in a facility when family is unavailable. It is important for these patients to have access to people who speak the same language and have similar cultural experiences to enhance reality orientation and correctly assess cognitive function.

GOOD TO KNOW

Family members must be provided information on being a caregiver and how to cope with the long-term emotional strain. This should be part of all patients' plan of care.

Tool Box

The 36-Hour Day: A Family Guide to Caring for People Who Have Alzheimer Disease, Other Dementias, and Memory Loss, 7th Edition (2021) by Mace and Rabins is a must-read for family caregivers.

Classroom Activity

Arrange a visit to a local facility that specializes in memory care. Interview the staff to learn how they do this work every day.

Identify local resources such as support groups or adult day care for people with dementia.

CRITICAL THINKING QUESTION

In report, you are told that your 90-year-old patient with moderate dementia has been awake all night, pacing the floor. In the morning, you find him sound asleep at 10 a.m. What should be your plan for the day shift?

The next day, this patient is very agitated and repeatedly insists on walking out the unit door. The health-care provider leaves an order for soft restraints to prevent wandering. Before applying these, what interventions should you try?

Key Points

- Delirium is a frequent diagnosis in the acute hospital setting due to complex medical conditions, medication side effects, and sensory overload.
- Delirium is usually reversible once the underlying cause is identified; dementia is usually irreversible.
- Alzheimer's disease is by far the most common form of major neurocognitive disorder.
- Alzheimer's disease is a terminal illness, which has a tremendous effect on the patient's family and society.
- Other causes of dementia include vascular insufficiency, substance abuse, and Parkinson's disease.

- Medications such as antianxiety medications and antipsychotics often have a side effect of confusion and should be chosen carefully for use in people with neurocognitive disorders.
- Medications are chosen to treat specific behaviors; they are not a substitute for more direct interventions.
- Care of the patient with dementia should focus on maintenance of safety, prevention of infection, and family support.

Safe and Effective Nursing Care

Provide a safe environment that is free of hazards.

Prevent falls.

Provide adequate supervision for safety and to maintain the patient's dignity.

Utilize swallowing precautions for anyone at risk for aspiration.

Allow the patient to move through their environment, but prevent wandering and leaving the safe environment unsupervised.

Provide adequate identification in case the patient does leave the facility or home without warning.

Use alternative interventions before considering use of physical restraints.

CASE STUDY

Mrs. G is an 84-year-old widow who lives alone. She has episodes of anxiety and paranoia. She calls her son at odd hours, telling him that a neighbor is spying on her. Despite these episodes, she seems to function normally and is able to care for herself. Her son reports that her memory seems to be getting poorer, and he notices that she leaves notes to herself around the apartment, reminding herself to lock the door, brush her teeth, or water the plants. He also notices that she looks as though she has lost weight recently, although she tells him she is eating well. He looks in her refrigerator and sees very little food. He asks her what she eats, and she says, "Yogurt." She cannot think of anything else. She reports fear of using the stove, so she eats only cold foods. He looks at her mail and notices a past-due notice on her water bill. She says she is sure she paid that. The son is getting concerned and takes her to a health-care provider who specializes in gerontology for an evaluation.

The health-care provider does a complete assessment in the office and orders an MRI. A diagnosis of early- to moderate-stage Alzheimer's disease is made.

1. What actions would you suggest the patient and her son institute at this time?
2. How would you differentiate between dementia and depression?
3. What safety measures need to be implemented?

Review Questions

1. You are working the night shift in your surgical unit. Ms. Y, who is 1 day postoperative for a total hip replacement, is taking several medications for pain, along with an antibiotic. She is 70 years old and presented as alert and oriented before surgery. She lives independently. Ms. Y suddenly begins screaming and thrashing in bed, begging you to "Get the spiders out of my bed!" What is the best explanation for Ms. Y's behavior?

   a. Delusions
   b. Delirium
   c. Dementia
   d. Sepsis

2. The best nursing intervention for you, the licensed practical nurse (LPN)/licensed vocational nurse (LVN), to help Ms. Y is to:

   a. Inform the charge nurse and doctor immediately.
   b. Turn on the light and ask her where the spiders are.
   c. Stop her pain medications.
   d. Check her medical record for a diagnosis of mental illness.

3. Mr. H has been admitted to your nursing home with late-stage Alzheimer's disease. His wife is crying and says to you, "Nurse, when will he get better? I don't know what I will do without him at home. Why can't the doctor fix him?" Your best response to Mrs. H is:
   a. "Hopefully with time he will improve."
   b. "Maybe you should stop visiting for a few days, and then you'll feel better."
   c. "You sound really worried. Tell me what the doctor has told you about his condition."
   d. "Mrs. H, your doctor has explained that Mr. H will not get better. You need to make a plan for the future."

4. Donepezil (Aricept) is a medication approved for the treatment of symptoms of Alzheimer's-type dementia. Nurses must be alert to which of the following side effects?
   a. Tachycardia
   b. Insomnia
   c. Mania
   d. Weight gain

5. Which statement is *not* true about Alzheimer's disease?
   a. It is a dementia disorder.
   b. It may occur in middle to late life.
   c. It is a chronic disease.
   d. It is caused by hardening of the arteries.

6. Which of the following would you expect to see in a patient who is diagnosed with a neurocognitive disorder?
   a. Intact memory
   b. Appropriate behavior
   c. Disorganization of thought
   d. Orientation to person, place, and time

7. Cholinesterase inhibitors are used in treatment of Alzheimer's disease. Which of the following are cholinesterase inhibitors?
   a. Haloperidol and chlorpromazine
   b. Donepezil and rivastigmine
   c. Memantine and donepezil
   d. Haloperidol and galantamine

8. Your patient, who is recovering from an exacerbation of an AIDS-related infection, is opting to be treated by family and friends at home. The family has expressed concern because they sense a change in the patient's cognitive abilities. Part of the discharge teaching for this family might include:
   a. "It's nothing, really. Patients sometimes get confused in the hospital."
   b. "Keep an eye on him. You don't want him to start wandering."
   c. "You're concerned about the change in his ability to remember things? Let me call the doctor for you. This is something that you need to discuss together."
   d. "I thought something was strange!"

9. Mr. F is brought in by a family member who expresses concern over his memory loss. The physician diagnosed the patient with vascular dementia (multi-infarct dementia). You realize this disorder:
   a. Is irreversible
   b. May progress rapidly or slowly
   c. Indicates the patient has most likely experienced more than one stroke
   d. All of the above

10. The use of reality-orienting techniques would be helpful with which patient?
    a. One in the advanced stage of Alzheimer's disease
    b. One with advanced vascular dementia
    c. An older patient who is confused and screaming out for her mother
    d. One who is recovering from delirium and seems more relaxed when reminded of where she is

REVIEW QUESTIONS ANSWER KEY 1. b, 2. a, 3. c, 4. b, 5. d, 6. c, 7. b, 8. c, 9. d, 10. d

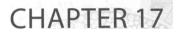

CHAPTER 17
Substance Use and Addictive Disorders

KEY TERMS

Addiction
Alcohol abuse
Alcohol use disorder
Alcoholism
Binge drinking
Codependent
Co-occurring disorder
Delirium tremens
Detoxification
Dysfunctional
Intoxication
Psychoactive drugs
Substance abuse
Substance dependence
Substance use disorder
Tolerance
Withdrawal

CHAPTER CONCEPTS

Addiction
Behaviors
Cognition
Family
Health promotion
Mood and affect
Safety
Self

LEARNING OUTCOMES

1. Describe substance use disorder and how it affects society.
2. Define codependency.
3. Define co-occurring disorders.
4. Identify common medical treatments for addictive disorders.
5. Identify nursing interventions for patients with addictive disorders.

Mind- or mood-altering substances have been used throughout human history. Today, these substances include alcohol, sedatives/hypnotics, narcotic analgesics, stimulants, hallucinogens, and cannabis as well as **psychoactive drugs** (any drug that alters mood, perception, mental functioning, and/or behavior). Most of these categories of substances can be and are used legally and therapeutically. However, they all have the strong potential to be abused and potentially addictive. Taken in excess, these substances activate the brain's reward system and can lead the user to neglect normal activities in favor of seeking out the substance again and again.

People use these substances for a variety of reasons: relief of physical and emotional pain, relaxation, elevation of mood, enhancement of socialization, improved alertness, and alteration in perceptions of reality. Alcohol and caffeine are probably the most-used socially acceptable psychoactive substances. Tobacco was also part of that group, but in recent years, its use has become much less acceptable in U.S. society (FIG. 17.1).

Substance abuse is a major health problem in the United States. Substance abuse contributes to higher health-care costs, significant disability, and even suicide attempts (Cook & Alegría, 2011). **Substance use disorder** (SUD) is a cluster of cognitive, behavioral, and physiological symptoms indicating that the person continues

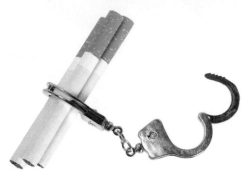

FIGURE 17.1 Nicotine is an addiction, and it can be the most difficult one to overcome.

to use the substance despite significant substance-related problems (American Psychiatric Association, 2022).

In the past, substance abuse and **substance dependence** were traditionally separated as two distinct diagnoses. Because these two designations were sometimes confusing and difficult to differentiate, the *Diagnostic and Statistical Manual of Mental Disorders,* 5th ed., known as DSM-5 (American Psychiatric Association, 2013), combined abuse and dependence into substance use disorder, with a graded clinical severity of mild, moderate, and severe. In addition to SUD, other diagnostic categories include substance-induced **intoxication** (a state of disturbance in cognition, perception, and other functions directly attributable to the effects of the substance) and **withdrawal** (the body's readjustment that accompanies the discontinuation of a substance). Each category has specific criteria that allow diagnosis for each substance. However, because the terms abuse and dependence are so common in today's culture, they will still be used throughout this chapter along with substance use disorder.

People with psychiatric disorders commonly abuse drugs and alcohol as a way to self-medicate to reduce anxiety, insomnia, depression, loneliness, rapid thoughts, frightening hallucinations, and other distressing symptoms. Considered a **co-occurring disorder** (also called dual diagnosis), this form of SUD adds additional complications to the psychiatric diagnosis; it makes daily management, treatment, and recovery more difficult. Co-occurring disorders are the rule rather than the exception for patients with psychiatric disorders. Which comes first—the substance abuse or the psychiatric disorder? Co-occurring disorders can start with a patient self-medicating to treat symptoms of a psychiatric diagnosis, or substance abuse can be the initial

---

Tool Box

The National Survey on Drug Abuse and Health conducts an annual survey of Americans' use of alcohol and other substances and provides the following data from 2020:

• In 2020, 21.4% of people aged 12 or older (59.3 million people) used illicit drugs in the past year. Marijuana remains the most widely used drug that remains illegal in some states. Illicit drugs include marijuana/hashish, cocaine (including crack), heroin, methamphetamines, hallucinogens, inhalants, or prescription-type psycho-therapeutics used nonmedically.
• 40.3 million people aged 12 or older (or 14.5%) had an SUD in the past year, including 28.3 million with alcohol use disorder, 18.4 million with an illicit drug use disorder, and 6.5 million with both alcohol use disorder and an illicit drug use disorder.

National Survey on Drug Use and Health: Summary of national findings: https://www.samhsa.gov/data/sites/default/files/2021-10/2020_NSDUH_Highlights.pdf

---

diagnosis that leads to other psychiatric disorders as a complication (FIGS. 17.2 and 17.3). Also, prolonged use of substances increases the *underlying risk* for mental illness (Greenstein, 2017). Outcomes for treatment are more effective when the substance use treatment is integrated into the treatment for the psychiatric disorder (NAMI, 2020).

Health-care professionals are not immune to problems with alcohol and drugs. In fact, they are somewhat more likely than the general population to abuse alcohol or prescribed drugs. Stressful jobs, access to controlled substances, and ineffective coping strategies are contributing factors. In nurses, medication errors, high absenteeism, and poor concentration are some of the signs of substance use, and all of these put patients and coworkers at risk. Because they do not fit the typical image of a substance abuser, nurses as well as their coworkers can more easily deny the problem. Coworkers may even avoid reporting suspicion of a problem in order to protect the nurse. Some states have mandated reporting that requires observers to report substance-abusing nurses. Many states have developed drug-diversion programs to provide confidential

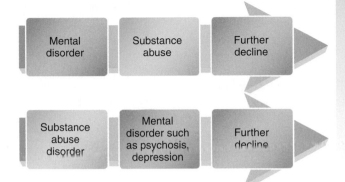

FIGURE 17.2 Common pathways in co-occurring disorders.

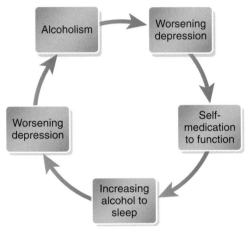

FIGURE 17.3 An example of the cycle of decline in co-occurring disorders.

treatment and rehabilitation for doctors, nurses, and other health-care workers.

Classroom Activity

Investigate your state's policy on drug diversion programs for nurses.

GOOD TO KNOW

Generally, substance use becomes a problem when it

1. interferes with normal functioning
2. continues despite negative consequences
3. hurts others

CRITICAL THINKING QUESTION

You are working in an outpatient mental health clinic. A new patient with a long history of schizophrenia tells you he needs to leave the clinic for an hour to meet someone who gives him "special medicines" to help him sleep. What concerns would you have? What action would you take?

GOOD TO KNOW

All psychiatric patients should be screened for SUDs.

Classroom Activity

• Movies that address SUDs include *Days of Wine and Roses, Lost Weekend, I'm Dancing as Fast as I Can, 28 Days, Flight, The Gambler, Beautiful Boy, Leaving Las Vegas, Trainspotting, A Star Is Born.*

Some of the characteristics of progressive SUD include (American Psychiatric Association, 2013; 2022):

• The essential feature of a substance use disorder is a cluster of cognitive, behavioral, and physiological symptoms indicating that the individual continues using the substance despite significant substance-related problems.
• A need for markedly increased amounts of the substance to achieve intoxication or desired effect **(tolerance)**
• Markedly diminished effect with continued use of the same amount of the substance (tolerance)

- Characteristic withdrawal syndrome for the substance
- The same (or a closely related) substance is taken to relieve or avoid withdrawal symptoms (e.g., alcohol and tranquilizers reduce symptoms of alcohol withdrawal)
- The substance is often taken in larger amounts or over a longer period than was intended (analgesics originally used for pain relief then continued when source of pain resolved)
- A persistent desire or unsuccessful effort to cut down or control substance use
- A great deal of time is spent obtaining the substance (e.g., visiting multiple doctors or driving long distances to a source), using the substance, or recovering from its effects
- Important social, occupational, or recreational activities are given up or reduced because of substance use (e.g., quitting school, giving up a favorite sport)
- The substance use is continued despite knowledge of having a persistent or recurrent physical or psychological problem that is likely to have been caused or exacerbated by the substance (e.g., current cocaine use despite recognition of cocaine-induced depression or continued drinking despite recognition that an ulcer was made worse by alcohol consumption)
- Failure to fulfill major role obligations at work, school, or home (e.g., repeated absences or poor work performance related to substance use; substance-related absences, suspensions, or expulsions from school; neglect of children or household)

- Recurrent substance use in situations in which it is physically hazardous (e.g., driving an automobile or operating a machine when impaired by substance use)
- Recurrent substance-related legal problems (e.g., arrests for substance-related disorderly conduct)
- Continued substance use despite having persistent or recurrent social or interpersonal problems caused or exacerbated by the effects of the substance (e.g., arguments with spouse about consequences of intoxication, physical fights)

ALCOHOL

As the most commonly abused substance worldwide, alcohol is readily available in most cultures and is often included in important occasions and religious ceremonies. Roughly 8.5% of Americans over 18 years old have an **alcohol use disorder** (American Psychiatric Assocation, 2013). The National Survey on Drug Abuse and Health (2020) found that 12.8% of current alcohol users meet the criteria for heavy drinkers. Alcohol is quickly absorbed in the body, with initial effects of intoxication producing relaxation, euphoria, and loss of inhibition. In most states, intoxication is legally defined as having a blood alcohol level of 0.08 g/dL. Higher blood alcohol levels (levels greater than 0.4 g/dL) depress the central nervous system (CNS), leading to staggering gait, labile emotions, incoherent speech, poor judgment, belligerent/aggressive behavior, and eventually coma and respiratory depression. Alcohol content varies with the type of beverage. The same amount of alcohol is present in:

- 12 ounces of most beers (5% alcohol)
- 5 ounces of wine
- 1.5 ounces of 80-proof distilled spirits such as whiskey or vodka

GOOD TO KNOW

For most adults, low-risk alcohol use—up to 14 drinks per week for men and 7 drinks per week for women and older people—causes few, if any, problems (National Institute of Alcohol Abuse and Alcoholism "Rethinking Drinking").

Alcoholism is defined as a chronic illness characterized by compulsive and uncontrolled consumption of alcoholic beverages usually to the detriment of the drinker's health, personal relationships, and

Cultural Considerations

Substance abuse crosses all cultures and ethnic groups. Some groups are known to have a higher incidence that may reflect genetic risk and/or cultural patterns. For example, Native Americans have a high rate of alcoholism. Genetic factors predispose this population to poor metabolism of alcohol while social factors, such as high rates of unemployment and poverty, also contribute to the problem. On the other hand, people of Asian descent have a lower-than-average rate of substance abuse. Genetic intolerance for alcohol creates an unpleasant sensation when alcohol is consumed and may be a factor in the lower incidence of alcoholism in this population (Townsend, 2017).

social standing. **Addiction** to alcohol has been referred to as alcohol dependence, alcohol abuse, and now alcohol use disorder.

Given the same amount of alcohol, women have higher blood-alcohol concentrations than men, even with body size taken into consideration. Differences in fat and body water content lead to women being more prone to long-term effects of heavy alcohol use (Fig. 17.4) (National Institute of Alcohol Abuse and Alcoholism, 2021).

Early signs of serious problems with alcohol use in men and women can include:

- drinking in secret
- drinking first thing after waking up
- gulping the first drink
- preoccupation with alcohol
- onset of blackouts (lapses in memory resulting from persistent heavy drinking)

Binge drinking is a pattern of drinking that brings blood alcohol concentration (BAC) levels to 0.08 g/dL. This typically occurs after women consume four drinks and men consume five drinks in about 2 hours. Binge drinking can lead to serious health consequences from alcohol poisoning (when alcohol reaches toxic levels), as well as risky behaviors when under its influence. Binge drinking is a serious issue particularly in the adolescent and college-aged population. The Youth Risk Behavior Survey from the Centers for Disease Control and Prevention (CDC) found that 1% of high schoolers participated in binge drinking in the past 30 days (2019).

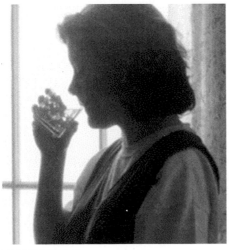

FIGURE 17.4 The use—and abuse—of alcohol occurs in persons of all ages, races, and cultural backgrounds, and in women as well as men.

> **GOOD TO KNOW**
> Binge drinking in college-age adults may be seen as a rite of passage for many, but it can lead to serious damage and even death. Students and parents need to be advised of the effects of toxic levels of alcohol. Many colleges now provide specific information to students about the risk of alcohol poisoning from binge drinking.

> **GOOD TO KNOW**
> Any alcohol use in children and teens is a cause for concern. This population may access alcohol from their homes or the homes of acquaintances, at parties, or by buying it with fake identification or from older friends. Seeing their parents drinking may give a double message to children or teens who are eager to grow up. Adolescents commonly experiment with alcohol, and it is difficult to know which ones will develop a lifetime of struggles with it. A high percentage of adult alcoholics started drinking as teenagers, so any sign of alcohol use by a child or teen must be addressed.

Effect on the Family

Family members and friends often develop protective behaviors to control, hide, or deny the alcoholic's behavior to maintain a sense of normality for the family. Such **codependent**, or enabling, behaviors can include making excuses for the drinker's alcohol use, covering up the drinker's unacceptable behavior, and self-blame for the drinking. Codependency may be seen in families of users of other substances besides alcohol.

Alcoholism is a family disease. Nearly half of all adults have a family history of alcoholism or problem drinking, and one in five children grow up in a home where someone drinks too much (National Institute of Alcohol Abuse and Alcoholism).

> **CRITICAL THINKING QUESTION**
> Your patient is a 16-year-old girl admitted from the emergency department (ED) with moderate injuries from a car accident. She was the driver. The other teens in the car were also injured. The patient is awake and tells you that her parents cannot know that she had a "couple of drinks" at a party just before driving her friends home. How would you respond? Should her parents be told? Are you an enabler if you choose not to share this information?

Tool Box

Adult Children of Alcoholics (ACOA) has support groups for people who grew up in a family made **dysfunctional** by alcoholism: www. adultchildren.org/

Alcohol's Impact on Health

Alcoholism is the third leading cause of preventable death in the United States (National Institute of Alcohol and Alcoholism, 2020). Because alcohol use is a frequent factor in chronic illness, nurses will see patients who are known to abuse alcohol but do not yet have the diagnosis. Heavy drinking contributes to heart disease, some cancers, liver failure, and stroke as it affects most organs in the body. In addition, alcoholism leads to more complications in the presence of diabetes. Impaired judgment related to alcohol use also contributes to countless traffic accidents, falls, incidents of domestic violence, suicides, participation in risky activities, industrial accidents, and other unsafe activities.

Alcohol abuse is often unrecognized and undertreated in the over-65 age group. Whether a lifelong pattern or a new coping mechanism in facing problems, heavy drinking in this population can be confused with dementia and can mask depression. Alcohol use can also contribute to falls or fires in the home and contribute to adverse reactions to many medications. Finally, alcohol in a pregnant woman's bloodstream can be passed to her unborn child. Fetal alcohol spectrum disorder (FASD) is characterized by physical and mental problems as well as learning disabilities in a child exposed to alcohol in utero.

Tool Box

The National Institute on Alcohol Abuse and Alcoholism has research on the current picture of alcohol use in the United States: http://niaaa. nih.gov/

GOOD TO KNOW

Long-term alcohol abuse can contribute to a form of dementia in later life.

Tool Box

Use the CAGE questionnaire, a four-question tool, to identify problems with alcohol use. CAGE stands for:

- Have you felt you should **C**UT down your drinking?
- Are you **A**NNOYED by others who criticize your drinking?
- Do you feel **G**UILTY about your drinking?
- Have you **E**VER had a drink first thing in the morning to steady your nerves?

The CAGE questionnaire is found at: https://www.hopkinsmedicine.org/johns_ hopkins_healthcare/downloads/CAGE%20 Substance%20Screening%20Tool.pdf

Etiology of Alcohol Abuse

Alcoholism runs in families. Biological offspring of parents with an alcohol abuse history have a significantly greater incidence of alcoholism than offspring of parents who did not abuse alcohol. These data support the genetic theories of alcoholism. The link between depression and alcoholism also suggests biological factors. These facts support the view of alcoholism as a disease. Recent developments in medications to treat alcoholism demonstrate the role of altering brain chemicals to treat the disease. Lifestyle and family dynamics are also a factor. Social factors, stress, and the ready availability of alcohol may contribute to progression of the disorder in some individuals. Growing up in a home where alcohol is used as a coping mechanism for stress also puts a person at risk. But just because alcoholism tends to run in families does not mean that a child of an alcoholic parent will automatically abuse alcohol. Likewise, some people develop alcoholism even though no one in their family has a drinking problem.

Alcohol Withdrawal

Nurses need to be able to recognize the signs of alcohol withdrawal. Signs include:

- autonomic hyperactivity (high blood pressure, tachycardia, fever)
- hand tremor
- insomnia
- nausea and/or vomiting
- anxiety

• transient visual, tactile, or auditory hallucinations or illusions
• early signs of delirium
• tonic-clonic (grand mal) seizures

Withdrawal symptoms can occur 4-12 hours after reduction of alcohol intake following prolonged heavy drinking (American Psychiatric Association, 2022). Analgesics and recovery from anesthesia can precipitate a withdrawal reaction. Withdrawal may look like classic delirium, so it is vital to screen patients about alcohol use as part of the routine admission assessment in the hospital.

GOOD TO KNOW
The U.S. Preventative Services Task Force (2018) recommends that primary care providers screen for alcohol abuse in all adults and pregnant women to identify problem drinkers earlier.

Questions that can be asked routinely on admission to identify patients at risk for withdrawal include:

• How often do you drink alcohol?
• How much do you usually drink?
• When was the last time you used alcohol or any drug?
• Have you had any problems because of drinking or drug use?

GOOD TO KNOW
The routine admission questions noted previously can also be used to screen for use of other substances.

Tool Box
The Clinical Institute Withdrawal Assessment for Alcohol Scale, known popularly as *CIWA-Ar*, is a tool used by many hospitals to monitor patients at risk for withdrawal syndrome. The CIWA-Ar is available at https://umem.org/files/uploads/1104212257_CIWA-Ar.pdf.

Withdrawal symptoms are generally most intense on the second day of abstinence. A **detoxification** regimen to prevent or reduce the uncomfortable effects of withdrawal may be ordered. Withdrawal from alcohol is very uncomfortable but generally not life threatening. Historically, withdrawal has been managed with longer-acting CNS depressants such as diazepam (Valium) and chlordiazepoxide (Librium), which have anticonvulsant actions and are relatively safe. A newer approach is to use shorter-acting agents, like lorazepam (Ativan), to decrease the risk of oversedation. These medications are given more frequently and are easier to titrate than the longer-acting ones. Anticonvulsants may also be added. These are administered routinely and tapered down over several days. Fluids, vitamins (especially thiamine [vitamin B$_1$]), and electrolyte replacement are also part of the treatment plan. For patients with liver disease, it is important to use shorter-acting benzodiazepines such as oxazepam (Serax) as well as lorazepam.

Withdrawal can induce an extreme form of delirium, sometimes referred to as **delirium tremens** or DTs, evidenced by impaired consciousness and memory as well as hallucinations and severe tremors.

Classroom Activity
Role play with classmates how to ask patients about their alcohol and drug use.

Clinical Activity
Any patient who indicates a history of problems with alcohol should be monitored for withdrawal.

CRITICAL THINKING QUESTION
Your 80-year-old patient is 2 days postop recovering from a fractured hip. Until now, her recovery has been routine. She calls you to her bedside and looks anxious and trembling. She tells you that a glass of wine would help make her more comfortable. What would you do?

GOOD TO KNOW
An individual desperate for alcohol may take alcohol-based medications like cough syrup to control withdrawal.

DIFFERENTIAL DIAGNOSES

• sedative, hypnotic, or anxiolytic use disorder
• nonpathological use of alcohol
• co-occurring disorders such as depression or bipolar disorder where alcohol is used to manage symptoms

Treatment of Alcohol Use Disorder

Treatment for alcohol use disorder usually begins with some form of detoxification to remove the alcohol from the body. This may be done during a short-term hospitalization or in an outpatient setting. This is followed by some form of rehabilitation to maintain abstinence from alcohol. Alcoholics Anonymous (AA) provides a treatment approach for rehabilitation. AA is based on the 12 Steps Program (Table 17.1). In a group setting where only first names are used, individuals must acknowledge their powerlessness over alcohol to begin the healing process. Following the 12-step program, the individual participates in the groups, which are run by the members themselves. These meetings are available in most communities. Together, group members discuss the struggles and challenges of living without alcohol. Individual support is provided to new members by other group members who act as sponsors.

There are corresponding groups for families of the alcoholic (Al-Anon) and a special group for teenagers (Alateen). Adult Children of Alcoholics (ACOA) is a branch of AA formed for people who are now adults but grew up in an alcoholic home and were not able to get help at the time. These groups all follow a similar model. Other 12-step groups serving other dependency needs, such as narcotics, cocaine, and gambling, have modeled themselves after AA.

GOOD TO KNOW

AA is usually a lifetime commitment. It is known internationally, and the person can reach out to any group when away from home.

Tool Box

A variety of education materials, including videos on addressing alcohol addiction, can be found at www.aa.org.

Classroom Activity

Though most AA meetings are private, at times local groups will identify open meetings where interested observers can attend. Attend an open meeting of AA and identify how the meeting provided support to the attendees.

Additional forms of alcohol treatment include family therapy as well as individual and group therapy to learn new coping mechanisms. Life without drinking presents many challenges to the individual experiencing alcohol use disorder, including finding different friends and social activities and repairing family relationships. Pharmacological therapy is growing as an important component of treatment (see Pharmacology Corner). Generally, abstinence from alcohol is part of most treatment programs. Some studies have reported that certain individuals are able to return to low-risk drinking during and after treatment and do not escalate back to heavy drinking (Witkiewirz et al., 2017).

CRITICAL THINKING QUESTION

Your friend stopped drinking about 1 year ago after she was in a car accident in which she was driving impaired with her 3-year-old in the car. She has been attending AA regularly. She is now going through a divorce and tells you she is so stressed and depressed that she has no more energy to get to the AA meetings. What would be your concerns? How can you help her?

CRITICAL THINKING QUESTION

Your 35-year-old patient is being treated for alcohol-related liver disease. He tells you he stopped drinking last month but is worried about his relationship with his fiancée, who is a heavy drinker. What would be your concerns? What suggestions can you make?

Table 17.1

The 12 Steps and 12 Traditions of Alcoholics Anonymous

The 12 Steps of AA	*The 12 Traditions of AA*
1. We admitted we were powerless over alcohol—that our lives had become unmanageable.	1. Our common welfare should come first; personal recovery depends on AA unity.
2. Came to believe that a Power greater than ourselves could restore us to sanity	2. For our group purpose, there is but one ultimate authority—a loving God as He may express Himself in our group conscience. Our leaders are but trusted servants; they do not govern.
3. Made a decision to turn our will and our lives over to the care of God as we understood Him	3. The only requirement for AA membership is a desire to stop drinking.
4. Made a searching and fearless moral inventory of ourselves	4. Each group should be autonomous except in matters affecting other groups of AA as a whole.
5. Admitted to God, to ourselves, and to another human being the exact nature of our wrongs	5. Each group has but one primary purpose—to carry its message to the alcoholic who still suffers.
6. Were entirely ready to have God remove all these defects of character	6. An AA group ought never endorse, finance, or lend the AA name to any related facility or outside enterprise, lest problems of money, property, and prestige divert us from our primary purpose.
7. Humbly asked Him to remove our shortcomings	7. Every AA group ought to be fully self-supporting, declining outside contributions.
8. Made a list of all persons we had harmed and became willing to make amends to them all	8. AA should remain forever nonprofessional, but our service centers may employ special workers.
9. Made direct amends to such people wherever possible, except when to do so would injure them or others	9. AA, as such, ought never be organized; but we may create service boards or committees directly responsible to those they serve.
10. Continued to take personal inventory and when we were wrong, promptly admitted it	10. AA has no opinion on outside issues; hence, the AA name ought never be drawn into public controversy.
11. Sought through prayer and meditation to improve our conscious contact with God, as we understood Him, praying only for knowledge of His will for us and the power to carry that out	11. Our public relations policy is based on attraction rather than promotion; we need always maintain personal anonymity at the level of press, radio, and films.
12. Having had a spiritual awakening as the result of these steps, we tried to carry this message to alcoholics and to practice these principles in all our affairs	12. Anonymity is the spiritual foundation of all our traditions, ever reminding us to place principles before personalities.

Source: The 12 Steps and 12 Traditions are reprinted with permission of Alcoholics Anonymous World Services, Inc. (AAWS). Permission to reprint the 12 Steps and 12 Traditions does not mean that AAWS has reviewed or approved the contents of this publication, nor that AA agrees with the views expressed herein. AA is a program of recovery from alcoholism only—use of the 12 Steps and 12 Traditions in connection with programs and activities that are patterned after AA but address other problems, or in any other non-AA context, does not imply otherwise.

Pharmacology Corner

Four drugs have been approved by the Food and Drug Administration (FDA) to treat alcoholism. Many other approaches are being researched.

1. *Disulfiram (Antabuse)* was the first medicine approved for the treatment of alcohol abuse and alcohol dependence. It works by causing a severe adverse reaction when someone taking the medication consumes alcohol. This reaction includes palpitations, nausea and vomiting, severe headache, and shortness of breath with exposure to any alcohol. This drug is contraindicated in the presence of severe heart disease.

2. *Naltrexone* works by blocking the high that people experience when they drink alcohol or take opioids. It is available in oral formulation (Revia) as well as an extended-release injectable form (Vivitrol). The patient must be opioid-free to take naltrexone.

3. *Acamprosate* (Campral) works by reducing the cravings for alcohol for someone who is in recovery. This medication is an alternative to naltrexone in the presence of liver disease.

4. *Topiramate* (Topamax) is an anticonvulsant that has shown promise in reducing alcohol intake and cravings.

See Table 17.2 for medications commonly used to manage withdrawal.

Table 17.2

Commonly Used Medications for Withdrawal Management of Alcohol and Other Substances

Alcohol Withdrawal

Lorazepam (Ativan)
Oxazepam (Serax)
Nutritional supplements (vitamins, magnesium, thiamine [B$_1$])
Anticonvulsants such as carbamazepine, valproic acid
Serotonin reuptake inhibitors (SSRIs) such as paroxetine, sertraline to treat anxiety and depression

Opioid Withdrawal

Naltrexone (Vivitrol)
Naloxone (Narcan)
Buprenorphine
Buprenorphine and naloxone (Suboxone)
Clonidine (Catapres)

Heroin Withdrawal and Maintenance

Methadone hydrochloride (Dolophine)

Stimulants

Chlordiazepoxide (Librium)
Antipsychotics

GOOD TO KNOW

Any patient on disulfiram (Antabuse) must be advised to avoid taking any substance with an alcohol base, including cough syrups and mouthwashes. Patients should at all times carry information that they are taking this drug so that it is available to emergency personnel.

Some patients taking disulfiram may skip a dose for a day or two so they can plan when they can drink. This can precipitate a reaction in some. This is also what makes this drug less useful.

OTHER SUBSTANCES

A wide variety of substances are abused. See Table 17.3 for a summary of the effects of commonly abused substances. Signs and symptoms of SUDs vary depending on the type of drug. Poly drug use is common and can create a confusing clinical picture. The individual may use one drug to counteract or enhance the effects of the first drug. In addition, drugs are often combined with alcohol. For example, cocaine users commonly use alcohol to get to sleep or calm down. Many drug and alcohol combinations have a synergistic effect that can be life threatening. Older adults are likely to abuse prescription tranquilizers, sedatives, and analgesics rather than illegal opioids.

The DSM-5 now categorizes each substance by substance-induced intoxication and withdrawal disorders. Each disorder has its own criteria for diagnosing based on the specific substance used. A diagnosis of SUD is based on a pattern of continued use despite substance-related problems.

Use of opioid drugs for nonmedical purposes is an urgent problem in the United States. Nonmedical purposes can include the use of pain medication to achieve a high or to relax rather than for physical pain relief. Desperate actions such as stealing drugs from

Table 17.3

Comparing Commonly Abused Substances

Drug	Intoxication	Overdose	Withdrawal	Nursing Considerations
Amphet-amines, including Dexedrine, Ritalin, Provigil, Adderall, metham-phetamine (crystal meth)	Signs: Euphoria, high energy, impaired judgment, anxiety, weight loss, anorexia, increased libido, aggressive behavior, paranoia, panic disorders, insomnia, elevated blood pressure (BP), dilated pupils, and delusions (especially with long-term use)	Signs: Ataxia, high temperature, seizures, hypertension, arrhythmias, respiratory distress, cardiovascular collapse, coma, brain damage, death Treatment: Supportive	Signs: Depression, agitation, anxiety, insomnia, confusion, vivid dreams followed by extreme lethargy Treatment: Antidepressants, counseling, suicide precautions	• Crystal meth is made from ephedrine & pseudoephedrine products • Tolerance can develop fairly rapidly. • User often also uses alcohol and other substances to relax • May cause a paradoxical reaction in children • May be used initially to lose weight • Crystal meth users prone to dental problems • Withdrawal is difficult and relapse is common • Remains in urine for up to 3 days • Therapeutic uses for some include narcolepsy, attention deficit-hyperactivity disorder (ADHD) in children
Cannabis, marijuana, hashish	Signs: Euphoria, intensified perceptions, impaired judgment and motor ability, increased appetite, weight gain, sinusitis and bronchitis with chronic inhalation, anxiety, paranoia, red conjunctiva. Oral ingestion slows absorption and has longer-lasting effects	Signs: Extreme paranoia, psychosis, delirium Treatment: Antipsychotics	Signs: Irritability, anxiety, insomnia, anorexia, restlessness, tremors, fever, headache Treatment: Supportive	• Most widely used illicit drug, although legal in some states (recreational and/or medical) • Impaired judgment may contribute to accidents. • Respiratory damage from inhaled substances can occur • Comes in a variety of formulations (gels, inhalers, edible, etc.) • Remains in urine for up to 7 days • May exacerbate psychiatric symptoms in mentally ill patients • May negatively affect fertility • K2 (also called *spice*) is a synthetic version of THC that is sometimes added to cannabis

Continued

Table 17.3

Comparing Commonly Abused Substances—cont'd

Drug	Intoxication	Overdose	Withdrawal	Nursing Considerations
Cocaine, including crack	Signs: Euphoria, grandiosity, sexual excitement, impaired judgment, insomnia, anorexia, nasal perforation associated with inhaled route, psychosis associated with long-term abuse	Signs: High temperature, pupil dilation, tachycardia, seizures, arrhythmias, transient venospasms possibly causing myocardial infarction or stroke, coma, death Treatment: Supportive	Signs: Fatigue, vivid dreams, depression, anxiety, suicidal behavior, bradycardia Treatment: Support, counseling, antidepressants	• Crack is smoked or injected IV and has a rapid onset and high dependency rate. • Tolerance develops rapidly. • Cocaine is inhaled, "snorted," or injected IV. • High risk of acquiring HIV, hepatitis, bacterial endocarditis, and osteomyelitis from shared IV needles or unprotected sex • May be used to control appetite
Hallucinogens, including LSD, psilocybin, ketamine, and mescaline	Signs: Dilated pupils, diaphoresis, palpitations, tremors, enhanced perceptions of colors and sounds, depersonalization, grandiosity	Signs: Panic, suicidality, psychosis with hallucinations, cerebral tissue damage, seizures, hyperthermia, death Treatment: Diazepam or chloral hydrate, quiet environment, antipsychotics	Signs: Reexperiencing perceptual symptoms Treatment: Supportive	• Flashbacks can occur for up to 5 years. • Could precipitate a psychiatric disorder in susceptible persons • Ketamine is used by some law enforcement to control violent suspects. • Ketamine is sometimes used as date rape drug.
Inhalants, including glue, gasoline, cleaning solutions, aerosol propellants like deodorants or hair spray, and paint thinner	Signs: Euphoria, impaired judgment, belligerence, blurred vision, unsteady gait, nausea/vomiting, wheezing, nystagmus, hypoxia	Signs: CNS depression, cardiac arrythmia, death Treatment: Supportive	Signs: None	• Most available substance for younger children • Intoxication period is brief (15–45 minutes). • Can cause permanent CNS damage • Death from aspiration of emesis can occur. • May be difficult to detect specific substance used • Particularly irritating and/or flammable substances can cause trauma and burns in nose, mouth, and airways.

Table 17.3

Comparing Commonly Abused Substances—cont'd

Drug	Intoxication	Overdose	Withdrawal	Nursing Considerations
Nicotine, including cigarettes, chewing tobacco, and nicotine gum or patch	Signs: Produces a sense of anxiety reduction, relief from depression, and satisfaction	Signs: Tachycardia, hypertension, abnormal dreams Treatment: Clonidine, benzodiazepines	Signs: Insomnia, depression, irritability, anxiety, poor concentration, increased appetite Treatment: Transdermal nicotine patches in decreasing doses, nicotine gum, nicotine nasal spray, Varenicline (Chantix) and bupropion hydrochloride (Zyban), behavioral modification. Long-term smokers may need to remain on nicotine therapy for some time.	• Monitor for weight gain. • Monitor for hypotension with clonidine, benzodiazepines. • Hospitalized smoker may need nicotine replacement to control withdrawal.
Opioids, including heroin, morphine, meperidine, OxyContin, fentanyl, hydrocodone, and codeine	Signs: Euphoria, analgesia, slurred speech, drowsiness, impaired judgment, constricted pupils	Signs: Dilated pupils, respiratory depression, seizures, cardiopulmonary arrest, coma, death Treatment: Naloxone, supportive	Signs: Yawning, insomnia, anorexia, irritability, rhinorrhea, muscle cramps, chills, nausea and vomiting, feelings of doom and panic Treatment: Detoxification, possibly with clonidine for severe anxiety and methadone, naloxone, and/or buprenorphine to block euphoria	• High risk of acquiring HIV, hepatitis, bacterial endocarditis, or osteomyelitis from shared IV needles • May be obtained illegally or through prescription abuse • At high risk for overdose after detox if the same predetox dose is taken • Monitor for hypotension with clonidine. • Abuse of Suboxone is a growing problem. • Fentanyl, the synthetic opioid, is being found in illegal opioid products, which greatly increases overdose potential.

Continued

Table 17.3

Comparing Commonly Abused Substances—cont'd

Drug	Intoxication	Overdose	Withdrawal	Nursing Considerations
Phencyclidine (PCP, angel dust)	Signs: Impulsive behavior, impaired judgment, belligerent/assaultive behavior, ataxia, muscle rigidity, nystagmus, hypertension, numbness or diminished response to pain	Signs: Hallucinations, psychosis, seizures, respiratory arrest, CVA Treatment: Gastric lavage, cranberry juice or ammonium chloride to acidify urine (if awake), quiet environment, haloperidol or diazepam, fluids	Signs: None	• Have adequate staff available because behavior is unpredictable, and patient may become violent. • Drugs remain in urine for several weeks. • Avoid using phenothiazines because they can potentiate the effects of PCP. • Delayed onset of delirium can occur.
Sedatives, hypnotics, and antianxiety drugs, including barbiturates and benzodiazepines	Signs: Relaxation, slurred speech, labile mood, inappropriate sexual behavior, loss of inhibitions, drowsiness, impaired memory	Signs: Hypotension, nystagmus, stupor, cardiorespiratory depression, renal failure, seizures (barbiturates), coma, death Treatment: Benzodiazepine antagonist (flumazenil), induce vomiting if awake, activated charcoal, cardiorespiratory support	Signs: Insomnia, tachycardia, hand tremor, agitation, panic disorder, nausea and vomiting, anxiety, tinnitus (with benzodiazepines), seizures, and cardiac arrest Treatment: Detoxification using gradually reduced dosages of a similar drug, anticonvulsants, and support and counseling	• Abrupt barbiturate withdrawal can be life threatening. • Alcohol will potentiate drug effects and can contribute to overdose. • Cross-tolerance may develop between alcohol and other CNS depressants. • Shorter-acting benzodiazepines have a greater risk of producing addiction and more severe rebound anxiety than longer-acting ones.
Club drugs, including flunitrazepam (Rohypnol), gamma hydroxybutyric acid (GHB),	Signs: Euphoria, muscle relaxation, poor judgment, relaxed inhibitions, increased sociability	Signs: Strong sedative effects leading to confusion, sedation, slurred speech Treatment: Supportive	Signs: Not physiologically addictive, but psychological dependence can cause depression, flashbacks	• Can cause memory loss • Often taken in combination with alcohol and other drugs • Rohypnol is called the "date rape" drug as it is slipped into drinks of an unsuspecting victim who becomes incapacitated and unable to resist sexual advances.

Table 17.3

Comparing Commonly Abused Substances—cont'd

Drug	Intoxication	Overdose	Withdrawal	Nursing Considerations
Continuation of list of club drugs: MDMA (Ecstasy)/ketamine may be included in this category (see hallucinogens)				• MDMA can induce serotonin depletion syndrome several days after ingestion.

Source: Adapted from Saunders et al. (2016); Townsend (2015), Morgan & Townsend (2021), and APA (2013).

family members or friends, forging prescriptions, and seeking out multiple doctors for prescriptions (called "doctor shopping") are signs that the person needs help. People with chronic pain who regularly take analgesics may be at increased risk for misusing prescribed medications at times of stress, with the new onset of more medical problems, and when experiencing mental health issues. This population needs to be educated on the appropriate use of these medications and monitored closely (Pergolizzi et al., 2012).

Patterns of drug use vary as new substances are discovered. Nurses should be aware of newer drugs that may be used by their patient population. For example, in some communities, methamphetamines are a problem, as are "club drugs" such as flunitrazepam (Rohypnol) (Fig. 17.5). Another new drug found in some communities is kratom. It is a naturally occurring substance from a tropical tree that has properties of both opioids and stimulants. Reports of abuse are now occurring as individuals may use it in place of or in combination with opioids. It is known to be addictive on its own. Using it to treat or reduce withdrawal symptoms has been reported though there is no evidence this is effective.

Marijuana is the most widely used psychotropic drug in the United States after alcohol. With the increase of legalization around the United States as well as the legal use of medical marijuana in many states, it is becoming increasingly readily available. Medical marijuana is used for treating pain, insomnia, and depression, and to stimulate appetite, among other things.

Substance abuse can be a contributing factor in child abuse as well as intimate partner abuse (see Chapter 22). The ripple effect of damage to the

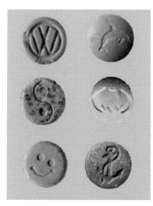

FIGURE 17.5 "Homemade" methamphetamine tablets *(courtesy of Drug Enforcement Agency, U.S. Department of Justice, Washington, D.C.).*

individual, the couple, and children can have many consequences, including disruption of the home environment and may even lead to foster placement.

Tool Box

The National Institutes of Health National Center for Complementary and Integrative Health provides a summary of data on how effective medical marijuana is for various symptoms: https://www.nccih.nih.gov/health/cannabis-marijuana-and-cannabinoids-what-you-need-to-know

DIFFERENTIAL DIAGNOSES

- other substance use disorder, intoxication, or withdrawal
- alcohol use disorder
- Co-occurring disorders such as depressive disorder, bipolar disorder

Substance Use in Children and Teens

Children and teens can also be at risk for substance disorders. The use of inhalants ("huffing"), including household items such as hair spray and aerosol whipped cream, is most common in children. These easily obtained substances can contribute to sudden changes in behavior. Cough syrups and prescription drugs from parents are other sources for children and teens. Signs of substance use in children and teens can include:

- change in functioning at school
- loss of interest in sports
- change in sleep patterns
- increased isolation
- irritability
- mood swings

Lifelong struggles with substance use often begin in childhood and adolescence. Younger brains are thought to be more vulnerable to the addiction cycle. Therefore, intervention with young people is essential to prevent addiction. Children and teens are still developing judgment and decision-making skills, so they may be swayed to try things as part of peer pressure or to self-medicate.

Vaping, the use of a device to heat and release chemicals that can then be inhaled, is a popular trend. Electronic cigarettes, also known as *e-cigarettes*, were initially introduced in 2007 with limited regulation on their use. Initially developed as a way to help people wean themselves off cigarettes, flavored vaping products were developed to appeal to teens and young adults. In addition to tobacco, THC (the active ingredient in marijuana) is also vaped. In 2020, 19.6% of high school students (3.02 million) and 4.7% of middle school students (550,000) reported current e-cigarette use (Wang, Neff, Perk-Lee, Ren, Cullen & King, 2020). In the summer of 2019, public health authorities identified an outbreak of a deadly vaping-related lung injury. The U.S. CDC later named the condition *EVALI* — e-cigarette, or vaping, associated lung injury. Once the scope of the potential harm from these products was identified, a number of regulations were put in place by the FDA and some states to limit the sale and use of some of these products.

Tool Box

The American Academy of Pediatrics recommends the use of the Screening to Brief Intervention (S2BI) for adolescents to identify substance abuse: https://www.adolescentsubstanceuse.org/screening-instruments/

GOOD TO KNOW

Infants born to mothers who are addicted to some drugs such as cocaine or heroin can have neonatal abstinence syndrome known as NAS. These infants often have low birth weights, feeding difficulties, and seizures.

CRITICAL THINKING QUESTION

Your 15-year-old nephew has been arrested for possession of a prescription analgesic that he stole from a friend's parent's medicine cabinet. You noticed that recently he has had more mood swings than usual, has been doing poorly in school, and is increasingly irritable. What other signs would you look for that he is using these drugs? What concerns would you have for his future?

Tool Box

The Drug Abuse Screening Tool, known as *DAST*, is used in some settings. The 20-question self-screening tool is available at https://cde.drugabuse.gov/sites/nida_cde/files/DrugAbuseScreeningTest_2014Mar24.pdf

---

Etiology of Substance Use Disorders

The causes of substance use disorders are similar to those of alcohol abuse, but with the wide variety of drugs abused, there can be some differences. Biological theories look at the role of specific brain dysfunction and view addiction as a brain disease. A drug will stimulate a specific brain pathway that induces an altered state; over time, the drug causes brain changes leading to craving this drug again. Cocaine has been studied the most, and it is believed that cocaine abusers have a deficiency of dopamine and norepinephrine that creates more craving. Other mind-altering drugs may be influenced by different pathways.

Psychological factors include use of drugs to relieve feelings of depression, anxiety, and low self-esteem. Sociocultural theories look at the effects of peer group and culture on those who use specific drugs.

Treatment of Substance Use Disorders

As with alcohol use disorder, 12-step programs provide important treatment and support for the individual with SUD. The same philosophy of acknowledging one's powerlessness over a substance and the importance of group support are the foundations of these programs.

In addition, some people benefit from inpatient drug rehabilitation programs, which can include detoxification, depending on the drug. Family therapy, individual psychotherapy, peer counseling with former addicts, and group therapy can be helpful in many cases. Cognitive behavior therapy (CBT) can also be useful. This approach is a short-term therapy that emphasizes learning the connection between stressors and symptoms, teaching new coping skills, and challenging distorted thinking. Most substance abuse programs involve the family in the treatment plan. Heroin addiction may be treated with methadone maintenance in which a long-acting opioid is taken daily to avoid the withdrawal symptoms without the high from taking other opioids. See the Pharmacology Corner for other medications used to treat addictions and withdrawal.

It is now commonplace for employers to request drug screening as a condition of employment or as a routine test while employed. Many companies have struggled with drug abuse with their employees and have found drug screening to be a deterrent.

In the hospital setting, awareness of a patient's past substance use history is important information to prevent or control withdrawal syndromes. In addition, a recovering substance abuser may be hesitant to take analgesics or tranquilizers for fear of returning to a past lifestyle. It is important to work with the patient to address these fears and identify alternative interventions if possible.

Cultural Considerations

Treatment for substance-related disorders is not equally available to all individuals. Members of some ethnic groups and individuals of lower socioeconomic status typically have more difficulty accessing treatment (Cook & Alegría, 2011).

People who take drugs intravenously (IV) are at risk of HIV, sexually transmitted infections, and hepatitis from infected needles. Treatment for substance abuse should include a medical work-up for these potential problems as well as education on prevention.

Clinical Activity

- Review the medical record for what substances your patient was abusing, the last time they were used, and the potential complications.
- Your patient who is an IV drug abuser should be screened for HIV, sexually transmitted infections, and hepatitis.
- Education may need to be provided on prevention of these diseases.

Classroom Activity

Identify resources for drug abusers in your community, such as methadone maintenance programs and halfway houses for recovering addicts.

CRITICAL THINKING QUESTION

You work at a methadone clinic and see the same patients daily for their medication dose. You notice that one patient arrives disheveled with slurred speech. What actions should you take?

CRITICAL THINKING QUESTION

You are asked to submit a urine test as a condition of employment for a new job at a local hospital. What is your response to this request? What are the pros and cons of drug testing for the employer and employee?

Pharmacology Corner

A variety of medications are used in the treatment of SUDs. Pharmacology can, in some cases, replace the illicit substance (e.g., methadone for heroin addiction) or reduce cravings by interacting with the drug's receptor system in the brain (e.g., buprenorphine and naloxone for opioid addiction). These substances also reduce the physical signs of withdrawal.

Medications are used in detoxification programs for many drugs, including opioids, barbiturates, sedatives, and tranquilizers. They are used to control withdrawal symptoms and discourage continued use of the abused substance. Most medications are used for only short periods until withdrawal is complete; however, in some cases, they may be used for longer periods to control cravings for the drug.

Methadone, a synthetic narcotic that resembles morphine and heroin but does not produce the euphoric effects, is used daily on a long-term basis to treat heroin addiction. Methadone to treat opioid addiction is used only in federally licensed opioid-treatment programs. Both physical and psychological dependence are maintained on methadone, but the euphoric effects of heroin are blocked. Patients usually make daily trips to a methadone clinic to obtain the drug. Buprenorphine, an opioid with agonist and antagonist action, has been used as an alternative to methadone. It can usually be given in an office-based setting, providing an alternative to the methadone clinics. Naltrexone also reduces the euphoric sensation from narcotics. Opioid withdrawal may be treated with a combination of buprenorphine and naloxone (Suboxone) that is available in oral, extended-release and long-acting injectable forms. Buprenorphine alone (Subutex) is also used to treat opioid withdrawal. Addiction specialists must be certified to prescribe buprenorphine. Patients on this medication must be monitored closely if they have conditions that require use of analgesics. Administering analgesics could precipitate a withdrawal syndrome. Clonidine (Catapres) is also used to suppress opioid withdrawal symptoms. It can serve as a bridge to eventually stop methadone maintenance.

The easy availability of fentanyl found in illegal drugs today has contributed to the rise in deaths from overdoses nationally. Because of this increase, there is a movement for emergency medical personnel to stock naloxone (Narcan, a form of naltrexone with shorter onset) to provide lifesaving reversal of respiratory depression in an overdose. In 2015, the FDA approved an intranasal form of naloxone hydrocholoride to use in potential opioid overdoses. This intranasal form is being used both by first responders and by friends and family members of addicts to prevent overdose-related deaths. Although administering these narcotic antagonists will potentially prevent death, it will induce acute withdrawal symptoms in anyone who is opioid dependent.

Benzodiazepine and sedative withdrawal are risky because of the potential for seizures and delirium. Tapering the dose of the abused drug (or one similar) while administering anticonvulsants, long-acting benzodiazepines, and antidepressants is the usual protocol.

Withdrawal from stimulants may require use of tranquilizers and antidepressants. These individuals are also at risk for suicide during withdrawal.

Bupropion and varenicline (Chantix) work in combination with behavioral treatments to help with nicotine withdrawal in addition to nicotine replacement in the form of gum or patches.

Herbs and plant products, such as chamomile, valerian, kava kava, and St. John's wort may be helpful in treating distressing withdrawal symptoms. However, St. John's wort is contraindicated if the patient is taking antidepressants, narcotics, or amphetamines.

Commonly used medications to treat withdrawal are covered in Table 17.2.

Clinical Activity

• Review agency policy on the management of drug-withdrawal regimens.
• Identify coping mechanisms your substance-abusing patient uses to cope with stress now that they are not using.
• Monitor for potential complications during detoxification.

CRITICAL THINKING QUESTION

Your 19-year-old patient is admitted for surgery after he broke his ankle in a car accident. His sister confides in you that he has been taking frequent doses of his mother's prescription tranquilizer, lorazepam. The patient has asked his sister to bring these to the hospital. The patient's sister has them but now wonders if giving them to him is the right thing to do. What concerns would you have about this drug? What action should you take?

NURSING CARE OF PATIENTS WITH SUBSTANCE USE DISORDERS (INCLUDING ALCOHOL)

Common nursing diagnoses in patients with substance-related disorders include the following:

• coping, ineffective
• denial, ineffective
• family coping: compromised
• injury, risk for
• sleep pattern, disturbed
• thought processes, disturbed
• violence, risk for

People who abuse drugs, alcohol, and other substances often use similar coping mechanisms to deal with their problems. See Table 17.4 for a list of common coping styles used by substance users. Understanding these coping mechanisms can help professionals understand behaviors and identify appropriate interventions.

General Nursing Interventions

Caring for patients with a variety of SUDs requires patience, knowledge, teamwork, and compassion. These patients present many challenges as there can be many complications related to the substance itself and/or the withdrawal process. In addition, the patient is often still using the same coping mechanisms they have used for years to hide the addiction and the problems it created. These can include denial,

Table 17.4
Common Coping Styles of Substance Abusers

Coping Style	Definition	Behaviors
Denial	Person minimizes or does not acknowledge the problem or the results of the problem even when strong evidence is presented.	• "I only have two drinks a day; I could stop any time." • Refuses to admit drug problems that are obvious to others. • Family may participate in denial by covering up the problems created by the abuser.
Projection	Blames others for their drinking and substance abuse	• Avoids taking responsibility for own unacceptable behavior. • "My brother is the one with the problem. He drinks more than I do." • "I'd stop if everyone would leave me alone."

Continued

Table 17.4

Common Coping Styles of Substance Abusers—cont'd

Rationalization	Justifies intolerable behavior by giving plausible excuses	• Excuses reinforce denial. • "I drink to fit in at parties." • "I never drink alone."
Minimizing	Avoids conflict by reducing the effect of the behavior	• Places less value on the behavior and the effects of the problem • "You worry too much." • "I'm not hurting anyone."
Manipulation	Plays one person against another in order to get one's way or cover up or avoid a problem	• Convinces one or two people that condition will improve if they will help • If they fail, it is the fault of the helper.
Grandiosity	Maintains a sense of superiority and irresponsibility particularly evident when intoxicated.	• Lacks concern for others' feelings.

Source: Adapted from Gorman and Sultan (2008). *Psychosocial Nursing for General Patient Care,* 3rd ed. Philadelphia: F.A. Davis Company, with permission.

manipulative behavior, and rationalization. The nurse may be in the role of limit setter and rule enforcer, which can be challenging. The nurse may also be faced with patients who are intoxicated on the substance. This can mean dealing with offensive, abusive behaviors that require maintenance of safety for all involved See Table 17.5 for specific interventions related to alcohol and drug abuse disorders. See Figure 17.6 for the Concept Map for the Patient Abusing Alcohol.

GOOD TO KNOW

Patients with a substance abuse history often refuse analgesics for fear this will lead to abusing the substance again. Trying alternate methods of pain control, ordering appropriate analgesics by the physician (e.g., long-acting oral opioids rather than injectable to reduce the high), and using nonopioid analgesics can be helpful.

Table 17.5

Problems With Substance Abuse: Symptoms and Nursing Interventions

Types	*Symptoms*	*Nursing Interventions*
Alcohol abuse	• Inability to cut down or stop using • Daily use common • Binges that last 2 days or more • Blackouts, which increase • Impaired social function • May use drugs in addition to alcohol to manage symptoms • Increase in alcohol tolerance • Drinking in "secret" • Preoccupation with alcohol • Gulping first drink • Inability to discuss problems	• Communicate honestly. • Assist patient in identifying thoughts and feelings. • Convey acceptance of individual. • Challenge rationalizations or denial with reality. • Encourage participation in support groups and maintain consistency with new behaviors learned in group. • Confront use of maladaptive defense mechanisms.

Table 17.5

Problems With Substance Abuse: Symptoms and Nursing Interventions—cont'd

Types	Symptoms	Nursing Interventions
	• Loss of control • Rationalization of drinking • Failure in efforts to control drinking • Grandiose and aggressive behavior • Trouble with family, employer • Self-pity • Loss of outside interests • Unreasonable resentment • Neglecting food • Tremors (hands) • Morning drinking • Prolonged intoxication • Physical and moral deterioration • Impaired thinking • Free-floating anxiety • Obsession with drinking • Constant use of alibis	• Support any acknowledgment of the abuse. • Support and give positive reinforcement of progress. • Set firm limits as needed. • Provide information about substance abuse, causes, and treatment. • Monitor for withdrawal syndromes and complications from substance abuse. • Support drug/alcohol-free lifestyle. • Recognize that patient may have setbacks with drinking but encourage to restart treatment. • Avoid any enabling of patient's bad behavior.

Substance use	• Similar to alcohol abuse with addition of:
	  • Red, watery eyes
	  • Runny nose
	  • Hostility
	  • Paranoia
	  • Needle tracks on arms or legs
	  • Erratic, unpredictable behavior
	  • Risky behaviors including stealing, lying to obtain drug
	  • May use alcohol, too, to self-medicate for symptoms
	  • Other symptoms depending on drug being used
		• See "Alcohol Abuse."
		• Encourage patient to be tested for HIV if drug use included IV needles.
		• Monitor drug testing if ordered.
		• Be aware of attempts to manipulate you.

Codependence	• Significant others beginning to lose their own sense of identity and purpose, existing solely for the abuser • Actions of significant others taking away opportunity for user to take responsibility for his or her own actions • Lowered self-esteem • Taking part in actions that are self-destructive and reinforce drug seeker's/drinker's problems	• Encourage participation in assertiveness classes. • Promote self-care and problem-solving. • Encourage attendance at support groups. • Challenge rationalizations of or denial about substance abuser. • Help person identify self-destructive patterns. • Encourage activities to promote self-esteem and individuality.

GOOD TO KNOW

Recognize that maintaining sobriety or abstinence from drugs or alcohol is a lifelong process. During periods of stress or illness, the urge to use these substances can increase. The patient needs added support at these times.

GOOD TO KNOW

People with a history of drug abuse may have learned to use charm and manipulation to get the drugs they are seeking. Family, friends, and health-care providers who have been taken advantage of in the past may have difficulty trusting these patients in recovery.

The nursing care plan for a patient abusing alcohol is provided in Table 17.6.

CRITICAL THINKING QUESTION

Your 45-year-old patient is admitted to the hospital with multiple injuries that she states she sustained in a fall at home. When the husband of the patient arrives, he smells of alcohol, is belligerent, and demands his wife be released. After security asks him to leave, the wife tells you that he has never acted like this before and she is sorry she upset him by telling him their son acted out in school. She denies he hurt her and says that she tripped on the stairs because she left some of the younger son's toys there. You wonder if the wife is covering up her husband's drinking problem. What would you consider as a possible nursing diagnosis for this patient? If the husband comes back, what actions should you consider?

GOOD TO KNOW

Denial is a powerful coping mechanism common in alcohol and substance use disorders that gets reinforced by the effects of the substance. Patients may minimize the effects of the substance abuse even when presented with objective data like a blood alcohol level or toxicology screen. Look for slightest indication of insight and emphasize that rather than support the denial.

Evidence-Based Practice

Clinical Question: What concerns do nurses have in caring for patients with a history of misusing opioids?

Discussion: Negative attitudes toward patients with a history of abusing opioids can present challenges for nurses. This study involved interviewing obstetrical nurses as to their perceptions of their patients who were misusing opioids.

Evidence: Four themes were derived from the interviews: needing more knowledge, feeling challenged, expressing concern for mother and infant, and knowing the truth. The interview process helped identify a number of areas where the nurses felt they could improve patient care. The nurses expressed several ideas for intervention development, including continuing education offerings relevant to caring for mothers who misuse opioids, collaborating with providers to design education, reevaluating pain-management philosophies and practices at all levels, and working with social workers to explore available and needed community resources.

Implications for Nursing Practice: Recognizing the challenges presented by this population as well as one's own attitudes can lead to efforts to improve patient care.

Shaw, M. R., Lederhos, C., Haberman, M., Howell, D., Fleming, S., Roll, J. (2016). Nurses' perceptions of caring for childbearing women who misuse opioids, *The American Journal of Maternal/Child Nursing.* 41(1): 37–42. doi: 10.1097/NMC.0000000000000208

GOOD TO KNOW

The American Psychiatric Association DSM-5-TR has proposed criteria for internet gaming disorder. Proposed criteria include persistent and recurrent use of the internet to engage in games leading to clinically significant impairment or distress.

Table 17.6

Nursing Care Plan for Patients Abusing Alcohol

Assessment/Data Collection	Nursing Diagnosis	Plan/Goal	Interventions Nursing Actions	Evaluation Criteria
• History of heavy drinking • Minimizes negative effects of drinking • Denies concern about recent erratic behavior • Blames his spouse for recent argument	Ineffective denial	Acknowledges drinking is out of control by third AA meeting Asks for help	Demonstrate acceptance by avoiding criticism or judgment of his behavior. Identify recent inconsistencies in his behavior. Help patient identify feelings/ events that led to recent binge. Foster problem-solving to identify new ways to cope with stress. Provide information about AA. Set limits on manipulative behavior. Promote taking responsibility for hurting spouse's feelings.	Patient acknowledges need for help. Patient attends AA meeting. Patient shares one emotion. Patient will be able to define their triggers for drinking.

Patient/Family Education

• Provide information on the effects of the substance being abused.
• Ensure follow-up resources for support programs, counseling, and detoxification are scheduled.
• Provide information to family members on substance use and the effect family and friends can have.
• Ensure any pharmacological treatment for withdrawal or maintenance has follow-up appointments in place to ensure compliance with the regimen.

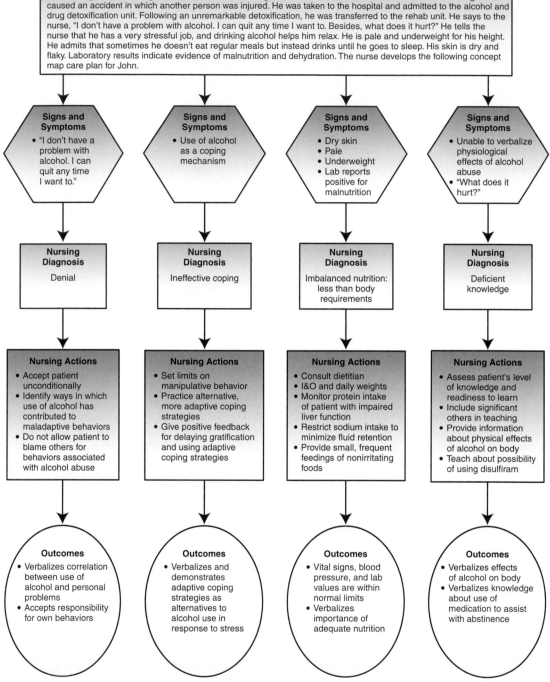

Clinical Vignette: John, age 56, was arrested for driving while under the influence of alcohol. He ran a red light and caused an accident in which another person was injured. He was taken to the hospital and admitted to the alcohol and drug detoxification unit. Following an unremarkable detoxification, he was transferred to the rehab unit. He says to the nurse, "I don't have a problem with alcohol. I can quit any time I want to. Besides, what does it hurt?" He tells the nurse that he has a very stressful job, and drinking alcohol helps him relax. He is pale and underweight for his height. He admits that sometimes he doesn't eat regular meals but instead drinks until he goes to sleep. His skin is dry and flaky. Laboratory results indicate evidence of malnutrition and dehydration. The nurse develops the following concept map care plan for John.

Signs and Symptoms
- "I don't have a problem with alcohol. I can quit any time I want to."

Signs and Symptoms
- Use of alcohol as a coping mechanism

Signs and Symptoms
- Dry skin
- Pale
- Underweight
- Lab reports positive for malnutrition

Signs and Symptoms
- Unable to verbalize physiological effects of alcohol abuse
- "What does it hurt?"

Nursing Diagnosis
Denial

Nursing Diagnosis
Ineffective coping

Nursing Diagnosis
Imbalanced nutrition: less than body requirements

Nursing Diagnosis
Deficient knowledge

Nursing Actions
- Accept patient unconditionally
- Identify ways in which use of alcohol has contributed to maladaptive behaviors
- Do not allow patient to blame others for behaviors associated with alcohol abuse

Nursing Actions
- Set limits on manipulative behavior
- Practice alternative, more adaptive coping strategies
- Give positive feedback for delaying gratification and using adaptive coping strategies

Nursing Actions
- Consult dietitian
- I&O and daily weights
- Monitor protein intake of patient with impaired liver function
- Restrict sodium intake to minimize fluid retention
- Provide small, frequent feedings of nonirritating foods

Nursing Actions
- Assess patient's level of knowledge and readiness to learn
- Include significant others in teaching
- Provide information about physical effects of alcohol on body
- Teach about possibility of using disulfiram

Outcomes
- Verbalizes correlation between use of alcohol and personal problems
- Accepts responsibility for own behaviors

Outcomes
- Verbalizes and demonstrates adaptive coping strategies as alternatives to alcohol use in response to stress

Outcomes
- Vital signs, blood pressure, and lab values are within normal limits
- Verbalizes importance of adequate nutrition

Outcomes
- Verbalizes effects of alcohol on body
- Verbalizes knowledge about use of medication to assist with abstinence

FIGURE 17.6 Concept Map of the Patient Abusing Alcohol. (From Morgan & Townsend (2021). Essentials of Mental health Psychiatric Nursing. FA Davis.)

Safe and Effective Nursing Care

Anticipate withdrawal symptoms in anyone suspected of substance use.
Provide a safe environment free of hazards for the impaired individual.
Provide adequate supervision for any individual who is impaired to prevent further complications or overdoses.
Prevent falls.
Communicate a caring environment with appropriate limit setting on behavior around the substance use.

Key Points

- Substance abuse and dependence are growing disorders in the United States, with wide-ranging effects on health, safety, and family life.
- Polydrug use is common as the user tries to self-medicate to decrease discomfort from another drug. Use of multiple drugs contributes to more complications and possible synergistic effects that can be life threatening.
- Dependence on a substance occurs when one is unable to control its use, even while knowing that it interferes with normal functioning, and more of the substance is required to produce the desired effects.
- The presence of substance abuse with a psychiatric disorder is called a *co-occurring disorder* or *dual diagnosis*. It is commonly seen in the psychiatric population and needs to be included in the screening.
- Codependency is often seen in family and friends of substance abusers as they try to help the person by covering up or enabling addictive behaviors.
- Serious complications from alcohol abuse include heart disease, liver failure, and some cancers.
- Acute withdrawal is commonly seen in the acute hospital setting when the patient is without the abusing substance for hours or days.
- Nursing management of patients with SUDs requires keen observation, setting limits, involvement of the family, and compassion.

CASE STUDY

Jim is a 26-year-old first-year resident in medicine at a large university hospital. His father and mother are both physicians, and he felt pressure to graduate from medical school with high honors. He struggled throughout medical school to maintain passing grades but achieved more success in his last year as he realized how much he wanted to be a doctor when he was working with patients. After graduation, he ranked high enough to be selected for a residency at a prestigious hospital. During medical school, he was in a car accident that left him with residual back pain, which he managed with yoga and occasional ibuprofen.

Once his residency began, he was working long hours on his feet, and his back pain increased. He no longer had time for yoga, and ibuprofen was no longer helping. He had an old prescription for acetaminophen and hydrocodone, which he took at night when he was not on call. It helped him sleep and be more rested to function well at the hospital. He obtained a prescription for more from a doctor friend, based on his back pain. As time went on, Jim needed more pain medication to sleep and then started taking a pill during his shift when he felt jumpy.

Colleagues reported that at times Jim was irritable, and at other times almost euphoric. Jim was called in by his supervisor when he made a prescribing error. Jim felt he needed more opioids to function so that he would not make errors. Then Jim's friend said he could not write any more prescriptions for him. This friend suggested he pursue a pain-management referral. Jim was not interested and pursued other routes to get pain medication, including writing his own prescriptions to a fake patient. He had a minor car accident when he fell asleep at the wheel. When he returned home from work one day, the police arrived with a warrant for unlawful prescription

Continued

CASE STUDY—cont'd

writing. A local pharmacist had become suspicious and reported Jim's activity to the police.

Jim was now in police custody. Jim's father and his hospital supervisor arrived and proposed a drug treatment program. Jim agreed.

1. Upon Jim's entering the drug treatment facility where you work, what information would you want to know about Jim's drug use?

2. In reviewing Jim's case study, at what point did the drug use turn from therapeutic to substance abuse?

3. Identify two interventions you would use initially to support Jim.

Review Questions

1. The defense mechanism most frequently demonstrated by the substance-dependent person is:
   a. Undoing
   b. Rationalization
   c. Denial
   d. Reaction formation

2. Nurses know that alcohol functions as a:
   a. CNS depressant
   b. CNS stimulant
   c. Major tranquilizer
   d. Minor tranquilizer

3. The patient who is experiencing delirium tremens (DTs) is most likely to exhibit which of the following symptoms?
   a. Tremors
   b. Auditory hallucinations
   c. Confusion
   d. All of the above

4. Sally and Susie are twins. They are 20 years old. Susie has a habit of drinking too much when they go out, and this has become more frequent. They were out celebrating their birthday last night, and this morning Susie is vomiting. Sally calls her sister's professor. "Susie is really ill. I think she has the flu; anyway, she can't come to class today. She said she has a test today and an assignment that she was supposed to pick up. I can come in and get the assignment for her. When can she make up the test?" Sally's behavior might indicate:
   a. Collaboration
   b. Compensation
   c. Lying
   d. Codependency

5. You are Sally and Susie's friend. A therapeutic response to them might be:
   a. "Sally and Susie, you are really going to get in trouble if you keep partying like that. It's bad for you."
   b. "Sally and Susie, I care for you both; but, Susie, you misuse alcohol. You both need help. Sally, you are not helping Susie by 'taking care' of her; she needs to do it herself."
   c. "Sally, why do you keep lying for Susie? Just because she's in trouble doesn't mean you have to cover up for her."
   d. "Susie, this is just a stage you're going through. Everybody does it; it's not a big deal. You're young! Have fun!"

6. Sally and Susie seek treatment. Susie is treated as an inpatient, and Sally as an outpatient. The nurse planning discharge teaching from their programs will encourage them to:
   a. Attend weekly AA and Al-Anon meetings
   b. Check back into the hospital unit weekly
   c. Attend weekly sessions with the psychologist
   d. Attend weekly Adult Children of Alcoholics (ACOA) meetings together

7. Your patient admits to using an illegal substance daily, thinking about it when not actually using it, and spending a lot of time figuring out where to get it. This patient could have:
   a. A delusion
   b. The DTs
   c. An addiction
   d. Dementia

8. One of the major skills a person or family can learn during substance abuse treatment is:
   a. Honest communication
   b. Codependency
   c. Denial
   d. Scapegoating

9. Your spouse, an alcoholic for many years, was sober for the last 2 years but has recently begun drinking again. To keep your spouse from driving drunk, you begin acting as their chauffeur. You are displaying what kind of behavior?
   a. Dry drunk
   b. Codependent
   c. Compassionate
   d. Tough love

10. Which of the following medications is most likely to be ordered for a patient experiencing alcohol withdrawal?
    a. Haloperidol
    b. Chlordiazepoxide
    c. Methadone
    d. Chlorpromazine

11. Your patient just attended her first AA meeting. Which statement reflects that she understands the purpose of AA?
    a. "Once I dry out, I know I can have an occasional drink."
    b. "If I lose my job, AA can help me find another one."
    c. "AA is only for people who have hit bottom."
    d. "AA can help me stay sober."

12. A patient is suspected of methamphetamine abuse. What symptom would you be most likely to see?
    a. Weight loss
    b. Incontinence
    c. Weight gain
    d. Gastrointestinal (GI) bleed

REVIEW QUESTION ANSWER KEY 1.c, 2.a, 3.d, 4.d, 5.b, 6.a, 7.a, 8.a, 9.b, 10.b, 11.d, 12.a

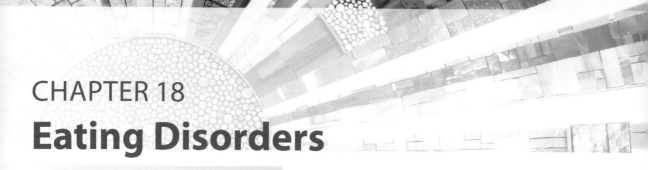

CHAPTER 18
Eating Disorders

KEY TERMS

Anorexia nervosa (also called anorexia)
Binge eating disorder
Body image
Body mass index (BMI)
Bulimia nervosa (also called bulimia)
Morbid obesity
Obesity
Purging

CHAPTER CONCEPTS

Family
Growth and development
Mood and affect
Nutrition
Safety
Stress and coping

LEARNING OUTCOMES

1. Define anorexia.
2. Describe the similarities and differences between anorexia and bulimia.
3. Define morbid obesity.
4. Discuss bariatric (also called weight loss) surgery.
5. Identify populations at risk for eating disorders.
6. Identify possible causes of eating disorders.
7. Describe nursing interventions for patients with eating disorders.

Dieting is a national obsession in the United States, especially among women. Fitness clubs are filled with individuals trying to attain the "perfect," thin, muscular body. The Barbie® doll has represented the idealized female body shape for several generations. It has almost become accepted behavior to be obsessed with body weight and shape and to view food as a source of stress. Self-esteem and happiness in young girls are often linked to weight and body shape. Men are not immune to this obsession. When this social influence is combined with certain biological, psychological, and family dynamic factors, an eating disorder, such as **anorexia nervosa** or **bulimia nervosa**, can result (Yager & Andersen, 2005). Binge eating disorder is now recognized as a diagnosis on its own in the *Diagnostic and Statistical Manual for Mental Disorders,* 5th ed., also known as the DSM-5 (American Psychiatric Association, 2013). Eating disorders have little to do with simply not eating enough or overeating. Rather, they are psychiatric disorders with substantial emotional and physical consequences. Americans have a 9% chance of having an eating disorder in their lifetime (Strategic Training Initiative for the Prevention of Eating Disorders, 2020). Obesity and morbid obesity, although not considered eating disorders or psychiatric diagnoses, often lead to emotional distress.

Classroom Activity

Discuss with classmates their experiences with eating disorders that either they or friends have had.

GOOD TO KNOW

People with some types of eating disorders are at higher risk for drug and alcohol abuse.

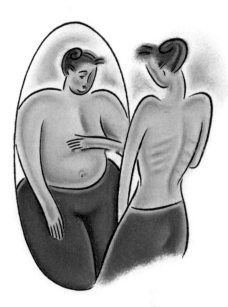

FIGURE 18.1 In anorexia nervosa, patients view their bodies in a distorted way *(photograph by Stockbyte).*

 ## ANOREXIA NERVOSA

The term anorexia (as used in anorexia nervosa) is really a misnomer because this condition has very little to do with reduced appetite. It has more to do with the person's morbid fear of obesity, causing anxiety and obsessive worry about losing control of food intake. In fact, persons with anorexia are often hungry and view the discomfort of hunger as a reminder of the deprivation they need to inflict on themselves. Only in the late stages of this disorder is appetite actually lost. Distorted **body image** causes patients to see themselves as fat even though they appear emaciated to bystanders (FIG. 18.1). No amount of weight loss relieves the anxiety, causing this deadly cycle to continue. Complications can continue for years, even after successful treatment.

GOOD TO KNOW

Body image is a very personal issue. When working with patients with eating disorders, take the time to learn about how they view their bodies. Avoid stereotyping and reacting emotionally to their appearance. The fact that they look thin to you does not mean that is how they see themselves.

Anorexia nervosa crosses all ages and genders with a lifetime prevalence of 2.4% to 4.3% (Call, Attia, & Walsh, 2017). It is much more common in females, but the rate in males has been increasing in the last few years (Woolridge & Lemburg, 2016). Onset generally peaks in the early to late teens (Anderson & Yager, 2009). For a young person this leads to delays in physical and psychosexual development. Poorer prognosis is associated with older age of onset, a lower minimum weight, and vomiting. Anorexia nervosa has the highest rate of death of any psychiatric disorder (Arcelus, Mitchell, Wades, & Nielson, 2011). Suicidal ideation is common and completed suicides are the second leading cause of death in this population (APA, 2022).

Many experts view anorexia nervosa as a struggle with autonomy and sexuality. Patients with anorexia nervosa will go to great extremes to deprive themselves of food. They will also use methods such as excess exercise and purging to rid themselves of calories to maintain control of any weight gain and emotionally attempt to control personal feelings and issues. **Purging**, which causes electrolyte imbalance and arrhythmias through inducing vomiting or overuse of laxatives, is usually combined with compulsive exercise to accelerate weight loss, making a lethal combination. Successful treatment of anorexia is measured by weight gain, return of menstruation (usually absent in anorexic women), and reduction of compulsive behaviors. Full recovery is evidenced by return of weight, growth and development, menstruation, and normal eating behaviors. Increased awareness of this disorder is leading many patients to receive earlier treatment, which improves the prognosis.

SYMPTOMS OF ANOREXIA NERVOSA

Some of the behaviors, signs, and symptoms associated with anorexia nervosa are listed in Box 18.1.

Tool Box

The National Eating Disorders Association has an eating disorders screening tool at https://www. nationaleatingdisorders.org/screening-tool

Box 18.1

Behaviors, Signs, and Symptoms of Anorexia Nervosa

Initial signs
- extremely restricted eating
- extreme thinness (emaciation)
- a relentless pursuit of thinness and unwillingness to maintain a healthy weight
- intense fear of gaining weight
- distorted body image, a self-esteem that is heavily influenced by perceptions of body weight and shape, or a denial of the seriousness of low body weight

Long-term effects
- electrolyte imbalances
- lanugo (fine body hair)
- amenorrhea (absence of menstruation)
- thinning of the bones (osteopenia or osteoporosis)
- mild anemia and muscle wasting and weakness
- brittle hair and nails
- dry and yellowish skin
- severe constipation
- low blood pressure
- slowed breathing and pulse
- damage to the structure and function of the heart
- brain damage
- multiorgan failure
- drop in internal body temperature, causing a person to feel cold all the time
- lethargy, sluggishness, or feeling tired all the time
- infertility

National Institute of Mental Health. (2021). Eating disorders. Available at https://www.nimh.nih.gov/health/topics/eating-disorders/index.shtml

Cultural Considerations

Once thought to be a disorder of higher socioeconomic groups, anorexia nervosa crosses across all levels of society.

Patients with anorexia usually hide their extreme weight loss to avoid exposure of their illness. The individual may wear baggy clothes, move food around on the plate to give the impression of eating, exercise in secret, not eat unless certain demands about food combinations are met, or give excuses for not eating, such as having snacked before dinner. Once weight loss is exposed, the individual often objects to treatment and denies the seriousness of the condition in an effort to continue to control the illness.

GOOD TO KNOW

The "proana" (proanorexia) movement supports the anorexic culture and teaches these individuals ways to hide their illness. Nurses should be aware of this movement as patients may be utilizing this type of support on social media to reinforce their disorder.

Etiology of Anorexia Nervosa

Causes of anorexia nervosa include biological factors and genetics, along with psychological factors. Biological factors include alterations in regulation of neurotransmitters like dopamine and dysfunction of the hypothalamus. Calorie restriction can result in release of endogenous opioids that produce a euphoric response to not eating. Psychological theories include the child's fear of maturing and unconscious avoidance of developmental tasks. By not eating, the person forestalls sexual development and remains a child in the family. Other dynamics include overly demanding and disturbed parental relationships. Anorexia can represent a way to maintain control over parental figures. The person with anorexia experiences a strong need to control their intake, thereby counteracting feelings of loss of control and reducing conflict. A traumatic event such as sexual abuse or bullying has been known to trigger anorexia in individuals who are already at risk for the condition.

DIFFERENTIAL DIAGNOSES

- medical condition contributing to weight loss such as hyperthyroidism, inflammatory bowel disease-ulcerative
- major depressive disorder
- bulimia nervosa
- substance use disorders
- schizophrenia
- obsessive-compulsive disorder

TREATMENT OF ANOREXIA NERVOSA

Treatment of anorexia generally requires a collaborative approach among providers in the following health-care areas: internal medicine; behavior modification; nutrition; individual, group, and family therapy; and pharmacology (see Pharmacology Corner). Specialized inpatient treatment programs are available in some areas.

The mortality rate for anorexia can be high, with serious complications including bone loss, heart failure, serious arrhythmias, and electrolyte imbalances. Suicide risk can also be higher. Close medical monitoring is essential for the patient with this disorder. A patient with severe anorexia may require long-term hospitalization with some form of artificial nutrition if severely malnourished. Some people with anorexia do better with this approach as they are relieved that they no longer have to make decisions about food; however, the team must consider the ethics of involuntary refeeding. Every effort must be made for the patient to eat voluntarily (American Psychiatric Association, 2006). Other people with anorexia become more anxious and resentful with forced refeeding and try more drastic measures to take control of their intake. These people may, for example, hide objects in their clothes to feign weight gain or change drip rates on tube feedings. Parenteral nutrition can be associated with many complications, so it is usually avoided if possible.

Behavioral programs for people with anorexia often include rewards for weight gain and restrictions for weight loss, as well as keeping a food diary. Therapeutic approaches should focus on increasing socialization and self-esteem. Cognitive behavior

therapy (CBT) can be useful to challenge negative feelings associated with eating. Family therapy is a key part of treatment. Suicide prevention may need to be incorporated in the plan for some patients. The main goal of treatment is to normalize eating patterns and behaviors to support weight gain. Additionally, working to address distorted beliefs and thoughts that maintain abnormal eating patterns will lead to normalization. Successful treatment focuses on the goals of returning to a healthy weight, stopping abnormal eating behaviors, dismantling unhealthy thoughts, treating comorbidities, and planning for relapse prevention (Anderson & Yager, 2009). The recommended dietary regimen generally promotes slow, steady weight gain of no more than 3 pounds per week (Yager & Anderson, 2005). Inpatient psychiatric hospitalization may be needed.

GOOD TO KNOW

Patients with anorexia often have a strong need to control their environment, which can lead to power struggles with the nurses.

GOOD TO KNOW

It is very stressful to care for a patient who refuses to eat. Nurses caring for these patients may experience frustration and anxiety as no matter what they do the patient will not eat. Collaborating with the interdisciplinary team is essential.

Classroom Activity

Obtain information about local eating-disorder treatment programs and review and discuss this information with your classmates.

Clinical Activity

Monitor electrolytes of your patient with anorexia nervosa.

CRITICAL THINKING QUESTION

Parents bring their 14-year-old daughter, Amanda, to your primary care office to seek help. Amanda appears pale and thin and is wearing a long, baggy dress. As you prepare Amanda for her physical examination by the nurse practitioner, you are shocked by her thin body. Her spine and ribs are prominent, she has no breasts, and her skin is dry with a fine layer of hair over her body. Amanda asks you if you think she is fat. How would you respond?

Pharmacology Corner

Anorexia

There are no medications to specifically treat anorexia, but medications can be useful to help manage some of its symptoms such as anxiety and depression as well as obsessive-compulsive behaviors. Fluoxetine (Prozac) as well as other selective serotonin reupdate inhibitors (SSRIs) have been used in some cases; however, side-effect profiles can be high due to the patient being severely underweight. Antianxiety medications given before meals have been useful for some patients. It should be recognized that symptoms of depression and cognitive changes can also be indications of malnutrition.

BULIMIA

Bulimia (also called bulimia nervosa) is binge eating generally followed by purging in an effort to control weight. Binging is eating large quantities of food at one sitting. In bulimia, the binge eating is followed by purging, usually in the form of self-induced vomiting, although laxatives and diuretics can also be used. The purging is often a result of shame and guilt brought on by the binge. To qualify for this diagnosis, the binging and purging must occur at least once per week for 3 months (American Psychiatric Association, 2022). A nonpurging form of bulimia including fasting or excessive exercise after a binge also exists. Bulimia was officially designated as a psychiatric disorder in 1980 and is harder to diagnose than anorexia. Many of the behaviors associated with bulimia are carried out in private, and the person may appear to be a healthy weight to others (FIG. 18.2). It is common that these behaviors are hidden for years.

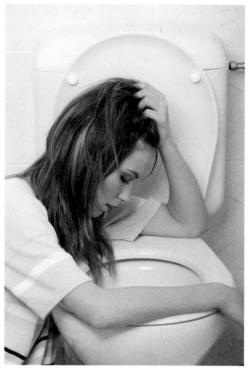

FIGURE 18.2 Bulimic woman vomiting after eating a large meal.

This disorder is much more common in females, with a lifetime prevalence of 2% (Call, et al, 2017), although it does exist in males (American Psychiatric Association, 2013). Those with bulimia rapidly consume huge amounts of food, especially food high in carbohydrates. As many as 8,000 calories in a 2-hour period several times daily can be consumed. Bulimia tends to be manifested during late adolescence to young adulthood. A higher risk occurs in the college years. The binge may be triggered by a stressful event, feelings about weight and appearance, hunger from dieting, or negative self-image. Many celebrities have acknowledged a history of bulimia, which has given this disorder more public attention. Some athletes, such as jockeys, gymnasts, and wrestlers, and others in the public eye, such as actors and fashion models, are at risk for bulimia due to pressure to maintain a specific weight. Abuse of alcohol as well as stimulants is more common in this population.

Cultural Considerations

Bulimia tends to occur in cultures where thinness is highly valued and where there is an abundance of food.

GOOD TO KNOW
People with bulimia often keep their disorder secret and are only found out when a friend or relative finds evidence of purging behaviors such as vomiting or laxative abuse.

Symptoms of Bulimia

Box 18.2 lists the most common symptoms of bulimia. Individuals with bulimia often are very self-conscious about their weight and appearance and may focus a lot of their time on dieting and controlling their weight. Their self-concept is closely tied to their appearance. There is a lifetime prevalence of substance use disorder, particularly alcohol or stimulant use, of at least 30% in this population (American Psychiatric Association, 2013). Suicide ideation is common in this population.

Etiology of Bulimia

Because bulimia has close ties to depression, individuals with this disorder may have abnormal levels of serotonin. An impaired satiety mechanism also could be a factor as the person may not recognize when he or she has had enough to eat. Psychological theories include low self-esteem, presence of

Box 18.2

Behaviors, Signs, and Symptoms of Bulimia

- rapid ingestion of high-calorie foods (binging)
- binge followed by abdominal discomfort, sleep, self-induced vomiting
- use and abuse of laxatives or syrup of ipecac (to induce vomiting), diuretics
- feeling of loss of control over binging behavior
- obsession with food and eating
- poor self-concept
- thoughts of harming self
- routine use of bathroom immediately after eating
- erosion of tooth enamel or hoarseness from vomiting
- extreme sensitivity to body shape and weight
- poor self-concept
- likely to appear at healthy weight or slightly overweight
- impulsive
- feeling depressed, guilty, worthless
- history of anorexia nervosa

Source: Morgan & Townsend (2021), National Institute of Mental Health. (2021). Eating disorders. Available at https://www.nimh.nih.gov/health/topics/eating-disorders/index.shtml

conflict in parental relationships, and a family history of alcoholism or abuse. A history of childhood obesity may be a contributing factor as well.

DIFFERENTIAL DIAGNOSES

- anorexia nervosa
- binge eating disorder
- major depressive disorder
- bipolar disorder
- borderline personality disorder
- substance abuse disorder
- hyperthyroidism
- medical conditions resulting in changes in weight such as thyroid disease

Treatment of Bulimia

Because people with bulimia hide the disorder from others and are typically of average weight, they may suffer in silence for years before acknowledging the need for treatment. Individual, group, and family therapy are important components of treatment to gain insight into the feelings that lead up to the need to binge as well as to treat depression or other disorders. Keeping a food diary with associated feelings is a common behavioral approach. Nutritional rehabilitation includes restoring healthy eating habits. Complications of bulimia include electrolyte imbalance, dehydration, erosion of tooth enamel, and tears in the gastric or esophageal mucosa from self-induced vomiting, which may require involvement of internal medicine and dentistry. The support group Overeaters Anonymous has been helpful for some people with bulimia. Usually, this disorder is treated in the outpatient setting.

CRITICAL THINKING QUESTION
Your friend Carole constantly talks about her weight. She needs frequent reassurance that she is attractive, but then she criticizes herself for being fat. She is not overweight in your opinion. She is part of a group that meets monthly at a restaurant for drinks and dinner. You notice that she eats a very large, high-calorie meal each time but visits the restroom two to three times during the evening. You are wondering if she has bulimia. What else would you look for to consider bulimia? What concerns would you have for her?

Pharmacology Corner

Bulimia

Because of the high correlation of bulimia with depression, patients diagnosed with bulimia are often given SSRI antidepressants. Some antidepressants, including fluoxetine (Prozac), paroxetine (Paxil), sertraline (Zoloft), and fluvoxamine (Luvox), are particularly helpful if there are obsessive-compulsive features with the bulimia. Fluoxetine has also been found useful even without depressive symptoms as it may help reduce cravings for carbohydrates. Antidepressants need to be given enough time (months) to determine their efficacy. Other medications to treat additional psychiatric disorders such as anxiety disorder, substance abuse, and bipolar disorder may be used as well.

BINGE EATING DISORDER

Now recognized as a disorder separate from bulimia, **binge eating disorder** is most often seen in individuals who are obese or who exhibit fluctuations in weight. This diagnosis is believed to be more common than anorexia, and the occurrence in males is more common than with either anorexia or bulimia (American Psychiatric Association, 2013). Binge eating disorder is characterized by eating large amounts of food rapidly when not hungry, eating alone, and experiencing feelings of disgust and guilt after overeating. Triggers to binging may include interpersonal stressors, low self-esteem, and boredom. The person with binge eating disorder generally does not purge. They may describe a sense of loss of control during the binge episode. For a person to receive this diagnosis, the binging must occur at least once per week for 3 months (American Psychiatric Association, 2022). The association with depression is high in this population. Binge eating disorder should be differentiated from obesity, as most overweight individuals do not engage in recurrent binge eating. Binge eating disorder is associated with more distress, poorer quality of life, and greater psychiatric comorbidity than for those with obesity (American Psychiatric Association, 2013). The etiology of binge eating disorder is uncertain. Treatment focus has been on CBT along with medication. Pharmacological treatment includes topiramate (Topamax) and the amphetamine Lisdexamfetamine (Vyvanse), which has been approved for short-term treatment of binge eating disorder. Antidepressants are also used.

DIFFERENTIAL DIAGNOSES

- bulimia nervosa
- major depressive disorder
- bipolar disorder
- borderline personality

MORBID OBESITY

Obesity is defined as a **body mass index (BMI)** greater than 30. **Morbid obesity** refers to a body weight more than 100 pounds above established norms for a person's height and sex. Obesity often leads to a lifetime of emotional, social, and physical problems, but obesity itself is not considered a mental disorder (American Psychiatric Association, 2013). Potential health problems include a wide range of chronic conditions, including hypertension, cardiac problems, diabetes, respiratory insufficiency, and joint and back disorders. Risk of death increases with a BMI greater than 30 (see Box 18.3 to determine BMI). Nutritional deficiencies are also extremely common because the obese person may lack a well-balanced diet or may experience protein deficiencies related to crash dieting. Again, obesity is not classified as a psychiatric disorder, but it may include features of binge eating disorder and depression.

Society often views morbidly obese individuals as undesirable. They may be abused by strangers and treated with contempt by family members. Even health-care providers may view them as emotionally disturbed, although there is no increased incidence

---

Box 18.3

Example of Body Mass Index Calculation

BMI = weight (in kilograms) ÷ height in meters squared

Example:

What is the BMI of a 180-pound woman who is 5 feet tall (60 inches)?

First, convert pounds to kilograms. Then, convert inches to centimeters and centimeters to meters:

180 pounds ÷ 2.2 = 81.81 kg

60 inches × 2.54 = 152 cm; 152 ÷ 100 = 1.52 m

$1.52 \times 1.52 = 2.31 \text{ m}^2$

$81.81 \text{ kg} \div 2.31 \text{ m}^2 = 35.41 \text{ BMI}$

of psychopathology in morbidly obese people. Others may view these individuals as lazy, unkempt, and lacking in self-control.

Weight stigma is defined as negative, prejudicial attitudes on the basis of body size; discrimination involves unequal treatment and biased behavior and has been documented in physicians, nurses, medical students, and other health-care professionals (Rubino, Puhl, Cummings, Eckel, Ryan, Mechanick, et al., 2020). Increased BMI has been associated with decreased utilization of the health-care system.

Cultural Considerations

Morbid obesity affects all ages and races, although it is much more common in lower socioeconomic groups. Obesity is equally distributed between men and women. Childhood obesity is considered a national health problem that can lead to a lifetime of chronic illnesses.

People who are morbidly obese face discrimination particularly in the workplace because they are viewed as less healthy, less diligent, and less intelligent than their thinner peers. Certainly, with this kind of reaction, it is no wonder that obese people often experience poor self-esteem, feelings of isolation and helplessness, and loss of control. Individuals who are morbidly obese often subject themselves to many weight-loss strategies only to regain the weight, which increases the stress on the body.

Health-care providers are in a key position to offer options for weight loss to their patients. However, these providers may not address the issue for a variety of reasons, including discomfort talking about the subject, lack of time to talk with the patient, lack of knowledge of options, limited reimbursement, and a belief that this recommendation will not make any difference (Lewis & Gudzune, 2014). Extremely obese people may avoid regular medical care because of shame about their weight. Many experts promote viewing individuals with obesity as having a chronic illness rather than a cosmetic problem.

Obesity in children and teens is a serious health concern in the United States and globally (CDC, 2021). Long-term emotional effects of obesity include depression, social isolation, poor self-esteem, and poor academic performance. These can lead to lifelong problems (Cornette, 2008).

All nurses will encounter patients who are morbidly obese in their practices. Sensitivity to the patient's fears, embarrassment, and coping mechanisms should be incorporated in the treatment plan. Having properly sized equipment like wheelchairs, beds, gowns, blood pressure cuffs, and scales can avoid embarrassment and help reduce the patient's anxiety. Having this equipment will also give the nurse confidence to better care for these patients.

Etiology of Morbid Obesity

Causes of morbid obesity are complex. Genetic predisposition is one factor. Abnormalities in the brain related to satiety, abnormalities of the thyroid gland, and decreased insulin production are some of the many physical factors that may contribute to morbid obesity. Psychological theories include tendency toward depression and use of food to comfort oneself related to past traumas such as sexual abuse. Overeating as a learned response to stress, tension, and boredom, along with a sedentary lifestyle and poor nutrition, may all contribute to obesity.

Treatment of Morbid Obesity

Obesity is a complex issue, and any weight-loss program needs to include a multidisciplinary approach. In 2018, the U.S. Preventative Services Task Force found that there is adequate evidence that behavior-based weight loss maintenance interventions are of moderate benefit and should be recommended for people with a BMI greater than 30. Behavioral approaches to address triggers for overeating can be part of counseling. Self-help groups like Overeaters Anonymous or Weight Watchers can be a major source of support and provide behavioral-based interventions. Web-based support programs to manage weight are increasingly popular.

When these measures have been unsuccessful, some people pursue surgical interventions, called bariatric surgery. The most common surgeries are adjustable gastric banding, gastric sleeve, and gastric bypass. The banding procedure creates restriction of the stomach using an inflatable band. When the band is pulled tight, it restricts the size of the stomach to accept food. This operation is performed laparoscopically. The gastric sleeve involves removing part of the stomach, creating a smaller reservoir for food. In gastric bypass, a small stomach pouch is created with a stapler device and connected to the distal small intestine. Generally, bariatric surgery is considered only for people with a BMI greater than 40 or for those with a BMI greater than 35 with serious medical complications related to the excess weight, such as diabetes. Surgery is not a miracle cure and requires ongoing support to adjust to life without eating as much. New coping mechanisms need to be developed and patients are encouraged to continue in behavioral support programs.

Clinical Activity

With the permission of participants, attend an Overeaters Anonymous meeting in your community.

Cultural Considerations

Some cultures are more accepting of obesity than others. Asking the patient about their family's or community's views on obesity can give you some insight into whether the patient considers his or her obesity a problem.

GOOD TO KNOW

The coronavirus disease 2019 (COVID-19) pandemic created increased stress for those with morbid obesity. Obesity was identified as a risk factor for severe viral disease. Individuals with morbid obesity may have avoided seeking out health care due to heightened stigma and perceived personal vulnerability, potentially contributing to more complications from the infection.

CRITICAL THINKING QUESTION

Your 35-year-old patient is in the hospital for complications from a recent abdominal surgery. This man weighs more than 400 pounds. He is withdrawn and appears depressed. When you bring in his dinner tray, he tells you to take it away. He does not want to eat because the doctor told him he has to lose 100 pounds quickly. How should you respond? What options can be given to this patient?

Pharmacology Corner

Morbid Obesity

The Food and Drug Administration (FDA) has approved several drugs for weight loss:

- Qsymia combines the appetite suppressant phentermine and the antiseizure/migraine drug topiramate. Phentermine was once widely pre-scribed as the "phen" part of the fen-phen weight-loss drug that was popular in the 1990s. Qsymia should not be used during pregnancy.
- Contrave is an extended-release form of two previously approved drugs: naltrexone and bupropion. Bupropion has antidepressant effects, and naltrexone, in addition to controlling addiction, can reduce food cravings and appetite. This medication should not be used in patients who are dependent on opioids or in treatment for drug or alcohol withdrawal.
- Liraglutide (Saxenda) is an injectable form of lira-glutide that regulates appetite. In lower dosage, it is used to treat diabetes and is known as *Victoza*.
- Xenical works by blocking the enzyme that breaks down fats in the diet. Undigested fats pass out of the body in stool. Xenical is sold over the counter in a lower dosage as Alli®.

NURSING CARE OF PATIENTS WITH EATING DISORDERS

Common nursing diagnoses in patients with eating disorders include the following:

- body image, disturbed
- coping, ineffective
- nutrition, imbalanced: less than body requirements
- powerlessness
- self-esteem, disturbed
- nutrition, imbalanced: more than body requirements

General Nursing Interventions for Patients With Eating Disorders

1. *Promote positive self-concept:* Gaining the patient's trust and giving positive reinforcement for the progress the patient makes will help the patient learn to change their lifestyle.
2. *Promote healthy coping skills:* Nurses who understand that developing healthy coping skills

is time consuming and difficult for anyone with an eating disorder are able to demonstrate confidence that the patient can change. Empathy for the depth of these disorders will help gain the patient's trust and cooperation. Be careful not to be manipulated into negative behaviors by the patient with anorexia. Setting limits on behavior is part of the plan of care. Having the patient consistently stay within those limits is part of teaching new lifestyle behaviors.

3. *Promote adequate nutrition:* The health-care provider and dietitian or nutritionist will meet with the patient to discuss calorie and nutrient requirements. Most of these patients will have nutritional deficiencies—even those who are overweight. Nurses are responsible for monitoring the patient's ability and willingness to consume the specified amount of food. Usually, smaller and more frequent meals are tolerated better than the traditional three larger meals. For a person with an aversion to food, presenting a large tray of food can be overwhelming and discouraging. Positive reinforcement for complying with caloric intake can be helpful. NOTE: When implementing this type of behavior modification, praise the caloric intake or the healthy food choices, *not* the weight change. How you word the reinforcement can be crucial to the patient's willingness to continue the plan of care (Crisafulli, Von Holle, & Bulik, 2008; Silber, Lyster-Mensh, & DuVal, 2011).

4. *Promote self-acceptance:* Anxiety over their body image is a frequent contributor to distress in these patients. Promoting self-acceptance and realistic expectations is important. Encourage the patient to think about accomplishments unrelated to body weight.

See Table 18.1 for specific interventions for each eating disorder.

The nursing care plan for patients with eating disorders is provided in Table 18.2. (See Figure 18.3 Concept Map: Anorexia Nervosa.)

GOOD TO KNOW

Movies that address eating disorders include *The Best Little Girl in the World* (anorexia nervosa), *Super Size Me* (obesity), *To the Bone* (anorexia nervosa), *A Secret Between Friends* (bulimia), and *Sharing the Secret* (bulimia).

Evidence-Based Practice

Clinical Question: Caring for patients with anorexia nervosa presents many challenges for the nurse. What have patients who are receiving treatment for anorexia nervosa found useful in their recovery process?

Evidence: A group of 21 women undergoing specialist treatment for anorexia nervosa were asked what they found helpful in their treatment. The following answer clusters were found: (1) shifts in control, (2) experience of transition, (3) importance of supportive staff relationships, (4) sharing with peers, and (5) process of recovery and self-discovery.

Implications for Nursing Practice: Bringing awareness to what these patients found helpful in their recovery process brings knowledge and hope to nurses caring for them. This provides a framework for interventions the nurse can utilize in caring for these patients.

Smith, V., Chouliara, Z., Morris, P. G., Collin, P., Power, K., Yellowlees, A., Grierson, D., Papageorgiou, E., & Cook, M. (2016). The experience of specialist inpatient treatment for anorexia nervosa: A qualitative study from adult patients' perspectives. *Journal of Health Psychology, 21*(1), 16–27. https://doi.org/10.1177/1359105313520336

Patient/Family Education for Eating Disorders

- Provide information on the particular eating disorder.
- Regularly monitor weight and medication side effects.
- Provide information on managing depression, anxiety, suicidal thoughts.
- Ensure that referrals are in place for individual, group, and family therapies as well as eating-disorder programs.
- Help identify triggers for destructive eating behaviors and help patient identify effective coping mechanisms such as relaxation techniques and problem-solving skills.

Table 18.1

Nursing Interventions for Eating Disorders

Disorder	Nursing Interventions
Anorexia nervosa	• Promote positive self-concept and healthy body image. • Promote healthy coping skills. • Promote adequate nutrition. • Support patient being open about fears and concerns. • Report any evidence of patient sabotaging treatment plan. • Encourage patient to talk about their body image and promote realistic image. • Allow patient some control in decision making. • Monitor patient during meal times and right after for support for anxiety as well as to control sabotage. • Monitor for hiding food. • Establish goals with patient and team for weight gain. • Establish appropriate behaviors in terms of exercise and food preparation. • Avoid focusing on food all the time. Encourage other interests.
Bulimia nervosa	• Approach with positive, realistic expectations of food intake. • Help patient identify feelings when they get the urge to binge or purge. • Encourage eating in public. • Monitor for eating in secret. • Provide support during meals and discourage use of bathroom after eating. • Promote a realistic body image by discussing how patient views self. • Help patient identify feelings associated with eating. • Incorporate ways to promote improved self-concept.
Morbid obesity	• Work with patient, family, health-care provider, and dietitian to formulate healthy meal plans. • Encourage patient to participate in groups to promote acceptance of self and development of self-esteem. • Make efforts to promote improved self-concept. • Respect privacy. • Work with patient to identify small, achievable goals in weight-loss plan. • Encourage keeping a diary of food intake. • Discuss feelings associated with eating. • Work with team to develop a realistic exercise regimen. • Help patient look at weight loss in small increments rather than total weight-loss goal. • Promote dignity by being sensitive to patient's appearance in public. • Plan ahead to right-size equipment available, such as wheelchairs. • Promote positive self-image and acceptance of body by emphasizing personal traits other than weight. • Continue to provide support and education after weight-loss surgery.

Table 18.2

Nursing Care Plan for Patients With Anorexia

Assessment/Data Collection	Nursing Diagnosis	Goal	Interventions	Evaluation
Emaciated patient describes self as fat; wears baggy clothes.	Body image disturbance	Patient refers to her body in a more positive way.	Avoid overreacting or insincere response to self-deprecating comments.	Patient makes one positive or less negative comment about herself.
			Rather, listen to patient and then comment on how you see her. Encourage discussion of positive traits.	

CRITICAL THINKING QUESTION

You are caring for a 21-year-old woman with anorexia nervosa. She is in the hospital receiving enteral feedings due to extreme weight loss. She just started eating small amounts of food as well. When you walk in the room, you see the patient staring at her food tray and looking very anxious. She asks you to take the tray away. How should you respond? What factors might have triggered this reaction?

Safe and Effective Nursing Care (SENC)

Provide a safe environment with appropriate equipment to provide care.

Recognize and address patient's distress around meal time.

Maintain structured activities to keep patient engaged in therapies.

Recognize patient need to maintain control. Provide opportunities for patient to exert some control of their environment.

Classroom Activity

• If caring for a patient with anorexia, review the care plan so that consistent behavioral approaches are followed.

• Review recommendations from the nutritionist for the patient with bulimia.

• For the morbidly obese patient, identify ahead of time what resources are available to assist in patient care; for example, scale, bed, proper size wheelchair, and proper size patient gown.

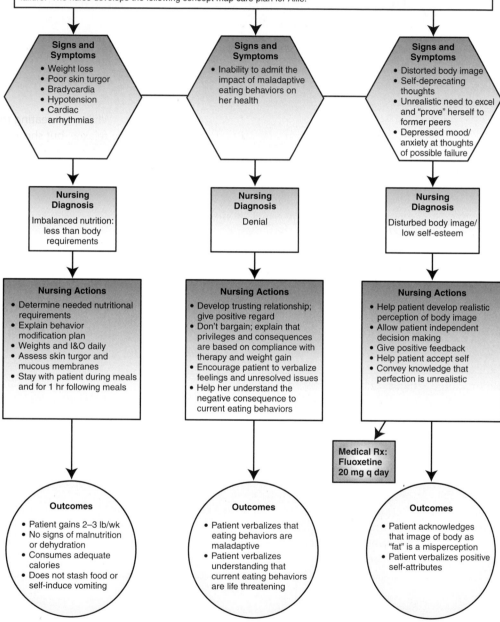

Clinical Vignette: Allie, age 18, graduated from high school 6 months ago. She is 5'10" tall and had frequently been teased by her peers because of her height. She lived in a rural community and was often ridiculed for her plan to become a model after graduation. But Allie was determined, and instead of going to college, she moved to New York City to pursue her dream. However, at the first modeling agency, she was told that she would never be accepted for modeling at her weight (140 pounds) and to come back when she had lost at least 15 pounds. She was devastated but steadfast in her determination to succeed. She cut her calories to 500 a day, exercised relentlessly, took over-the-counter laxatives and diuretics, and engaged in self-induced vomiting when she ate more than she felt she should. She became weak and chronically fatigued but persisted, until yesterday when she collapsed at the gym and the owner called 911. She was admitted to the psychiatric unit weighing 118 pounds, with poor skin turgor, blood pressure 75/45, and pulse 60 and irregular. She tells the nurse, "I can't be a model unless I get thin! Everyone at home will think I'm a failure!" The nurse develops the following concept map care plan for Allie.

Signs and Symptoms
- Weight loss
- Poor skin turgor
- Bradycardia
- Hypotension
- Cardiac arrhythmias

Signs and Symptoms
- Inability to admit the impact of maladaptive eating behaviors on her health

Signs and Symptoms
- Distorted body image
- Self-deprecating thoughts
- Unrealistic need to excel and "prove" herself to former peers
- Depressed mood/anxiety at thoughts of possible failure

Nursing Diagnosis

Imbalanced nutrition: less than body requirements

Nursing Diagnosis

Denial

Nursing Diagnosis

Disturbed body image/low self-esteem

Nursing Actions
- Determine needed nutritional requirements
- Explain behavior modification plan
- Weights and I&O daily
- Assess skin turgor and mucous membranes
- Stay with patient during meals and for 1 hr following meals

Nursing Actions
- Develop trusting relationship; give positive regard
- Don't bargain; explain that privileges and consequences are based on compliance with therapy and weight gain
- Encourage patient to verbalize feelings and unresolved issues
- Help her understand the negative consequence to current eating behaviors

Nursing Actions
- Help patient develop realistic perception of body image
- Allow patient independent decision making
- Give positive feedback
- Help patient accept self
- Convey knowledge that perfection is unrealistic

Medical Rx: Fluoxetine 20 mg q day

Outcomes
- Patient gains 2–3 lb/wk
- No signs of malnutrition or dehydration
- Consumes adequate calories
- Does not stash food or self-induce vomiting

Outcomes
- Patient verbalizes that eating behaviors are maladaptive
- Patient verbalizes understanding that current eating behaviors are life threatening

Outcomes
- Patient acknowledges that image of body as "fat" is a misperception
- Patient verbalizes positive self-attributes

FIGURE 18.3 Concept map: anorexia nervosa. (Morgan & Townsend, [2021]. Essentials of Psychiatric Mental Health Nursing. FA Davis.)

Key Points

- Eating disorders affect large numbers of people in the United States.
- Although more common in women, anorexia and bulimia are becoming increasingly common in men.
- Bariatric surgery is more common now than in years past. There are many physical and emotional considerations required when caring for patients undergoing this surgery.

- Eating disorders are serious and can be fatal as a result of malnutrition and electrolyte disturbances.
- Eating disorders may be related to emotional or physical causes. Obesity may have genetic and emotional causes.
- Nursing interventions for eating disorders center on promoting self-esteem and trust.

CASE STUDY

Penny is a 22-year-old woman who recently graduated from college. She has struggled with her weight all her life. She frequently refers to herself as "fat" and "unattractive" although her weight appears average for her height. Friends frequently encourage her to be more accepting of herself. She is currently job hunting and spends most days at a coffee shop searching for jobs on her computer. She rarely eats during the day, but while alone in her apartment at night she becomes increasingly anxious. Penny keeps bags of cookies and potato chips hidden and often eats entire packages of these items. While she is eating these items, she reports feeling relaxed; but shortly after, her stomach aches, and she feels anxious and guilty. She often reduces her anxiety by sticking her finger down her throat to induce vomiting. After vomiting, she collapses in bed and often cries herself to sleep.

1. What disorder is Penny most likely suffering from?
2. How could Penny get help for her eating disorder?
3. If Penny came to your mental-health clinic, what nursing interventions should be considered?

Review Questions

1. The eating disorder that is characterized as an aversion to food is called:
   a. Morbid obesity
   b. Bulimia nervosa
   c. Anorexia nervosa
   d. Pica

2. Your patient with anorexia is admitted to your medical surgical unit for malnutrition. She tells you she does not want to eat when her tray is delivered. Which statement is the best response?
   a. "The doctor said you will need a feeding tube if you don't eat."
   b. "Tell me what happens to you when you see the food tray."
   c. "I will ask the doctor to order an appetite stimulant."
   d. "You have to eat, or you will starve."

3. Your 19-year-old patient has a diagnosis of anorexia nervosa. You notice that she seems to spend more time playing with her food than eating it. You know that patients with anorexia:
   a. Will eat normally if ignored
   b. Fear being fat
   c. Have an accurate body image
   d. Will binge and purge

4. An appropriate nursing diagnosis for a patient with anorexia might be:
   a. Altered nutrition; less than required amount, as evidenced by distress in eating
   b. Altered nutrition; more than required amount, as evidenced by eating meals of 2,000 calories or more, six to seven times per day
   c. Altered body image as evidenced by stating the need to gain weight
   d. Fluid excess related to weight gain

5. A key nursing intervention to help patients with eating disorders is:
   a. Let the patients know they will be watched closely at mealtimes
   b. Have the patients chart their own intake and output
   c. Lock the patient's bathroom door for 2 hours after meals
   d. Encourage the patients to express their underlying feelings about food, body image, and self-worth

6. Bulimia nervosa is characterized by all of the following *except:*
   a. Binging on food
   b. Purging the food after eating it
   c. Being able to control eating pattern
   d. Having an obsession with body shape and size

7. Donald has just been admitted to your surgical unit after undergoing stomach-stapling surgery. You prepare your list for postoperative care and include therapeutic communication statements such as:
   a. "You must be so relieved to be on your way to being thin."
   b. "What is the first meal you plan to eat?"
   c. "I'm interested to know if the rest of your family is also heavy."
   d. "I'm here to help you in any way I can."

8. It is Donald's second postoperative day. He is scheduled to have his first oral liquids. As you check on his progress at lunch, you note he has not touched his beverage. "I'm afraid to," he tells you. Your response might be:
   a. "It's OK for you to drink now. You won't choke."
   b. "Tell me more about your fear."
   c. "It's important that you drink that, or the doctor may need to order the intravenous (IV) feedings again."
   d. "Why are you afraid to eat?"

9. Your new admission, a 14-year-old female, presents with multiple symptoms including recent extreme dieting, use of laxatives and diuretics, thoughts of suicide, impulsive behavior, and erosion of the enamel on her teeth. The patient's medical diagnosis most likely is:
   a. Anorexia nervosa
   b. Binge eating
   c. Bulimia nervosa
   d. Morbid obesity

10. In bulimia, purging is done to achieve which of the following?
   a. To gain feelings of euphoria at getting rid of the food
   b. To gain attention
   c. To release tension followed by depression and guilt
   d. To gain control

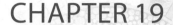
CHAPTER 19
Childhood and Adolescent Mental Health Issues

KEY TERMS

Attention deficit-hyperactivity disorder
   (ADHD)
Autism spectrum disorder (ASD)
Bipolar disorder
Bullying
Conduct disorder
Cyberbullying
Disruptive mood dysregulation disorder
Hyperactivity
Impulsivity

CHAPTER CONCEPTS

Family
Growth and development
Mood and affect
Stress and coping

LEARNING OUTCOMES

1. Identify child and adolescent populations at risk for mental health disorders.
2. Describe the effect of autism spectrum disorder on the family.
3. Define three mental health conditions commonly seen in children and adolescents.
4. Identify mental health treatment modalities used in children and adolescents.
5. Identify two medications used to treat attention deficit-hyperactivity disorder.
6. Identify age-appropriate nursing care for two selected mental health issues of children and adolescents.

Today, children are displaying behaviors and being diagnosed with mental disorders that two or three generations ago were nonexistent or at least not so readily observed in society. Many factors have contributed to these diagnoses, including greater access to mental health information by parents and teachers. However, stresses on children today are much different than in previous generations and are contributing as well. The fast pace of life, the internet, social media, continuous exposure to news, instant access to information, and exposure to violence at a young age all lead to children growing up more quickly and having to deal with many issues that previous generations never had to address until they were much older. **Bullying** and especially **cyberbullying**, in which peers use the internet to embarrass or shame a victim, is another stressor that young people may encounter.

Children and adolescents are at risk for developing many of the same mental health disorders as adults. A family history of substance abuse, schizophrenia, or bipolar disorder predisposes children and adolescents to the development of mental health problems. Family dynamics influence the development of many disorders as well. Diagnosing a psychiatric disorder in a child requires taking into account how the child copes, adapts, and relates to others and the world in the context of their developmental stage as well as chronologic age (Linnard-Palmer & Coats, 2017). The Centers for Disease Control and Prevention reports that being mentally healthy during childhood means reaching developmental and emotional milestones, as well as learning healthy social skills and how to cope when there are problems. Mentally healthy children have a positive quality of life and can function well at home, in school, and in their communities (CDC, 2021).

Mental health disorders among children are a serious national issue, with the CDC reporting 13% to 20% of children experiencing a mental disorder in a given year (Danielson, Bitsko, Ghandour, Holbrook, Kogan, & Blumberg, 2018). The most commonly reported disorders are attention deficit-hyperactivity disorder (ADHD) and conduct disorders, followed by anxiety and depression. Mental disorders in children can lead to a lifetime of problems, including poor peer relationships, problems in school, substance use, and risk-taking behaviors as well as being more likely to develop a chronic psychiatric illness. Of special concern is the fact that many children do not get adequate early treatment, perhaps due to denial on the part of parents and teachers; lack of mental health services, especially in the schools; lack of funding for treatment; and the stigma that can come with having a mental health problem. Teens with a mental health condition are more likely to drop out of school early. Strong social connections, parental understanding of normal child-development stages, adequate parenting skills, and family support all are factors that can help to keep a child grounded when going through crises such as a mental health disorder (Parsons, 2016). This chapter will discuss depression, bipolar disorder, suicide, ADHD, autism spectrum disorder (ASD), and conduct disorder in children and adolescents.

The coronavirus disease 2019 (COVID-19) pandemic has had a significant mental health effect on children and teens, as their worlds were turned upside down when they were not able to attend school in person. Stressors included social isolation, parental angst, and uncertainty (Wagner, 2020). These, along with the economic effect of the pandemic on many families, created high levels of stress and anxiety. As plans and schedules were disrupted, many young people were left with less structure and support as parents tried to cope with the pressures of children learning virtually and working remotely or being unemployed.

Tool Box

The CDC Morbidity and Mortality Report for November 13, 2020, identified the effect of the pandemic on children's mental health. The report is available at https://www.cdc.gov/mmwr/volumes/69/wr/mm6945a3.htm

Tool Box

Information for parents from the National Institute of Mental Health entitled *Children and Mental Health* is available at https://www.nimh.nih.gov/health/publications/children-and-mental-health/index.shtml

GOOD TO KNOW

The parents of children with any mental health disorder are under tremendous stress. This stress may be expressed as frustration, irritability, extreme fatigue, depression, and increased use of alcohol or drugs.

GOOD TO KNOW

When there is a mental health disorder in children, siblings in the home are at high risk for acting out. They may feel ignored because of the extra attention their sibling with the mental health disorder receives. Siblings have also been exposed to some of the same stressors as their brother or sister with the disorder.

Classroom Activity

Participate in or volunteer at a pediatric camp for children and teens with emotional problems.

Clinical Activity

Review the patient's medical chart for family history and social worker's notes on family dynamics and coping when caring for a child with mental health issues.

DEPRESSION, BIPOLAR DISORDER, AND SUICIDE IN CHILDREN AND ADOLESCENTS

Depression

Children and adolescents can exhibit symptoms of major depressive and persistent depressive disorders. The symptoms seen in children are very similar to those in adults (see Chapter 11). In addition to the classic general symptoms of depression, children may exhibit a change in their school routines, such as truancy or dropping extracurricular activities, changes in sleep habits, and extreme irritability. Other signs specific to the younger age group are social isolation, boredom, irritability, complaints of physical illness, and poor concentration (American Academy of Child and Adolescent Psychiatry, 2018). Children may become inattentive, experience a drop in grades, and lose interest in or become anxious about being at school. Adolescents who become depressed may show all of the classic symptoms of depression as well as those connected with childhood, while trying to deal with changing bodies, social roles, and peer groups. Adolescent symptoms of depression may include rebellion, intense ambivalence, anger, irritability, rage, pessimism, self-destructive behaviors, and low self-esteem (FIGS. 19.1 and 19.2). The diagnosis of persistent depressive disorder in children occurs when symptoms have been present for 1 year as opposed to 2 years in adults (American Psychiatric Association, 2022). Estimates are that 17% of youths between ages 12 and 17 suffer from major depression, with girls at more than twice the risk of boys (SAMHSA National Survey on Drug Use and Health, 2020). In children, it is believed that the major factor in development of depression is family influence. If parents are depressed, the children are three times more likely to be depressed than their age mates. Environment and biochemical imbalances in the brain are also possible causes.

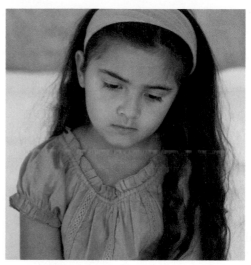

FIGURE 19.2 Children who are depressed may seem bored and unusually irritable.

GOOD TO KNOW

Depression in children and teens may appear as withdrawal, antisocial behavior, avoidance of school, irritability, or loss of confidence.

DIFFERENTIAL DIAGNOSES

- substance use disorder
- bipolar disorder
- other medical conditions
- disruptive mood dysregulation disorder
- social anxiety disorder
- autism spectrum disorder
- conduct disorder

Bipolar Disorder

Bipolar disorder is more difficult to diagnose in childhood and may be confused with conduct disorder or ADHD. Some experts think bipolar disorder has been over-diagnosed in children and teens in the past. For an adult diagnosis of bipolar disorder, the *Diagnostic and Statistical Manual of Mental Disorders,* known as the DSM-5 (American Psychiatric Association, 2013, 2022) requires the existence of distinct episodes of mania that differ from the baseline personality with or without depression episodes (see Chapter 12 for more information on adult bipolar disorder). Children with bipolar disorder generally do not have the typical cycling of mania to

Tool Box

National Institute of Mental Health information on adolescent depression: https://www.nimh.nih.gov/health/publications/teen-depression/index.shtml

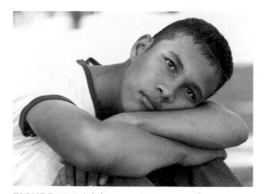

FIGURE 19.1 Adolescent symptoms of depression may include rebellion, intense ambivalence, anger, rage, pessimism, and low self-esteem.

depression seen in adults. Some behaviors associated with childhood mania include episodes of:

- hyperactivity
- extremes in emotional reactions
- flight of ideas
- grandiose delusions
- irritability
- rapid speech/racing thoughts
- reduced need and desire for sleep
- rapid mood swings
- grandiose delusions in children exist when such beliefs are present despite clear evidence to the contrary or the child attempts feats that are clearly dangerous and, most important, represent a change from the child's normal behavior

Ideally, more accurate diagnosis of bipolar disorder in children will lead to improved treatment. Childhood adversity (including early emotional trauma, parental psychopathology, and family conflict) is a known risk factor for bipolar disorder and appears to predispose to early onset of bipolar disorder (American Psychiatric Association, 2022). As with adults, the major contributor to bipolar disorder is family history. Any time a child or teen shows mood-related symptoms and there is a family history, bipolar disorder needs to be considered. Interestingly, in the past, children who were diagnosed with bipolar disorder (perhaps inaccurately) had a greater tendency toward anxiety and depression as adults rather than bipolar symptoms.

Tool Box

National Institutes of Health (NIH) brochure for children and teens and their parents on bipolar disorder: https://www.nimh.nih.gov/health/publications/bipolar-disorder-in-children-and-teens/index.shtml

---

In the *DSM-5*, **disruptive mood dysregulation disorder** (DMDD) was added as a diagnostic category under depressive disorders. DMDD is characterized by severe temper outbursts in children with irritable or angry mood, but no clear manic episodes, in at least two settings up to age 12. It is known now that children with this symptom pattern typically develop unipolar depressive disorders or anxiety disorders, rather than bipolar disorders, as they mature

into adolescence and adulthood (American Psychiatric Association, 2022). This diagnostic category may include some children who were previously diagnosed as bipolar. Substance use could also contribute to symptoms of this disorder.

DIFFERENTIAL DIAGNOSES

- major depressive disorder
- DMDD
- conduct disorder
- ADHD
- substance use disorder
- oppositional defiant disorder

Suicide

Suicide is the second leading cause of death in adolescents 14 to 18 years old (CDC Youth Risk Behavior Survey, 2019) (see FIG. 19.3). The frequency of suicide attempts in adolescents has

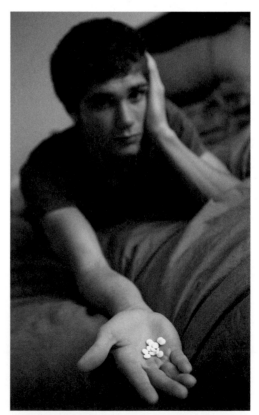

FIGURE 19.3 Suicides among teenagers are growing alarmingly. Many of the teens who attempt suicide state feelings of anger and frustration about not being listened to or not being taken seriously as the reason for their action.

increased alarmingly in recent years. The CDC Youth Risk Behavior Survey found that 18.8% of high school students contemplate suicide each year. Peer pressure, the increased use of social media, and bullying leave some vulnerable teens viewing their lives as hopeless. The stress created by the COVID-19 pandemic has also been recognized as contributing to suicidal behavior in children and teens (American Academy of Pediatrics [AAP], 2020). In addition, young people may romanticize suicide, which may be a contributing reason for taking part in suicide pacts. Depression and bipolar disorder are major contributors to suicide risk, but other factors, including substance abuse and ADHD, can also contribute. Younger children can also attempt suicide and may think of it as a magical way to "get back" at parents or others. LGBTQ+ youths are at especially high risk for suicide as they struggle to fit in with their peers. Gender dysphoria, which refers to psychological distress resulting from an incongruence between a person's sex assigned at birth and their gender identity, can increase the risk for depression and suicide. Children with autism spectrum disorder who have impaired social communication have a higher risk of self-harm with suicidal intent, suicidal thoughts, and suicide (American Psychiatric Association, 2022). ADHD is also a risk factor for suicidal ideation and behavior in children (see Chapter 13).

Signs of suicide risk can include:

- talking a lot about death
- asking questions about death
- giving away possessions
- creating artwork or engaging in play with death themes
- losing interest in friends or sports
- showing evidence of substance abuse
- having poor sleep habits
- expressing hopelessness or self-hate
- previously attempting suicide

Youth who consider suicide often act impulsively with a short interval between thought and action, so restricting access to items such as firearms and pills can be very helpful for parents to keep their children safe. Young people's methods of suicide may be similar to those of adults, for example, using firearms or hanging, but may also include impulsive acts (especially common in young children) such as jumping out of a window or running in front of cars. As with adults, children's talk about suicide and previous attempts must be taken as serious warnings.

GOOD TO KNOW

Children can be very sensitive to rejection, which can lead to suicidal thoughts and impulsive acts. Any time a child mentions thinking about suicide, investigate fully. Never minimize the child's concerns.

Clinical Activity

Be aware of your patient's changes in behavior that can signal exacerbation of depression, bipolar disorder, or suicidal intent.

Cultural Considerations

Children and adolescents of every racial and ethnic group have mental health disorders. In the past, these disorders were less frequently diagnosed in non-white young people, but now parents and those in the educational system are more informed, prompting earlier identification across all groups.

CRITICAL THINKING QUESTION

Your new patient is a 10-year-old boy who has just been admitted to the pediatric unit after being hit by a car. His injuries are not life threatening. A neighbor told the paramedics she saw the boy run into the street, right at the car. She thought he did it on purpose in a suicide attempt. The boy's parents report that he has been bullied by two older boys lately and has been very upset, but they refuse to consider this a suicide attempt. What other information would you want to know about the patient and his family? What interventions should the staff consider for this boy?

Treatment of Children and Adolescents With Depression, Bipolar Disorder, and Suicidal Behavior

Treatment of depression and bipolar disorder in children and adolescents is challenging. Group therapy, family therapy, individual psychotherapy, and partial or day-hospital programs have been shown to be helpful for many in this age group. Treatment should focus on strengthening coping skills and providing support. Parental involvement is essential for recovery. Psycho-education focuses on teaching patients and their parents life skills, effective communication techniques, problem-solving strategies, and ways to recognize early signs of relapse.

Any sign of suicide risk in a child or teenager requires immediate intervention, including psychiatric evaluation. See Chapter 13 for specific interventions.

GOOD TO KNOW

It is often difficult for parents, teachers, and health-care professionals to acknowledge suicidal behavior in children. Any sign of suicidal behavior needs to be addressed immediately.

Tool Box

Compassionate Friends is a national support program for parents whose children have died, including those who have died from suicide: https://www.compassionatefriends.org/surviving-childs-suicide/

Pharmacology Corner

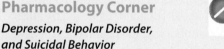

Depression, Bipolar Disorder, and Suicidal Behavior

Antidepressants must be used cautiously in children and teens. In September 2004, the Food and Drug Administration (FDA) of the United States recommended that a strong caution be placed on all antidepressant medications for children and teenagers due to increased risk of suicide. The caution that suicide can be a side effect of antidepressants led to the "black box warning" that is now on all antidepressants. Doctors and parents need to weigh the benefits of using these medications against their potential risks. Antidepressants that have been approved include the selective serotonin reuptake inhibitors (SSRIs) fluoxetine (Prozac) for children and adolescents and escitalopram (Lexapro) for adolescents.

Bipolar disorder in children and teens as well as in adults is treated with mood stabilizers and

some antipsychotics (see Chapter 12). Because children and adolescents may need to remain on medications for years, accurate diagnosis and long-term management of medication side effects are essential. A child or teen cannot be taking stimulant medication used to treat ADHD (see the following sections) if a bipolar diagnosis is being considered, as stimulants can exacerbate mania.

Suicidal behavior is treated with antidepressants and antianxiety medications (see Chapter 13). Close monitoring must be in place for any potentially suicidal child who is taking antidepressants.

When children are diagnosed with a serious psychiatric disorder early in life, the long-term side effects of effective medications are a major concern and must be weighed against the potential benefits. Parents may be faced with difficult choices and will need counseling and support to make the necessary decisions.

See Chapter 8 for more information on pharmacological treatment of mental health issues.

Tool Box

FDA "black box warning" information on antidepressant use in children and adolescents: https://www.fda.gov/forconsumers/consumerupdates/ucm413161.htm

GOOD TO KNOW

Ensure that parents are familiar with all potential side effects of medications as well as required monitoring for their child.

Nursing Care of Children and Adolescents With Depression, Bipolar Disorder, and Suicidal Behavior

Common nursing diagnoses for children and adolescents with depression, bipolar disorder and/or suicidal behavior include the following:

- anxiety
- coping, ineffective
- hopelessness
- injury, risk for
- self-esteem, low

General Nursing Interventions

1. *Communicate* honestly and effectively and at an age-appropriate level.
2. *Identify limits and boundaries.* Explain what is appropriate behavior and what is not acceptable. Be clear and concise. Place the emphasis on the positive; that is, what the person can do rather than what they must avoid doing. For example, to an angry individual a nurse might say, "You may hit the punching bag in the gym, but not another person."
3. *Focus on the child's or adolescent's strengths.* Identify skills and interests of the child.
4. *Support the individual;* encourage verbalization of feelings and thoughts. Do not minimize the child's fears and concerns. Young children especially can benefit from art therapy to express their feelings.
5. *Encourage the completion of simple tasks.* Give the child honest feedback on all successes.
6. *Provide a safe environment* where the child feels comfortable to share fears and concerns and has an outlet for pent-up energy and frustration.
7. *Respond to any self-destructive behavior* with concern and action to maintain safety. Encourage the child who has self-destructive thoughts to talk with an adult. Children should be taught to never keep secret another person's suicide plan.

See Chapters 11, 12, and 13 for more interventions for depressive disorders, bipolar disorders, and suicide. See the nursing care plan for a child with depression in Table 19.1.

CRITICAL THINKING QUESTION

The mother of your 14-year-old patient who has been admitted after a suicide attempt asks to talk to you. She is understandably quite distressed and asks you to make sure the doctor starts her son on an antidepressant. What does the family need to be taught about antidepressants and teens who have suicidal thoughts?

ATTENTION DEFICIT-HYPERACTIVITY DISORDER

Attention deficit-hyperactivity disorder (ADHD) is a pattern of behavior involving inattention and/or **hyperactivity/impulsivity**. For this diagnosis, the child must display symptoms in more than one setting—for example, at home, in church, at school, or while at the shopping mall. This disorder, which can lead to problems with social, educational, and/or work performance, is grouped under neurodevelopmental disorders in the *DSM-5*. The diagnosis is generally made by the age of 12; however, ADHD can continue into adulthood, and adults with ADHD often remember having behavior problems as children. About half of children with ADHD continue to have troublesome symptoms of inattention or impulsivity as adults.

Table 19.1

Nursing Care Plan for the Child With Depression

Assessment/Data Collection	Nursing Diagnosis	Plan/Goal	Intervention	Evaluation
Child is increasingly isolated, refusing to go to school, drops out of sports, is irritable, reports feeling unable to meet teachers' and parents' expectations.	Low self-esteem	Child will demonstrate increased feelings of self-worth.	Encourage the child to talk about his fears and insecurities in a supportive setting without judgment; plan activities that provide opportunities for success; avoid minimizing his fears; give immediate feedback on any successes.	Child returns to one activity he previously enjoyed; is able to verbalize his strengths and successes.

However, adults are often more capable of controlling behavior and masking difficulties. ADHD in children younger than age 7 is a bit more challenging to diagnose because the younger child is prone to a shorter attention span as a result of his or her developmental stage. The symptoms are often recognized in school. ADHD is more common in males than in females and does seem to have a pattern of running in families. About 10.8% of children between the ages of 5 and 17 have this disorder (CDC, 2020). Prevalence is higher in special populations such as foster children or correctional settings (American Psychiatric Association, 2022). The troublesome behaviors must be present for at least 6 months to a degree that is maladaptive and inconsistent with developmental level to confirm this diagnosis. The American Academy of Pediatrics (2019) emphasized the importance of considering ADHD as a chronic illness for which there are effective symptomatic treatments but no cure. Some individuals, however, attain the ability to compensate adequately as they mature. A diagnosis of ADHD in an adult is given only when it is known that some of the symptoms were present early in childhood.

The presentation of ADHD varies based on the age of the youth. In preschool, the main manifestation is hyperactivity. Inattention becomes more prominent during elementary school. During adolescence, signs of hyperactivity (e.g., running and climbing) are less common and may be confined to fidgetiness or an inner feeling of jitteriness, restlessness, poor planning, or impatience. In adulthood, along with inattention and restlessness, impulsivity may remain problematic even when hyperactivity has diminished (American Psychiatric Association, 2022).

The symptoms of ADHD are divided into inattention and hyperactivity/impulsivity (Box 19.1). Children can have one or both categories of symptoms to receive this diagnosis.

Cultural Considerations

Historically, ADHD has been diagnosed mainly in white children and under-recognized in those belonging to other racial and ethnic groups. The American Academy of Pediatrics reports that ADHD is still underdiagnosed in African American and Latino children (2019). Improved diagnostic tools and more awareness should aid in recognizing ADHD in all ethnic groups, but gaps in diagnosis and care continue and need to be addressed. Cultural norms also need to be taken into consideration when determining what is considered "normal" behavior for children within a particular group. Children need to be assessed in their native language to avoid confusion about their concerns.

Box 19.1

Symptoms of ADHD

Inattention symptoms:
1. Fails to give close attention to details or makes careless mistakes in schoolwork
2. Has difficulty keeping attention during tasks or play
3. Does not seem to listen when spoken to directly
4. Does not follow through on instructions and fails to finish schoolwork, chores, or duties in the workplace
5. Has difficulty organizing tasks and activities
6. Avoids or dislikes tasks that require sustained mental effort (such as schoolwork)
7. Often loses toys, assignments, pencils, books, or tools needed for tasks or activities
8. Is easily distracted
9. Is forgetful

Hyperactivity/impulsivity symptoms:
1. Fidgets with hands or feet or squirms in seat
2. Leaves seat when remaining seated is expected
3. Runs about or climbs in inappropriate situations
4. Has difficulty playing quietly
5. Is often "on the go," acts as if "driven by a motor"
6. Talks excessively
7. Blurts out answers before questions have been completed
8. Has difficulty waiting for his or her turn
9. Interrupts others

Source: Adapted from American Psychiatric Association (2022). *Diagnostic and Statistical Manual of Mental Disorders* (5th ed.), Text Revision.

Because children with ADHD put great demands on adults in their life, they may be at higher risk for punishment from parents and teachers, which can increase these children's distress. The presence of ADHD puts the child at risk for a lifetime of maladaptive behaviors and impaired social relationships, so early identification and treatment are important. In addition, children with ADHD are prone to substance abuse, depression, anxiety, conduct disorders, and learning disabilities. Children with this disorder are generally of average or above-average intelligence but do not always perform at their level of intelligence.

A definitive cause of ADHD has not been confirmed. Combinations of biological, genetic, and environmental factors may put a person at higher risk. It is common that parents of children with ADHD showed signs of hyperactivity in their childhoods, indicating a strong genetic component. Abnormal levels of neurotransmitters are associated with many of the symptoms of ADHD, as is abnormal brain function. Chaotic family life is also a factor. Some children have benefited from diet modifications such as eliminating foods like milk products or sugar. Environmental factors, such as lead exposure, may also be a factor for some.

Every child suspected of having ADHD should be carefully examined to rule out other possible conditions or reasons for the behavior before pursuing a diagnosis with other professionals such as teachers, psychologists, and other therapists. ADHD is a risk factor for suicidal ideation and behavior in children. Similarly, in adulthood, ADHD is associated with an increased risk of suicide attempt, when comorbid with mood, conduct, or substance use disorders (American Psychiatric Association, 2022).

DIFFERENTIAL DIAGNOSES

- oppositional defiant disorder
- disruptive mood dysregulation disorder
- conduct disorder
- bipolar disorder
- depression
- anxiety disorder
- medical conditions including hyperthyroidism, seizure disorders

---

Clinical Activity

Identify triggers in the environment that lead to the disruptive behavior of your patient with ADHD.

Treatment of Children and Adolescents With ADHD

For children younger than 6 years old, parent training in behavior management should be tried before prescribing ADHD medicine (AAP, 2019). Behavior management involves teaching the parents to use positive reinforcement, structure, and discipline. Children older than 6 years are generally given medications and behavior management techniques to use in the home as well as in the school environment. The child needs to learn the consequences of, and alternatives to, impulsive behavior and to practice and improve social skills. Close involvement of the child's teachers can help with learning and classroom behavior.

Parents need to develop skills, including a system of rewards and consequences, to address their child's disruptive behaviors. A structured school and home life can make a difference. Groups that help parents connect with others who have similar problems provide ongoing support.

Tool Box

National Institute of Mental Health ADHD publication (2021): www.nimh.nih.gov/health/publications/attention-deficit-hyperactivity-disorder/how-is-adhd-treated.shtml
    Parental training on behavior management: https://www.cdc.gov/ncbddd/adhd/behavior-therapy.html

---

GOOD TO KNOW

Children may be unwilling to take their medication out of fear or anger or to avoid side effects. They may pretend to take it in front of their parents or the school nurse, so close monitoring and open communication are important.

Nursing Care of Children and Adolescents with ADHD

Common nursing diagnoses for children and adolescents with ADHD include the following:

- coping, ineffective
- family coping, compromised

Pharmacology Corner

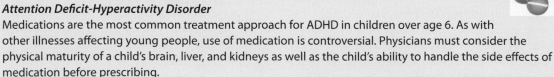

Attention Deficit-Hyperactivity Disorder

Medications are the most common treatment approach for ADHD in children over age 6. As with other illnesses affecting young people, use of medication is controversial. Physicians must consider the physical maturity of a child's brain, liver, and kidneys as well as the child's ability to handle the side effects of medication before prescribing.

Psychostimulants (also known as stimulants) are the most commonly used ADHD drugs. Although these drugs are called stimulants, they actually have a calming effect on people with ADHD by increasing the level of dopamine. These medications can increase the child's ability to concentrate and reduce their hyperactivity and impulsiveness. New, long-acting formulations, in both liquid and powder forms, can be sprinkled on food, and transdermal patches are available for some of these medications to help with compliance. Because these drugs are stimulants, they can cause major side effects, including overstimulation, restlessness, insomnia, anorexia, weight loss, headache, and irritability. Monitoring the dosage is important to manage side effects and also to ensure the youth is not increasing the dosage to gain more stimulation. Some of these stimulant medications are misused by teens and adults to achieve a high. Other categories of medications are approved for use in this disorder as well. See Table 19.2 for the common pharmacological treatments of ADHD.

Nursing considerations for children on stimulant medications include the following:

- Administer them after eating or with meals to reduce the effect on the child's appetite.
- Generally, administer them no later than 6 hours before bedtime to avoid interference with sleep.
- Before starting a stimulant medication, get a baseline weight, liver function studies, and vital signs. Then, monitor these routinely.
- The school nurse and teachers should be informed that the child needs the medications.
- Some schools require the school nurse to administer the medications.
- Monitor adolescents who may share medications or sell them to others.
- Prepare parents to monitor for the medication's effect on the child's growth.
- Educate parents that the child on stimulants should avoid caffeine, decongestants, and other substances that may potentiate the psychostimulant medication.

Table 19.2

Common Pharmacological Treatments for ADHD

Drug Category	Drugs
Psychostimulants	Dextroamphetamine/amphetamine (Adderall, Adderall XR) Methylphenidate (Ritalin, Aptensio XR, among other formulations) Methamphetamine (Desoxyn) Lisdexamfetamine (Vyvanse)
Nonstimulant	Atomoxetine (Strattera)
Miscellaneous	Bupropion (Wellbutrin), clonidine, guanfacine (long-acting) (Intuniv)

Source: Adapted from Morgan & Townsend (2021) and Antai-Otong & Zimmerman (2016).

- injury, risk for
- self-concept, alteration in
- self-esteem, disturbed
- social interaction, impaired

General Nursing Interventions

1. *Effective communication:* Therapeutic communication with the child or adolescent and the involved family members is always indicated. Teaching and modeling skills to assist with interpersonal family communication is helpful.

2. *Assist with behavior-modification tools:* Limit-setting, reward systems, and positive reinforcement may be helpful. Facilitate agreement between the parents and child or adolescent regarding what will be used as the reward, what is fair, and what the consequence to inappropriate behavior will be. Consistency among all parties is crucial in this modality.

3. *Promote self-esteem:* Help the child complete a task, and reward him or her with praise or other rewards. Give positive feedback for all appropriate behavior. Teach alternative behaviors. It can be helpful to break down tasks into small steps to reduce frustration from poor attention span. Reinforce socially acceptable behavior rather than giving a lot of attention to negative behaviors. Promote activities that encourage peer acceptance such as team sports and community activities.

4. *Low-stimulation environment:* Identify the signs when behavior is beginning to escalate, and intervene to reduce stimulation. Physical activity can be a good outlet for pent-up energy that can be done safely followed by a quiet environment.

5. *Reinforce information about medications:* The health-care provider should discuss the effects and side effects of any medications ordered. Family members may have further questions for nurses. Be prepared to assist with clarification about the medication(s). Stress the importance of compliance with the regimen to the child and parents.

6. *Promote a safe environment* as these children are susceptible to falls and accidents.

7. *Family support and education:* Living with a child with ADHD can be very stressful for a family. Encourage the family to let go of bitterness over the child's behavior. By trying to focus on the here and now rather than the past, parents can remain more positive.
See Figure 19.4 for Concept Map for Patient with ADHD.
(Pati, 2011; Primich & Iennaco, 2012; Antai-Otong & Zimmerman, 2016).

CRITICAL THINKING QUESTION
Your 6-year-old patient has recently been diagnosed with ADHD. The patient's mother tells you she has been giving him methylphenidate (Ritalin) at bedtime so that he will sleep better. What teaching would you provide to the mother to minimize side effects for the patient?

CRITICAL THINKING QUESTION
Your neighbor comes to you for advice about her 10-year-old child. He is failing in school because he is unable to concentrate and becomes very "antsy" in class. Your neighbor wants to change his school as she thinks the teacher is at fault. What suggestions would you make?

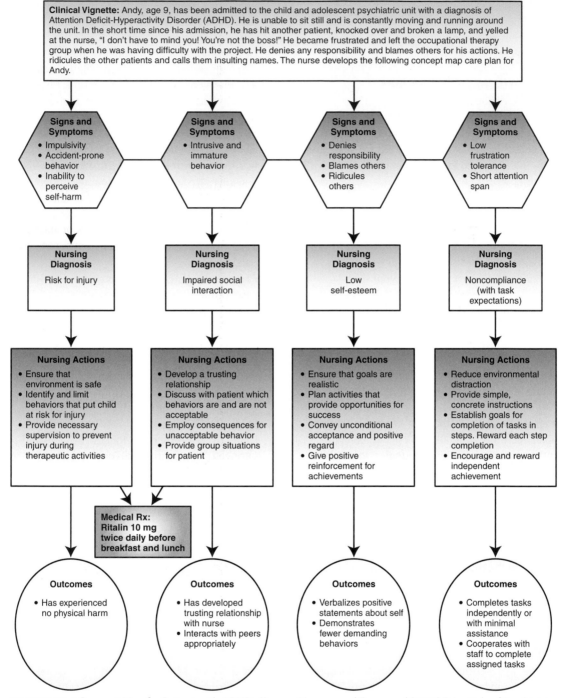

Clinical Vignette: Andy, age 9, has been admitted to the child and adolescent psychiatric unit with a diagnosis of Attention Deficit-Hyperactivity Disorder (ADHD). He is unable to sit still and is constantly moving and running around the unit. In the short time since his admission, he has hit another patient, knocked over and broken a lamp, and yelled at the nurse, "I don't have to mind you! You're not the boss!" He became frustrated and left the occupational therapy group when he was having difficulty with the project. He denies any responsibility and blames others for his actions. He ridicules the other patients and calls them insulting names. The nurse develops the following concept map care plan for Andy.

Signs and Symptoms
- Impulsivity
- Accident-prone behavior
- Inability to perceive self-harm

Signs and Symptoms
- Intrusive and immature behavior

Signs and Symptoms
- Denies responsibility
- Blames others
- Ridicules others

Signs and Symptoms
- Low frustration tolerance
- Short attention span

Nursing Diagnosis

Risk for injury

Nursing Diagnosis

Impaired social interaction

Nursing Diagnosis

Low self-esteem

Nursing Diagnosis

Noncompliance (with task expectations)

Nursing Actions
- Ensure that environment is safe
- Identify and limit behaviors that put child at risk for injury
- Provide necessary supervision to prevent injury during therapeutic activities

Nursing Actions
- Develop a trusting relationship
- Discuss with patient which behaviors are and are not acceptable
- Employ consequences for unacceptable behavior
- Provide group situations for patient

Nursing Actions
- Ensure that goals are realistic
- Plan activities that provide opportunities for success
- Convey unconditional acceptance and positive regard
- Give positive reinforcement for achievements

Nursing Actions
- Reduce environmental distraction
- Provide simple, concrete instructions
- Establish goals for completion of tasks in steps. Reward each step completion
- Encourage and reward independent achievement

Medical Rx:
Ritalin 10 mg twice daily before breakfast and lunch

Outcomes
- Has experienced no physical harm

Outcomes
- Has developed trusting relationship with nurse
- Interacts with peers appropriately

Outcomes
- Verbalizes positive statements about self
- Demonstrates fewer demanding behaviors

Outcomes
- Completes tasks independently or with minimal assistance
- Cooperates with staff to complete assigned tasks

FIGURE 19.4 Concept Map for Patient with ADHD. (Source Morgan and Townsend [2021] Essentials of Psychiatric Mental Health Nursing. FA Davis.)

AUTISM SPECTRUM DISORDER

Autism spectrum disorders (ASDs) are neurodevelopmental disorders, including several disorders such as classic autism and Asperger's syndrome. These disorders are now classified as ASD rather than treated as separate disorders (American Psychiatric Association, 2013). ASD is a complex developmental disorder of brain function that may be accompanied by intellectual and behavioral deficits. It is characterized by persistent difficulties in social communication and social interaction, problems in maintaining relationships, and repetitive patterns of behavior. ASD is called a *spectrum* disorder because it can be present in a mild form, with some peculiar behaviors and mild social isolation but otherwise normal behavior, or it can be a profound disability affecting all aspects of life. For a diagnosis of ASD, signs and symptoms must be present from infancy or early childhood; however, these signs and symptoms may not be detected until later because of infants' minimal social demands. In addition, parents and caregivers may step in to meet all the needs of young children so deficits in social functioning may be less obvious until the child is older.

Classroom Activity

View the movie *Rain Man* (1988) about an adult with autism or the streaming program *As We See It* about young adults on the autism spectrum coping with life on their own.

GOOD TO KNOW

In the *DSM-5*, ASD now includes what was previously known as Asperger's syndrome, although the latter term is still commonly used. Individuals with Asperger's have fewer problems with language and cognition than those with more severe forms of ASD. This syndrome was named after the Austrian pediatrician, Hans Asperger, who first described it. Sometimes, people with Asperger's syndrome are referred to as having high-functioning autism. These individuals often appear socially awkward with robotic speech characteristics.

Tool Box

Pediatric screening tools for autism at the CDC Autism Spectrum Disorders Web site: www.cdc.gov/ncbddd/autism/hcp-screening.html

---

The single most common symptom, or manifestation, of ASD is impaired social interaction. Learning disabilities, avoiding eye contact, and inability to make friends or respond to other people's emotions may be other symptoms. Children with this disorder may twirl their hair and/or perform self-injuring or self-mutilating behaviors, such as biting themselves or hitting their heads on objects. Repetitive patterns can include excessive adherence to routines, ritualistic behavior, and repetitive speech or motor patterns such as rocking or spinning. Children and especially adolescents with autism spectrum disorder have a higher risk of self-harm with suicidal intent, suicidal thoughts, and suicide plans (American Psychiatric Association, 2022).

Children with ASD commonly exhibit the following symptoms:

- no response to their name by 12 months of age
- not pointing at objects to show interest (e.g., not pointing at an airplane flying over) by 14 months
- not playing "pretend" games (e.g., pretending to "feed" a doll) by 18 months
- avoiding eye contact, physical contact
- having trouble understanding other people's feelings or talking about their own feelings
- delayed speech and language skills
- repeating words or phrases over and over (echolalia)
- giving unrelated answers to questions
- getting upset by minor changes
- obsessive interests
- flapping their hands, rocking their body, or spinning in circles
- unusually intense reactions to the way things sound, smell, taste, look, or feel
- appearing to be in their own world
  (Adapted from CDC Facts About ASD, 2020)

To make the diagnosis of ASD, health-care providers may also look at failure to meet certain developmental tasks, such as a baby not babbling or performing gestures (pointing, grasping, etc.) by age 12 months or a baby of any age losing language or social skills that had been acquired previously. Sometimes, the child may appear to have normal development and then stop gaining new skills. Several inventories administered by health-care providers, psychologists, or psychiatrists can help with diagnosis. Parents often notice the signs of ASD by age 2, when the child is not developing language skills and/or is showing difficulty with social interaction, such as not making eye contact or making repetitive nonpurposeful movements (American Psychiatric Association, 2022).

The incidence of ASD is on the rise. The CDC reports that 1 in 44 U.S. 8-year-old children have ASD (CDC Autism and Developmental Disabilities Monitoring Network, 2022). The number was 1 in 150 U.S. children in 2002. This tremendous increase in incidence reflects the increased awareness of parents and health-care providers to the early signs of ASD as well as the inclusion of Asperger's syndrome in the disorder. ASD affects males four times more frequently than it affects females. ASD is not curable, and many individuals will require lifelong treatment. Children with severe autism are considered disabled for life. Autism should not be confused with, or misdiagnosed as, schizophrenia, although some behaviors may be similar. Though disabling for some, ASD can be managed and many go on to have independent lives.

The causes of autism are suspected but not confirmed. Genetics, viral infections, and exposure to chemicals during pregnancy have been suspected causes for or contributors to the development of autism. For parents with one autistic child, there is an increased chance of having a second child with autism. Fragile X syndrome, congenital rubella, exposure to some medications in utero, and tuberous sclerosis (a genetic disorder characterized by benign tumors that can involve the brain) have been suggested as possible causes of ASD. Many people with ASD have disruptions in normal brain growth. The increased incidence of ASD has led to more emphasis on research.

Tool Box

NIH fact sheet on autism: https://www.ninds.nih.gov/Disorders/Patient-Caregiver-Education/Fact-Sheets/Autism-Spectrum-Disorder-Fact-Sheet

CDC fact sheet about ASD: www.cdc.gov/ncbddd/autism/facts.html

American Academy of Child and Adolescent psychiatry practice parameters for ASD: http://www.jaacap.com/article/S0890-8567(13)00819-8/pdf

GOOD TO KNOW

Some children with ASD demonstrate stimming behavior. This is a self-stimulating behavior, often involving repetitive motions or speech. Examples may include repetitive rubbing or clapping. This can be a soothing behavior to deal with sensory overload or uncomfortable situations.

Cultural Considerations

Historically, ASD has been underdiagnosed in the Latino and African American populations. This may have been due to inadequate research in these populations that identified it as a problem. This has led to later diagnosis and treatment in these populations in some cases. Previously viewed as a disorder mainly in white children, ASD is now known to exist in all racial and ethnic groups, so more resources are now available to identify and treat this disorder in other races.

GOOD TO KNOW

Some people continue to believe that autism is caused by childhood vaccines. This mistaken belief has led some parents to refuse vaccines for their infants, which can expose them to normally preventable illnesses and can contribute to the endangerment of others. *No credible evidence has linked autism to vaccines* (National Institutes of Health, 2022). If parents are concerned about vaccines, encourage them to discuss their concerns with their health-care provider before making any decisions.

Treatment of Children and Adolescents with ASD

Although there is no cure for autism at this time, early identification is important. Early intervention services help children from birth to 3 years old learn important skills and enhance development by taking advantage of the brain's ability to adapt.

Services can include therapies to help the child talk, walk, and interact with others. Many new treatment programs that incorporate intensive speech, occupational, and physical therapies, as well as behavioral training and management, may be appropriate for some children. These are home- and school-based intensive programs that have shown some success. Therapies may incorporate a structured reward system for responding to people. Each child must be evaluated individually for the best treatment. There are also many unproven treatments that parents may pursue in a desperate effort to treat their child.

GOOD TO KNOW
Having a child with ASD can create tremendous physical, emotional, and financial stress on the family. These families need information on all resources available in their community.

GOOD TO KNOW
Parents may be desperate for alternative treatments and may share approaches that you find questionable. It is important to maintain their trust and encourage them to be open to standard medical treatment and investigate thoroughly any alternative approach.

Pharmacology Corner
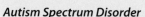

Autism Spectrum Disorder
Research trials for drugs to treat autism are ongoing, but so far there is no definitive pharmacological treatment. Health-care providers may prescribe medication for irritability, aggression, and/or deliberate self-injury. The FDA has approved the use of risperidone (Risperdal) and aripiprazole (Abilify) for children ages 6 to 17 with these symptoms (Earle, 2016; LeClerc & Easley, 2015). Patients on these medications require close monitoring. The dosage is based on the weight of the child and clinical response.

Clinical Activity
Review possible side effects of any medications your patient with ASD is taking. Reinforce education on medications to parents and the patient.

Nursing Care of Children and Adolescents With ASD
Common nursing diagnoses for children and adolescents with autism include the following:

- injury, risk for
- self-care deficit
- social interaction, impaired
- verbal communication, impaired

General Nursing Interventions
1. *Maintain safety:* Therapists may prescribe special equipment or even special clothing, such as helmets and arm covers, to help maintain safety. The goal of this intervention is to discourage and prevent self-destructive behavior. Assisting parents to identify situations that may trigger the unwanted behavior is also helpful in preventing or de-escalating the behavior. Monitor the child closely and remove any items in the environment that may cause injury.

2. *Reinforce medical and counselor teaching:* Work with the parents and child on social skills. Provide praise and positive reinforcement for both the parents and child. Technology is assisting with interventions for some patients. Virtual reality equipment and tablet computers are being used in some settings and with some success to help with teaching and behavioral training. The child may be able to relate more to these devices than through interaction with others. Pet therapy, where a child can interact with a dog, cat, or horse, has shown success.

3. *Maintain effective communication with all parties:* Speak to the child or adolescent in simple, direct, age-appropriate language. Ensure that the family and others involved in the day-to-day care of the patient feel comfortable discussing concerns.

4. *Maintain consistency of caregivers:* The child may do better with familiar people. Try to reduce the amount of stimulation from strangers. Keep expectations realistic, and recognize that progress is slow and regression to previous behaviors may occur, especially under stress. Support independence where possible.

5. *Avoid overstimulating the child:* Determine whether the child becomes more stressed with physical contact. The child may be

uncomfortable with being touched. Check with the family on what the child will accept.

6. *Establish a routine schedule* with the child that all staff follows as much as possible.

7. *Parental support:* Having an autistic child affects the entire family on a daily basis. They need support and resources.

See nursing care plan in Table 19.3.

Clinical Activity

• If your patient with ASD is hospitalized, encourage their family to bring in familiar objects and advise staff about usual routines.

• Talk with a social worker about potential support resources for the parents and siblings in the home.

CRITICAL THINKING QUESTION

An 8-year-old boy diagnosed with autism is admitted to your pediatric unit for an upcoming surgery. When you walk into his room, he is standing in the corner staring at one spot and does not respond to your greeting. Identify two approaches you would use to make contact with him.

Evidence-Based Practice

Clinical Question: How can nurses help parents support adequate sleep in their child with ASD?

Discussion: Two-thirds of children with ASD have chronic insomnia. This presents many challenges for parents who may be exhausted from providing care and need their own rest.

Evidence: The Sleep Committee of the Autism Treatment Network (ATN) has developed an evidence-based pathway to guide parents on how to help their child sleep. Interventions include sleep education, environmental changes, behavioral interventions, and exogenous melatonin.

Implications for Nursing Practice: Nurses caring for children with ASD need to routinely include education for parents on sleep hygiene, such as establishing a bedtime routine and encouraging behaviors that promote sleep, like setting up a quiet time the hour before bed, ensuring the bedroom is conducive to sleep, and encouraging the child to sleep alone.

Souders M.C., Zavodny S., Eriksen W., Sinko R., Connell J., Kerns C., Schaaf R., Pinto-Martin J. (2017). Sleep in children with autism spectrum disorder. *Current Psychiatry Reports.* 2017 Jun;19(6):34. doi: 10.1007/s11920-017-0782-x. PMID: 28502070; PMCID: PMC5846201

Table 19.3

Nursing Care Plan for the Child With Autism

Assessment/Data Collection	Nursing Diagnosis	Plan/Goal	Intervention	Evaluation
Eight-year-old autistic boy in the hospital is frequently banging his head on the wall and does not speak to any of the staff.	Impaired verbal communication	Child will demonstrate one alternative behavior indicating reaction to caregiver, e.g., facial expression, eye contact.	Assign consistent caregivers. Ask parents to bring in familiar objects from home and review usual routine. Give positive feedback for alternative behaviors.	Child has reduced frequency of head banging.

CONDUCT DISORDER

Conduct disorder is a disorder of childhood and adolescence that involves long-term (chronic) behavior problems associated with physical aggression, defiance, rule breaking, and disturbed peer relationships. Sometimes children with this disorder are viewed as "bad" or "delinquent" rather than having a psychiatric disorder. These children exhibit a repetitive and persistent pattern of behavior in which the basic rights of others or major age-appropriate societal norms or rules are violated. Conduct disorder is now categorized under disruptive, impulse control and conduct disorders in the *DSM-5*. The diagnosis of conduct disorder is based on the presence of a pattern of aggressive behavior to people and/or animals, destruction of property, deceitfulness, theft, and/or serious violation of rules. The diagnosis is much more common among boys than among girls. The onset can be in childhood or adolescence. For an accurate diagnosis, the behavior must be far more extreme than simple adolescent rebellion or boyish enthusiasm. It is a *pattern* of behavior; a one-time incident does not diagnose the condition. Some behavior patterns might be bullying, displaying or using a weapon, arson, lying, fighting, animal abuse, truancy from school, chronic rule breaking, and running away from home (FIG. 19.5).

If conduct disorder is suspected, careful screening and medical testing are important, as many changes are happening developmentally in this age group. The *DSM-5* notes several specific patterns that are sometimes seen in conduct disorder, including callousness and lack of remorse. When a person with conduct disorder has these traits, they are harder to treat. In some children, conduct disorder may be preceded by oppositional defiant disorder (ODD), which is a pattern of negativistic and hostile behavior toward authority figures. There is a risk of developing antisocial personality disorder (see Chapter 14) in adulthood.

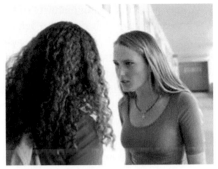

FIGURE 19.5 Recurrent bullying is a behavior that may indicate a conduct disorder, and it can be found among both boys and girls *(courtesy of U.S. Department of Health and Human Services, Office of Women's Health, Fairfax, VA).*

Causes of and contributing factors to conduct disorder include the following:

- victim of child abuse or neglect including harsh discipline
- early institutional living
- drug addiction or alcoholism in the parents
- ongoing family conflicts
- genetic defects
- alterations in neurotransmitters including norepinephrine and serotonin
- head trauma, brain disorder
- prenatal exposure to cocaine
- history of ADHD
- substance abuse

DIFFERENTIAL DIAGNOSES

- ADHD
- bipolar disorder
- mood disorders
- learning disabilities
- medical condition including traumatic brain injury, seizure disorder
- post-traumatic stress disorder
- substance use disorder
- oppositional defiant disorder

Treatment of Children and Adolescents With Conduct Disorder

Treatment includes counseling for the parents and family as well as the affected child. A child psychiatrist can work with the patient to address past traumas and anger issues. Parenting skills, consistency in limit setting, and progressing maturity of the child may, over time, lessen or eliminate the behaviors of conduct disorder, especially as the child moves out of adolescence. Parent-management training is an approach that teaches parents more effective ways to respond. Family therapy is often part of the treatment plan, and group therapy of some form can help the child relate more appropriately to their peer group.

Clinical Activity

When your patient has conduct disorder, recognize possible contributing factors, which can include a history of ADHD, child abuse, substance abuse, and lack of parental guidance.

GOOD TO KNOW

With children who have conduct disorder, it is important to maintain a calm but firm approach that does not communicate fear or avoidance. The child may have learned to use aggressive behavior to keep people away and maintain power over others.

Tool Box

The American Academy of Child and Adolescent Psychiatry has information on conduct disorder resources for families at: https://www.aacap.org/AACAP/Families_ and_Youth/Facts_for_Families/FFF-Guide/ Conduct-Disorder-033.aspx

---

GOOD TO KNOW

Parents of a child with conduct disorder are faced with many stresses as they must deal with others who are hurt by their child as well as with the child's behavior. They need legal, emotional, and financial resources to help them help their child.

CRITICAL THINKING QUESTION

Ben is 11 years old and was brought to your mental health clinic by his mother after the school expelled him for repeated bullying of younger children. One of the children attempted suicide after being repeatedly humiliated by Ben. Ben's mother is desperate for help and tells you she wants to turn Ben in to the juvenile authorities to institutionalize him. What would you say to this mother? What other options might be appropriate?

Pharmacology Corner

Conduct Disorder

There is no specific pharmacological treatment for conduct disorder. Medications are used to treat specific symptoms. The antipsychotic risperidone (Risperdal) can contribute to symptom control for extreme agitation. These medications work most effectively along with counseling. ADHD medications such as stimulants, along with antidepressants and clonidine, have been used with success for some patients with conduct disorder.

Nursing Care of Children and Adolescents With Conduct Disorder

Common nursing diagnoses for children and adolescents with conduct disorder include the following:

- coping, defensive
- injury, risk for
- other-directed violence, risk for
- self-esteem, disturbed
- social interaction, impaired

General Nursing Interventions

1. *Maintain safety:* Maintaining physical, psychological, and emotional safety is the primary nursing intervention for children and adolescents who have conduct disorder. In addition, maintaining the safety of those with whom these patients come in contact needs to be part of the care plan.
2. *Communicate honestly and effectively:* Communicate at an age-appropriate level the behaviors that are acceptable. Communicate the effect that inappropriate behavior has on

others around the child. Communicate the consequences of inappropriate behavior and, most importantly, be consistent with enforcing those consequences. Recognize that the child may have poor skills in social situations and may need coaching or positive reinforcement.

3. *Assist with behavior modification tools:* Limit setting, reward systems, and positive reinforcement may be helpful. Set realistic expectations according to the child's age and ability level. Consistency among all parties is crucial.

4. *Model the appropriate roles and educate the family about them:* In other words, parents need to be parents, and the child needs to be the child. The parents should be in control of the situation. The child has input; in fact, negotiation is healthy, depending on the age of the child; but the child does not always "win." When behavior limits are exceeded or violated, the consequences for the inappropriate behavior must be enacted. Parents may find this difficult and exhausting. They will need support and positive reinforcement from the nurse and medical or counseling staff. When the child is involved in hurting others or in risky behaviors, the adults must take control to stop these behaviors.

5. *Reinforce information about medications:* The health-care provider should discuss the effects and side effects of any medications ordered. Family members may have further questions for nurses. Be prepared to assist with clarification about medications.

6. *Reinforce the need for ongoing therapy:* Participation in behavioral therapy, psychotherapy, and family therapy is often part of the treatment plan. The child needs to learn how to handle feelings of anger.

Patient/Family Education for Children and Adolescents With Mental Health Issues

- Provide information on the specific diagnosis and signs of complications.
- Ensure all involved have adequate information on medication use and side effects.
- Provide information on support groups and counseling services available for the specific diagnosis.
- Promote involvement of teens and children, where appropriate, in their care and treatment.
- Provide information on providing a safe environment.

Safe and Effective Nursing Care (SENC)

Provide a safe environment to reduce the risk of harm to patient and others.

Identify risk factors that contribute to challenging behaviors.

Communicate effective strategies to care team for consistent approach.

Maintain appropriate limits.

Key Points

- Children and adolescents experience threats to their mental health. They have the same illnesses as adults but may manifest them in different ways. Some illnesses continue into adulthood.
- Medications and therapy are effective for a great many people in these age groups. Black box warnings are applied to certain antidepressants when used with children and adolescents; some antidepressants may actually increase the risk for suicide in these groups.

- The incidence of ASD has dramatically increased in the last two decades. ASD can be a serious disorder that has lifelong effects.
- Parents, family members, and other primary caregivers need to be involved in the treatment of children and adolescents with mental health disorders. Consistency of care is crucial. Parents may need counseling in order to become more effective in their role as parents.
- ADHD and conduct disorders present challenges to nurses working with children and teens.

CASE STUDY

Sharon, a 15-year-old girl, is brought to your family practice clinic by her mother. The mother explains that Sharon was suspended from school for assaulting a teacher and needed a "doctor's evaluation" before she could return to class. The history reveals that this is Sharon's tenth school suspension during the past 3 years. She has previously been suspended for fighting, carrying a knife to school, smoking marijuana, and stealing money from other students' lockers. When asked about her behavior at home, Sharon reports that her mother frequently "gets on my nerves" and at those times Sharon leaves the house for several days. The family history indicates that Sharon's father is incarcerated for auto theft and assault. Sharon's mother frequently leaves Sharon and her 8-year-old brother unsupervised overnight.

1. Given this information, what suggestions could be made to help this mother cope with the teen's behavior? How would you approach Sharon on first meeting her?
2. What possible diagnoses do you think would be considered?

Review Questions

1. An 8-year-old child is in the waiting room. This child has a diagnosis of conduct disorder. You call another patient to the examination room but notice this child beginning to act out inappropriately. Your first concern and nursing action would be:
   a. Ask the parent to take the child outside until they are called for their appointment.
   b. Provide an environment of safety for the child, parent, and others in the waiting room.
   c. Change the rooming order and take this parent and child ahead of the patient just called.
   d. Wait a few minutes; the child will probably calm down soon.

2. The child with autism has difficulty with trust. With this in mind, which of the following nursing actions would be most appropriate?
   a. Encourage staff to hold the child as much as possible.
   b. Support different staff caring for child so that she gets used to other people.
   c. Encourage the same staff person to care for the child each day.
   d. Avoid talking to the child so that she will not be fearful of you.

3. Your 5-year-old patient is not talking to you or the social workers. You suggest giving her some toys and drawing materials. Your rationale for this is:
   a. It gives you one less person to work with at the moment.
   b. You know children can be bribed.
   c. You think she might talk if she were distracted.
   d. Children often communicate feelings through their play.

4. Which of the following activities is most helpful for a child with ADHD?
   a. Checkers
   b. Pool
   c. Video games
   d. Volleyball

5. Which of the following groups of medications are most commonly used for patients with ADHD?
   a. Central nervous system (CNS) depressants
   b. CNS stimulants
   c. Antidepressants
   d. Antipsychotics

6. Martin is 7 years old and has a diagnosis of ADHD. He has broken his arm and requires surgery to have it set. You are the nurse doing the admission checklist with Martin and his family. You know that people with ADHD:
   a. Have normal or above-average intelligence
   b. Are impulsive
   c. Are inattentive or easily distracted
   d. All of the above

7. The single most common symptom of autism is:
   a. Strong ability to make friends
   b. Impaired social functioning
   c. Appropriate emotional responses
   d. Achieving and maintaining age-appropriate developmental tasks

8. The parents of 6-year-old Anna say, "Nurse, why us? The doctors tell us Anna has the most difficult of all childhood developmental disorders to cure. What did we do wrong? What can we do for her?" Your best response might be:
   a. "The doctors are correct."
   b. "Her medications should help calm her somewhat."
   c. "We have specialists here who can answer your questions. I will call someone."
   d. "Maybe she will outgrow the autism."

9. Which of the following would be most likely to predispose a child to conduct disorder?
   a. Overprotective parents
   b. Parents with very high expectations of academic excellence
   c. Chaotic home life with both parents being heavy drinkers
   d. One parent with a physical disability

10. What is the major concern in administering antidepressants to depressed children?
    a. The side effect of dry mouth may affect appetite.
    b. The child may not want to swallow these pills.
    c. The child is at higher risk for suicide.
    d. The child needs to stop drinking milk with these medications.

REVIEW QUESTIONS ANSWER KEY 1.b, 2.c, 3.d, 4.d, 5.b, 6.d, 7.b, 8.c, 9.c, 10.c

CHAPTER 20

Postpartum Issues in Mental Health

KEY TERMS

Postpartum blues
Postpartum depression
Postpartum psychosis

CHAPTER CONCEPTS

Family
Growth and development
Mood and affect

LEARNING OUTCOMES

1. Differentiate between postpartum blues and postpartum depression (PPD).
2. Define postpartum psychosis.
3. Discuss nursing interventions for new mothers who are feeling depressed.
4. Discuss possible side effects of taking psychotropic medications during pregnancy and breastfeeding.

Even though pregnancy and the birth of a child can be an exhilarating time for women, many experience feelings of sadness, anxiety, or inadequacy. The global term perinatal mood and anxiety disorders (PMAD) encompasses emotional problems experienced during pregnancy and up to 1 year after the birth. These problems can include **postpartum blues**, depression, anxiety, post-traumatic stress related to a past trauma, and even psychosis. New fathers can also be affected.

GOOD TO KNOW

Little research has been done on the effects of pregnancy and childbirth on fathers and other nongestational parents, such as the second parent in same-sex couples, parents who are pregnant through a surrogate, and adoptive parents. All are affected during the pregnancy and postpartum period.

Tool Box

The National Perinatal Association has a position statement on PMAD: http://www.national perinatal.org/resources/Documents/Position%20 Papers/2018%20Position%20Statement%20 PMADs_NPA.pdf

Cultural Considerations

Postpartum mental disorders cross all cultures. Each culture has expected behaviors of new mothers, and knowledge of these cultural expectations can make for more accurate screening of possible psychiatric disorders.

POSTPARTUM BLUES

Postpartum blues (sometimes called transient depressive symptoms) are an extremely common response to the sudden physiological changes immediately after childbirth. These "baby blues" occur in about 50% to 80% of new mothers (Massachusetts General Hospital Center for Women's Mental Health, n.d.#1). The major cause is believed to be the plummeting levels of the hormones estrogen and progesterone right after birth. Other factors include fatigue and stress of delivery along with the immediate postpartum responsibilities. Symptoms include crying spells, rapid mood shifts, sleep disturbances, forgetfulness, anxiety, and feeling overwhelmed (James, 2014). The symptoms typically peak at the fourth or fifth day after birth and resolve by day 10, but there is much individual variation (Massachusetts General Hospital Center for Women's Mental Health, n.d.#1). The disorder is generally self-limiting, does not reflect psychopathology, and does not affect the quality of care the mother is able to provide to the new baby. However, the presence of postpartum blues does increase the risk for postpartum major depression.

Treatment of Postpartum Blues

Postpartum blues require no psychiatric treatment. Families should be educated during the prenatal period about how frequently this transient condition occurs. Emotional support, compassion, and rest generally help resolve this problem in a matter of days. If the blues go on for a longer period of time (more than 2 weeks) and there is evidence the mother feels intense anxiety about the infant, agitated, inadequate, and overwhelmed most of the time, more intervention is needed. These behaviors could signal that postpartum blues have become postpartum depression.

CRITICAL THINKING QUESTION

Your postpartum patient is ready to be discharged home. Her family surrounds her, and they are all thrilled that she had a healthy baby boy. The new mother keeps crying and asks her family to leave her alone. They are shocked and wonder why she is not happy. What would you tell the family? How would you help the patient?

GOOD TO KNOW

New mothers and their families need to be prepared for postpartum blues and to be reassured that the mother's response is not abnormal. New mothers may not verbalize their feelings out of fear of appearing to be a bad mother.

Clinical Activity

• Incorporate support, reassurance, and rest in the care of the new mother.
• Provide education and resources, such as a lactation consultant, if needed, to this patient to help her gain confidence in caring for the infant.

Classroom Activity

Ask classmates who are mothers to discuss their feelings during the postpartum period.

POSTPARTUM DEPRESSION

Postpartum depression (PPD) is a serious disorder that occurs in about 1 in 8 women after delivering a baby (Centers for Disease Control and Prevention, 2020). It is sometimes referred to as perinatal depression to encompass depression that occurs during pregnancy as well as after delivery. Some researchers think that this condition is underdiagnosed and undertreated, particularly because depression in women in the general population peaks in the 25 to 44 age group. The symptoms of PPD are the ones typically seen in depression (see Chapter 11) with the addition of impaired ability to care for the baby. The majority of sufferers of PPD have had some type of mental health disorder earlier in life, such as depression. The American Psychiatric Association (2013) reports that 50% of postpartum major depressive episodes actually begin before delivery, referred to as peripartum onset. Postpartum onset of symptoms is typically later than those seen in postpartum blues and takes weeks to months to abate. The symptoms must occur within 1 year of delivery and be noticeable for at least 2 weeks to be given this diagnosis. Most of the time

PPD occurs within the first 3 months after delivery (Medline Plus, 2022). The new mother may hide her symptoms for fear of being viewed as a bad mother. This depression can lead to denial of the infant, inability to care for the infant, and even thoughts of hurting the infant, as well as suicidal thoughts or acts in rare, extreme cases.

The strongest risk factor for PPD is depression during a previous pregnancy or in the previous postpartum period. See Box 20.1 for symptoms of PPD and Box 20.2 for factors that contribute to PPD. Bipolar disorder can also be the cause of PPD. This should be considered if there is a family history of bipolar disorder or if the patient has atypical depression symptoms (Sharma, Doobay, & Baczynski, 2017).

Tool Box

The Edinburgh postnatal depression scale (EPDS) is a 10-item self-assessment tool used to monitor a mother's symptoms of depression after giving birth. The EPDS is sometimes used antepartum (before birth) as well. A score of 12 or more indicates the need for further evaluation.

https://psychology-tools.com/test/epds

Box 20.1

Symptoms of Postpartum Depression

- anxiety
- irritability
- loss of interest in new baby
- perception of infant as demanding
- withdrawal
- irrational guilt
- sleep disturbances
- loss of appetite
- inability to concentrate
- feelings of inadequacy in caring for baby
- lack of bond with or love of new baby
- excessive anxiety over baby's health
- feelings of worthlessness
- poor concentration
    Note: For a PPD diagnosis, the symptoms must persist for at least 2 weeks.

Sources: National Institute Mental Health (N.D.); Smith & Chichocki, 2017; Centers for Disease Control and Prevention, 2020.

Box 20.2

Contributing Factors to Postpartum Depression

- hormone fluctuations
- history of anxiety disorder
- personal and/or family history of depression or any mood disorder
- history of premenstrual dysphoric disorder
- stressful relationship with partner
- lack of social support
- major life stressors around the pregnancy
- ambivalence about the pregnancy
- sleep disturbance
- medical problems during the pregnancy or just after birth
- history of a troubled childhood
- pregnancy under age 20
- abuse of alcohol, illegal substances

Source: National Institute of Mental Health (N.D.); McCoy, 2011; Massachusetts General Hospital Center for Women's Mental Health, n.d. #1; Medline Plus, 2022.

Cultural Considerations

The EPDS is also available in Spanish: http://www.heardalliance.org/wp-content/uploads/2011/04/Postpartum-Depression-Edinburgh-Scale-Spanish.pdf

Cultural Considerations

A recent study evaluating the differences in PMAD for black, Latina, and white women found that while black women were less likely to express feelings of depression or anxiety, their rate of depression and anxiety was much higher than that of their white counterparts. The study also found that black and Latina women were less likely to seek support, treatment, and follow up after an initial psychiatric appointment. This suggests there may be an unmet need for culturally respectful and appropriate services for these communities. Additionally, when black and Latina women sought services, the time span between symptomatology and engagement with treatment was much longer than for white women (Keefe, Brownstein-Evans, & Polmanteer, 2016).

DIFFERENTIAL DIAGNOSES

- bipolar disorder
- adjustment disorder with depressed mood
- mood disorder due to another medical condition
- substance-induced depressive or bipolar disorder

Treatment of Postpartum Depression

PPD is a serious disorder that requires treatment. Early intervention is associated with a good prognosis. When the diagnosis of PPD is made, the mother is usually placed on antidepressants and begins some form of psychotherapy, including cognitive behavior therapy. If the mother is breastfeeding, she may be reluctant to take medications that are excreted in breast milk. See the Pharmacology Corner for more information on the potential risks associated with antidepressants. Discussion with the health-care provider and the pharmacist can be helpful to determine any risks to the baby. Some women may choose to continue with psychotherapy only, as well as pursue alternative treatments such as light therapy. Another option is to stop breastfeeding. The woman should be followed closely for at least 6 months after successful treatment of PPD. During treatment, the family must provide support and ensure safety of the baby and mother. Treatment will help with establishing a healthy bond between the mother and baby. If left untreated, this depression can continue for months or even years. The mother should be aware that, once she has been diagnosed with PPD, she is at high risk for recurrence of it with subsequent pregnancies.

A new mother who has any symptoms of or is at risk for PPD should take steps right away to get help. Some helpful tips if a mother is experiencing early signs of PPD include:

- asking for help in caring for the baby
- talking about these concerns with her health-care provider and nurses
- talking about her feelings
- avoiding making major life changes during pregnancy or right after delivery
- encouraging realistic expectations of herself
- taking time to get out of the house without the baby, visit with friends, spend time alone with her partner, or participate in an exercise program
- joining a support group with other new mothers
- ensuring adequate rest, for example, sleep when the baby is sleeping, arrange for child care so that she can sleep
- complying with any treatment recommendations for depression

CRITICAL THINKING QUESTION

You are working in a postpartum clinic. Your new patient is 4 weeks postdelivery. Her husband is concerned that his wife is extremely tired and irritable. On further questioning, he tells you she is in bed most of the day and that family members are caring for the baby. What would you ask the patient when you see her for the initial screening?

Clinical Activity

- Be aware of your postpartum patient's history and family history for psychiatric disorders.
- Review the patient's current and past psychiatric medications.

 POSTPARTUM PSYCHOSIS

Postpartum psychosis, sometimes called puerperal psychosis, is a psychiatric emergency It is rare, occurring in only about 0.1% to 0.2% of pregnancies (Hatters, Friedman, & Sorrento, 2012). The majority of women with this disorder have had symptoms of mental illness before pregnancy. It is most common in first pregnancies and is generally evident within a few weeks of delivery. This disorder occurs most frequently in women with a history of bipolar disorder prepregnancy. Postpartum psychosis can sometimes be an episode of bipolar illness (see Chapter 12 for detailed information on bipolar disorder). In fact, postpartum recovery time is considered a high-risk period for bipolar disorder recurrence in at-risk women (Sharma & Pope, 2012). Pregnancy and the postpartum period can exacerbate bipolar disorder symptoms. Any woman with a history of bipolar disorder should be monitored closely during pregnancy as recurrence of mania symptoms may occur. Women with a history of bipolar disorder are usually advised to discontinue lithium and some other bipolar medications due to possible adverse effects on the developing fetus. The absence of medication puts the woman at high risk for recurrence. See the Pharmacology Corner for more information.

The earliest signs of postpartum psychosis are:

- restlessness
- irritability
- insomnia

These can progress quickly to:

- rapidly shifting moods
- erratic or disorganized behavior
- delusions of grandeur or persecution
- extreme impulsivity
- disorganized speech and behavior
- hallucinations
- disorientation/confusion

Delusional beliefs are common and often center on the infant. For example, the mother may believe that the infant is evil or that the infant can read the mother's mind. Auditory hallucinations (sometimes referred to as command hallucinations) that instruct the mother to harm herself or her infant may also occur. The mother may deny the existence of the child, leading to not caring for the infant. Risks for infanticide and suicide are significant in this population (Massachusetts General Hospital Center for Women's Mental Health ,n.d. #2).

In addition to bipolar disorder, postpartum psychosis can also be categorized as brief psychotic disorder with postpartum onset in someone without a psychiatric history (American Psychiatric Association, 2013). This onset can be during the pregnancy or usually within 4 weeks of delivery for this diagnosis. PPD can also worsen to become a psychosis with paralyzing depression and, in rare cases, hallucinations and delusions.

Postpartum psychosis that occurs right after delivery needs to be differentiated from delirium. Delirium could be a reaction to many factors during delivery such as anesthesia or dehydration.

DIFFERENTIAL DIAGNOSES

- bipolar disorder
- major depressive disorder
- generalized anxiety disorder
- substance-induced bipolar or depressive disorders
- schizophrenia spectrum or other psychotic disorders

Treatment of Postpartum Psychosis

Immediate medical and psychiatric treatment must be instituted when postpartum psychosis is diagnosed (FIG. 20.1), and safety of the infant must be a priority. Severe hyperactivity and delusions may require rapid tranquilization of the mother by benzodiazepines and antipsychotic drugs. Mood stabilizing drugs, such as lithium, are useful in treatment and possibly for prevention of episodes in women at high risk (i.e., women who have already experienced manic or psychotic episodes). In some cases, electroconvulsive (electroshock) treatment is used. If the woman exhibits signs of psychosis during pregnancy, antipsychotic medications may need to be started at that time. The family needs to consult with experts about the possible risks to the fetus from these medications.

The question of where to treat a woman with postpartum psychosis is an issue, as her hospitalization is disruptive to the family. It is possible to treat moderately severe cases at home, where the sufferer can maintain her role as a mother and build up her relationship with the infant. Treatment at home requires the presence, around the clock, of a competent adult (such as the mother's partner or a grandparent) and frequent visits by professional staff. If hospital admission is necessary, there are advantages in conjoint mother and baby admission; however, multiple factors must be considered in the subsequent discharge plan to ensure the safety and healthy development of both the baby and mother. Discharge planning often involves a multidisciplinary team to follow up on the mother, the baby, their relationship, and the entire family. Family therapy is essential in the treatment process as family members may be traumatized by the patient's bizarre behavior.

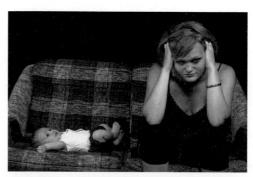

FIGURE 20.1 New mother with postpartum psychosis is hearing distressing voices.

CRITICAL THINKING QUESTION

You are doing a home health 6-week follow-up visit for a postpartum patient with a history of bipolar disorder. When you walk in the house, the patient is agitated and tells you that the baby is driving her crazy and that she wants to get rid of him. What do you do?

Pharmacology Corner

Treatment of PPD and postpartum psychosis usually requires psychoactive medications. Concern about the safety of these medications to the fetus during pregnancy and the infant during breastfeeding is a major issue in treatment. Informed decisions by the mother require thorough patient education about the burden and benefit of medications as well as consultation with a psychiatrist and pharmacist. Many women may consider stopping psychoactive medication abruptly after learning they are pregnant, but this can carry risks that need to be evaluated. There is limited research on effects of many of these psychoactive medications on the developing fetus and the breastfeeding infant, which presents a major challenge. The potential risks to the baby must be weighed against the potential benefits to the mother. Some concerns include the following:

- Some studies report the fetus is at increased risk for complications when exposed to certain antidepressants during pregnancy. Therefore, starting antidepressants during pregnancy, especially during the first trimester, must be discussed in detail before starting treatment. Exposure to antidepressant medication can happen in an unplanned pregnancy when a woman is being treated for depression.
- Antidepressants are excreted in breast milk, and the infant could be subject to the drug's side effects. If the decision is made to take antidepressants, the woman should be on the lowest dose possible and should time breastfeeding so that it does not occur when the concentration of the antidepressant is high. The infant should be monitored closely for side effects and normal growth. Alternate treatment strategies must be used if the decision is made to avoid pharmacological intervention due to potential risks to the baby.
- Because the risk for PPD and psychosis in women with a history of bipolar disorder is high, considerations about continuing mood stabilizers during pregnancy must be discussed and the risks and benefits weighed. Risks to the fetus may include congenital malformations involving the development of the cardiovascular system as well as other organ malformations especially in the first trimester. Unplanned pregnancies in which the fetus has been exposed to mood stabilizers in the first trimester must be evaluated. In addition, the pregnant woman on lithium is more vulnerable to lithium toxicity due to fluid shifts. A psychiatrist should be consulted for alternate medications if the woman wishes to become pregnant. For patients at risk for postpartum psychosis, lithium sometimes is started later in the pregnancy or shortly after delivery (Massachusetts General Hospital Center for Women's Mental Health, n.d. #2). However, the risks to mother and fetus in untreated bipolar disorder can include sleep deprivation, poor nutrition, risk for suicide, and risk for injury. Atypical antipsychotic medications may be used in place of mood stabilizers with less risk to the fetus (Massachusetts General Hospital, n.d. #2).
- For women with bipolar disorder, breastfeeding may be problematic for a number of reasons. First is the concern that on-demand breastfeeding may significantly disrupt the mother's sleep and thus may increase her vulnerability to relapse during the acute postpartum period. Second, there have been reports of toxicity in nursing infants related to exposure to various mood stabilizers (Massachusetts General Hospital Center for Women's Mental Health, n.d. #2).
- Antipsychotic and antianxiety medications may be needed to treat postpartum psychosis as well as PPD. The psychiatrist will identify those medications with less risk to the mother and the breastfeeding infant. These medications are used in place of mood stabilizers in some cases.

NURSING CARE OF WOMEN WITH POSTPARTUM MENTAL DISORDERS

Nursing diagnoses for women with postpartum mental disorders include the following:

- anxiety
- coping, ineffective
- injury, risk for
- sleep pattern disturbance
- thought processes, disturbed
- violence to self/others, risk for

General Nursing Interventions

1. *Safety:* Maintain safety of the patient and her infant. Any risk factors for this disorder need to be identified early in the pregnancy as a routine part of prenatal care. Anyone at risk should be monitored closely, and the patient and family educated on what to look for. If the patient or infant is at any risk, immediate action must be taken to protect them. Safety also involves educating the new mother about risks associated with psychiatric medications.

2. *Compassion and support:* Adequate support for the new family must be in place. Helping the family with options for the mother to get enough rest, resources for infant care, and support groups should be in place.

3. *Ongoing monitoring* for high-risk patients: Be aware that patients with any history of mental disorders, substance abuse, and family conflict are at higher risk for postpartum mental disorders. This information should be identified during pregnancy so that adequate support and prevention strategies can be implemented. Listen to family members who may observe the mother's behavior. Home-health visits should be arranged for any mother at high risk for postpartum psychiatric disorders.

The patient's psychiatrist needs to be involved in the treatment plan.

4. *Education:* The new family needs education about the stresses of pregnancy and childbirth. Education of the new family about postpartum blues and its transient nature should be included in childbirth classes and health-care provider visits. Also, education on infant care and breastfeeding can reassure the mother of her skills.

5. *Medication management:* Because the use of psychiatric medications in this population involves some risks, providing ongoing support and education is essential.

6. *Further interventions:* See Chapters 10, 11, 12, and 15 for specific interventions for anxiety, depression, mania, and psychosis.

GOOD TO KNOW

Monitor coping mechanisms and evidence of family conflict in prenatal visits. This will help provide information to anticipate the types of support and teaching that may be needed after delivery.

GOOD TO KNOW

Women often have unrealistic expectations of their ability to care for a new baby and assume that other women are better mothers.

GOOD TO KNOW

Lactation consultants can be helpful for a new mother who feels inadequate because she and her baby are having difficulty with breastfeeding.

Clinical Activity

- Obtain information on how psychiatric disorders are addressed in local obstetrical clinics.
- Obtain information on local support groups for new mothers.

The nursing care plan for patients with postpartum issues is provided in Table 20.1.

GOOD TO KNOW

Loss of an infant due to stillbirth, delivery complications, abortion, or severe abnormalities requires special support for the mother, father, and other family members. Acknowledging the loss is key to begin the grieving process. Resources are available at https://www.postpartum.net/get-help/loss-grief-in-pregnancy-postpartum/.

Evidence-Based Practice

Clinical Question: How did the coronavirus disease (COVID-19) pandemic affect pregnant women?

Discussion: Pregnancy during the pandemic added another layer of stress as women worried about the risks from the virus to their babies and themselves.

Evidence: The Edinburgh Postpartum Depression scale was given to a sample of women experiencing depression in the postpartum period during the pandemic. They found that women experiencing higher levels of stress as well as those having a history of an abortion experienced higher rates of PPD.

Implications for Nursing Practice: Recognizing the stress of the pandemic on pregnant women can lead to incorporating support services earlier during the pregnancy and in the postpartum period. This support needs to include education about the effect of the virus and prevention strategies.

An, R., Chen, X., Wu, Y., Liu, J., Dang, C., Liu, Y., Guo, H. (2021). A survey of postpartum depression and healthcare needs among Chinese postpartum women during the pandemic of COVID-19. *Archives Psychiatric Nursing.* 35: 172-177. https://doi.org/10.1016/j.apnu.2021.02.001

Table 20.1
Nursing Care Plan for Patients With Postpartum Disorders

Behaviors	Nursing Diagnosis	Goals	Interventions	Evaluation
New mother is avoiding caring for new baby for the first 6 weeks. She has verbalized feelings of inadequacy and lack of attachment to new baby. She cries frequently and expresses feelings that baby would be better off without her.	Ineffective coping	Patient will verbalize her feelings. She will spend more time caring for baby. She will verbalize optimism regarding caring for new baby. Family will maintain safe environment for patient and baby.	Provide support and reassurance. Communicate your observations to the health-care provider. Educate patient and family about PPD. Encourage patient to complete small tasks in caring for baby. Reinforce successes in baby care. Assist family in maintaining adequate caregiving for baby. Educate on treatment options for this depression.	Patient verbalizes feelings of competence in caring for baby. Patient and baby remain safe. Patient participates in treatment plan.

Patient/Family Education

• Include the signs and symptoms of psychiatric disorders in pregnancy in prenatal education.
• Provide prenatal education about what to expect in the immediate postpartum period so that postpartum blues are recognized as common and time limited.
• Provide information to the family about resources for support and psychiatric care if a psychiatric disorder is suspected.
• Ensure consultation with a pharmacist if the patient is considering psychotropic medications.
• Arrange for home health-care follow-up for any new mother at risk for postpartum psychiatric disorders.

Safe and Effective Nursing Care (SENC)

Provide a safe environment for the mother and infant.
Identify risk factors early during pregnancy to identify high-risk patients.
Provide support and education to the family to help them care for mother and infant.
Review potential side effects and risk factors for any psychiatric medication.

Key Points

• Postpartum blues (or "baby blues") are a very common reaction to plummeting hormones right after delivery. These blues generally do not require any psychiatric treatment.
• All new mothers should be screened for PPD.
• PPD is often associated with a previous history of mood disorders.
• Postpartum psychosis is a rare disorder and often associated with a history of bipolar disorder.

• Pharmacological treatment of these disorders may be associated with risks to the fetus during pregnancy and to the infant during breastfeeding.
• Any pregnant woman with a history of psychiatric disorders should have psychiatric follow-up during the prenatal and postpartum periods.

CASE STUDY

Janice is 21 years old and experiencing her first pregnancy. She lives with the father of the baby and has additional support from her mother and grandmother. Janice has a history of substance abuse, including cocaine and opioids, as well as depression, but she denies any drug use during the pregnancy. She is 32 weeks pregnant. Upon arrival at the clinic, she appears tearful, unkempt, and sad. Her boyfriend tells you that she has been sleeping for days and does not talk to him. He noticed a big change in her behavior 4 weeks ago when she became more withdrawn and tearful. The boyfriend says she told him that she does not want to think about the baby or participate in preparations for the baby. She told him she is too tired to think about it. The boyfriend works long hours to make ends meet and confides in you that he does not know what they will do when the baby comes, if she remains in this condition. He is considering having Janice's mother take the baby if this continues.

1. Given this information, what would be your primary concern for Janice?
2. What would you ask Janice when you go in to see her?
3. What support options should be recommended for the baby's father?

Review Questions

1. Which statement reflects postpartum psychosis?
   a. "I wish my baby had more hair."
   b. "My baby has evil eyes."
   c. "I don't think I will be good at breastfeeding."
   d. "I am exhausted and want to sleep rather than see the baby right now."

2. Which of the following statements best reflects postpartum blues?
   a. "I wonder if I will be good at breastfeeding."
   b. "I wish the baby had never been born."
   c. "I am exhausted, so I won't feed the baby this morning."
   d. "I can't stop crying every time I look at the baby."

3. Which of the following is true about postpartum blues?
   a. The blues start several months after the baby is born.
   b. The blues occur in the majority of women a few days after childbirth.
   c. The diagnosis of postpartum blues is a psychiatric diagnosis.
   d. The postpartum blues are usually a precursor to poor bonding with the infant.

4. What is the most important risk factor for PPD?
   a. History of depression in a previous pregnancy
   b. History of pre-eclampsia in a previous pregnancy
   c. History of conflict within the family during the pregnancy
   d. History of a previous baby born with multiple anomalies

5. Which of the following is a good nursing intervention for a new mother with postpartum blues?
   a. "Let your mother take care of the baby for the first few days."
   b. "Recognize that it is normal to feel very emotional right after the baby is born."
   c. "Let's ask the doctor to order an antidepressant to start today."
   d. "It is important to stop crying around your new baby."

6. Your new patient in the prenatal clinic confides that she used to be bipolar, but that was in the past. What would be your major concern?
   a. The baby is at high risk for bipolar disorder.
   b. Bipolar disorder can return in the postpartum period, causing postpartum psychosis.
   c. Depression in the prenatal period can contribute to poor nutrition.
   d. The mother's previous use of medications for bipolar disorder may cause genetic anomalies in the fetus.

7. Which of the following is a sign that postpartum blues is progressing to depression?
   a. The new mother is crying for the first 4 days after delivery.
   b. The new mother verbalizes anxiety and fear that she feels nothing for her new baby 2 weeks after delivery.
   c. The new mother tells you that she has heard from her deceased grandmother that the baby is evil.
   d. The new mother wants to sleep for long periods 2 days after delivery.

8. What is the major risk factor of mood stabilizers during pregnancy?
   a. Increased risk of pre-eclampsia
   b. Increased risk of malformations in the fetus
   c. Increased risk of PPD
   d. Increased cholesterol levels postpartum

9. Which of the following is true about PPD?
   a. It is more common than postpartum blues.
   b. It is less common in Hispanic women.
   c. It can be safely treated with antidepressants when proper precautions for the baby are in place.
   d. It can be improved with diet and exercise.

10. Which of the following is true about postpartum psychosis?
    a. It is a medical emergency.
    b. It may be evidence of bipolar disorder.
    c. It may compromise the baby's safety.
    d. All of the above

REVIEW QUESTIONS ANSWER KEY 1.b, 2.d, 3.b, 4.a, 5.b, 6.b, 7.b, 8.b, 9.c, 10.d

CHAPTER 21
Aging Population

KEY TERMS

Ageism
Aphasia
Cerebrovascular accident
Elder abuse
Elderly
Geriatrician
Geriatrics
Gerontology
Insomnia
Omnibus budget reconciliation act (OBRA)
Palliative care
Paranoia
Restorative nursing

CHAPTER CONCEPTS

Communication
Grief and loss
Health promotion
Mobility
Neurological regulation
Safety
Sensory perception

LEARNING OUTCOMES

1. Discuss concepts of aging.
2. Define ageism.
3. Discuss social trends in the aging population.
4. Identify five mental challenges of the older adult.
5. Identify medical treatment for the older adult.
6. Identify nursing actions for general care of older patients.

Gerontology, the study of older adults, is a specialty area within nursing. **Geriatrics** is the branch of medicine that focuses on caring for older adults, and a physician who specializes in treating older patients is a **geriatrician**. With more and more North Americans reaching age 65 and well beyond, understanding their needs is imperative. The best ways to assist this population is better planning and preparation. Although planning for the aging has been ongoing, the preparation has not always been sufficient. According to the Population Reference Bureau (PRB), the number of Americans aged 65 years and older will grow from 52 million to 95 million by 2060 (2019).

> **GOOD TO KNOW**
> Aging begins at the moment of birth. Aging happens to everyone, and nobody has control over it. It is a condition of time passing. It is also a condition that researchers are beginning to redefine.

CRITICAL THINKING QUESTION

What is your current perception of age? How do you define *young, young-old, old,* or *old-old?* What are you using to measure age? What is your view when you meet people in each of these groups?

Overall, life expectancy in the United States is increasing. According to MarketWatch, in the United States, people who were 65 years of age in 2018 are expected to live until the age of 84 (2018). This is a result of declines in cancer cases and drug overdoses that are fatal (Pesce, 2020). However, life expectancy is expected to decline post-coronavirus disease 2019 (COVID-19) in the black and Latino populations (Andrasfay & Goldman, 2021).

Classroom Activity

Define three age ranges in your class and describe what you have in common with the people in your age group.

The majority of people over age 65 are intellectually intact and able to care for themselves (FIG. 21.1). However, older people are at greater risk for developing dementia or Alzheimer's disease (Chapter 16). In 2013, approximately 5 million older people had some form of dementia; this number is expected to grow to 13.8 million by 2050 (PRB, 2019), as children of the 1950s and 1960s—the "baby boomers"–enter advanced age.

Of course, many challenges are associated with aging. People aging normally may experience diminished visual and auditory acuity. Many older

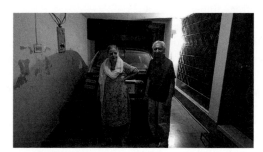

FIGURE 21.1 Most older adults are independent and fully able to care for themselves *(courtesy of Robynn Anwar).*

individuals live on fixed incomes that are not adequate to meet their needs for housing, food, and health care. Safety is also an issue. Criminals find older adults vulnerable and are robbing and scamming them in higher numbers than in generations past. Many older adults have more than one chronic illness and lack the funds to keep up with the rising cost of medication. For aging adults, facing their own death is a reality.

Certain illnesses become more prevalent as one ages. Alzheimer's disease may become more prominently manifested in an older person, rendering the individual incapable of caring for themselves and possibly requiring a move to a long-term care (LTC) facility or to a family member's home. Coronary artery disease, such as arteriosclerosis, and respiratory disorders, such as pneumonia, occur more frequently in this age group; and patients are less responsive to treatment than younger people are. Older people tend to have extended illness with excessive complications. Obtaining proper nutrition may also be a challenge. **Elderly** people may not be able to afford nutritious foods, or food does not taste as good as it once did because their taste buds are less sensitive; finances could also be a factor.

A phenomenon called ageism, which commonly occurs in the United States, is discrimination against people on the basis of their age. Ageism is the view that most older people are incapable of functioning in and contributing to society. Ageism is a misguided and hurtful prejudice toward a group of people, similar to sexism or racism. How common is ageism? What is your first thought when you see the car ahead of you being driven by an older person?

Classroom Activity

Answer the following questions and share your responses with your classmates:

• How will I look at 75 years of age?
• Will I be living independently at 75?
• What will I be doing at age 75?

Many people in the United States have postponed retirement as a result of a sluggish economy and changes to Social Security retirement benefits. To obtain full Social Security benefits, people who are currently in the workforce must work until they are 66 or older to receive full benefits. ***Provided their retirement funds are adequate,*** those who have retired can live a comfortable life (U.S. Social Security Administration, Retirement Planner: Full Retirement Age, 2016).

Unlike today's workers, who may change careers at least five times during their working years, older adults most likely had one or two jobs over their lifetime and worked 20 to 30 years at each job. For many individuals, being employed may have represented a large part of their identity and time; as a result, retirement may lead to feelings of low self-esteem and depression when the person has to redefine who they are without their work. Self-esteem, which may be tied to one's profession, is a human need according to Maslow and provides a sense of prestige and power (Green, 2000).

Retirees may live on a decreased and fixed income, which can have a negative effect on a person's lifestyle. Today, many older people on a fixed income must choose between buying groceries, paying their utility bills, or purchasing their prescribed medications.

Another loss that elders may experience is the loss of intimacy. The need for intimacy never leaves us. As human beings, the need to love and be loved is one of the primary needs for survival of the individual and the species (FIG. 21.2). Maslow's hierarchy of needs (Chapter 4) lists "love and belonging." As people age and spouses and friends die, older people may feel and actually be isolated and alone. Prospects for marriage are slim. Children and grandchildren may live on the opposite side of the country. Moving in with family members may be seen as the answer to an older relative's isolation and loneliness. However, this is not always an ideal situation. Older individuals are at risk for **elder abuse** (physical, emotional, and/or financial abuse) by their children or caregivers (Chapter 22). This is one reason for requiring a criminal background check for nursing students, healthcare providers, home health aides, and certified nurse aides (CNAs).

Aging has many challenges, yet most individuals are able to cope with the changes brought about by aging and progress through this life stage with dignity. They are proud of their families and their personal accomplishments. They can see the contributions that they have passed on to others. People who have learned to adapt to change throughout life have the best chances of progressing through old age with resilience.

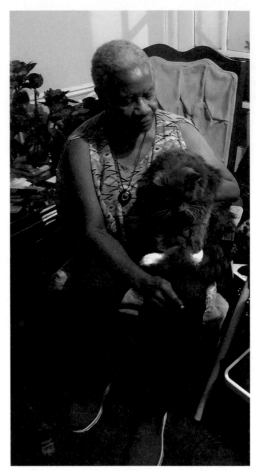

FIGURE 21.2 Pets can fulfill the need for companionship and intimacy in an older person's life *(courtesy of Robynn Anwar).*

Older adults with mental illness, whether the illness was diagnosed earlier in life or is a new diagnosis, face many challenges on top of the aging process. For example, an older person with schizophrenia, generalized anxiety disorder, or a personality disorder will need additional support as their health declines.

The **Omnibus Budget Reconciliation Act (OBRA)** is a federal act that provides standards of care for older adults residing in LTC facilities. Occupants in such facilities are known as *residents*. One of the provisions of OBRA is ensuring that residents receive proper care and assessment and are provided with a plan of care. In 1987, OBRA bylaws were required in all LTC facilities. Another provision of OBRA is that staff working in an LTC or an assisted-living facility receive proper education to care for its residents. OBRA standards are intended to reduce abuse and neglect and to ensure the provision of competent care.

Tool Box

Information about elders and mental health services: https://www.asaging.org/

Only a registered nurse (RN) may conduct or coordinate initial assessments of older adults admitted to an LTC, the same standard that applies to hospitals, acute care, and most other health-care facilities. The licensed practical nurse (LPN)/licensed vocational nurse (LVN) role is to assist the RN through active listening and competent observation. This responsibility is especially important in LTC facilities because the majority of the LPN/LVN responsibilities are administering medications and providing treatments.

RNs and LPNs/LVNs care for older individuals not only in health-care facilities but also increasingly in the privacy of the person's home (FIG. 21.3). In home health care, a multidisciplinary team assists and monitors the physiological and psychosocial needs of the older adult. It is believed people stay healthier and maintain more control of their lives if they remain at home, which has caused the home health-care industry to grow. One of the primary concerns for nurses and others caring for older adults is to help them maintain a good quality of life. Nurses caring for

patients in their homes need to be aware of some of the major mental and emotional disturbances they may encounter, as well as the physical diagnoses of the patient. Older patients may have been exposed to a number of major disorders that affect their emotional well-being. These are covered in the next sections (Box 21.1).

The Aging Brain

Studies have shown that as the brain ages there may be mild or severe changes to its size and vasculature. Both of these changes have an effect on the cognitive function of the individual's brain. According to Peters (2006), vascular changes occur normally with age, but if a younger individual develops these changes, the chances of dementia and/or a cerebrovascular accident (CVA) are increased. Changes in the person's cognitive ability may exaggerate a pre-existing mental illness. A person's white matter quantity also may decline with age. Other factors contribute to the mental changes, such as diminished glucose metabolism and lower hormone levels. Factors that are associated with vascular diseases linked to cognitive disabilities in the aged include:

- lack of exercise
- smoking
- damage to veins
- blood vessels affected by diabetes
- genetics

ALZHEIMER'S DISEASE AND OTHER COGNITIVE ALTERATIONS

By the time a person is diagnosed with Alzheimer's disease, the disease has most likely been progressing for many years. In its later stages, the debilitating effects are most observable. This disease may necessitate the person's leaving their home and even

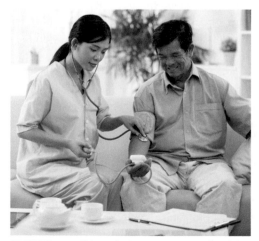

FIGURE 21.3 RNs and LPNs/LVNs caring for older individuals.

Box 21.1

Some Concerns of Aging Adults

Alzheimer's disease and other cognitive impairments
CVA (stroke or brain attack)
Depression
Medication issues
Paranoid thinking
Insomnia
End-of-life issues

living apart from their spouse. Socializing is curtailed because of the patient's inability to relate to others easily or to remember friends. Alzheimer's disease has an effect not only on the patient but also on all the people in the patient's life, including family, friends, and health-care providers.

CEREBROVASCULAR ACCIDENT (STROKE)

A **cerebrovascular accident** (CVA) (also known as a stroke or a brain attack) is a neurological deficit due to an interruption of the circulation of blood to the brain. This medical disorder has implications for mental health workers. A CVA is a devastating and frightening experience for the patient/resident and family. The probability of a CVA in the older population is higher than in the general population because of the vascular changes associated with aging. Depending on the location and size of the blood-vessel involvement, many physical and cognitive functions may be temporarily or permanently affected (FIG. 21.4). Two of the mental

Left-side infarct

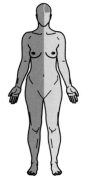

Right-side infarct

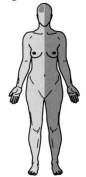

Right-sided weakness or paralysis

Aphasia (in left–brain-dominant clients)

Depression related to disability common

Left-sided weakness or paralysis

Impaired judgement/safety risk

Unilateral neglect more common

Indifferent to disability

FIGURE 21.4 The location of a stroke is a key factor in the physical and cognitive functions that may be affected. A stroke on the left side of the brain affects the right side of the body; a stroke on the right side of the brain affects the left side of the body *(from Williams and Hopper [2011]. Understanding Medical-Surgical Nursing, 4th ed. Philadelphia: F.A. Davis Company, with permission).*

health issues associated with CVA are depression and aphasia.

Depression Associated With CVA

Patients who have had a CVA realize that loss of mobility or speech may be associated with their stroke. They may not be able to express themselves verbally or physically, but they may realize that they cannot do things independently. Self-esteem decreases as the patient realizes they are incontinent, unable to eat independently, and unable to communicate with their family and friends. Depression may also develop. The patient may worry about the effect of their stroke not only on themselves but also on their spouse and other family members. Will the effects be permanent or temporary? Will another CVA happen? The patient may have sad or frightening memories of other family members or friends who have had a CVA.

As these worries become more pronounced, the patient may become more depressed. Health-care providers, nurses, and therapists will try to explain the course of recovery to the patient and family, but the resident/patient may still feel out of control of their destiny. Nurses may see the patient crying and refusing to perform tasks that they could do effortlessly before the stroke. The patient may avoid eye contact or refuse to interact with family members. All these behaviors may indicate depression in the patient who has had a CVA. By recognizing and confronting these behaviors, you can help the patient understand that you are really there to help and are concerned with the patient's thoughts and feelings.

Being honest and generous and providing positive reinforcement for attempts to overcome the feelings of depression will also be helpful in building the patient's confidence and self-esteem.

Aphasia

Aphasia, a speech disorder found in some patients who have had a CVA, is classified as expressive, receptive, and/or global (Chapter 2). A patient with aphasia may need to learn to talk all over again. Communication is such a basic human need that you and the patient *must* find a way to communicate. Give the person time to speak, write, or show what is needed, and praise them for all efforts to communicate. One communication technique that is effective, especially in expressive aphasia, is to associate the object with the word. The more senses a person can engage, the better the reinforcement for the learning.

GOOD TO KNOW

Patience is mandatory for anyone working with patients who have had CVAs. The goal of communicating with a person who has aphasia is to keep them involved in the recovery process.

The health-care provider and speech therapist will determine the proper plan of speech therapy. Closely follow this plan and document the patient's progress and emotional responses to speech therapy.

CRITICAL THINKING QUESTION

Consider the following scenario:

You are celebrating your retirement when the room goes dark. You wake up in a busy space with bright lights and noise and many people. You think you recognize some of them, and you try to call out, but they just stand there and look at you. Someone you do not know is saying something to you and keeps shining a flashlight in your eyes. Your life partner is crying. *What are you feeling now? What do you wish someone would do to help you?* Now think how your answers to these questions can enhance your care of a patient recovering from a CVA.

DEPRESSION IN THE OLDER ADULT

Depression is not a "normal" part of the aging process. Major depression in older adults can show itself differently than in other age groups. In addition to the signs of depression discussed in Chapter 11, collect subjective and objective data about physical symptoms that can mask depression in older people, for example, confusion, constipation, headaches, and other body aches. Often, older patients will discuss these physical symptoms rather than admit to being depressed.

Symptoms of depression are similar to other afflictions common in the older population, such as drug side effects (Box 21.2), electrolyte imbalances, and dementia. Gather accurate information, document it, and be certain that appropriate medical care is obtained to rule out other ailments.

Box 21.2

Common Drug Side Effects for Older Adult Patients

Dry mouth
Constipation
Orthostatic hypotension
Urinary complications
Confusion/disorientation/mental sluggishness
Fatigue
Mood swings/irritability

Clinical Activity

During clinical preconference at an LTC facility, determine how many residents have been diagnosed with depression. Develop a care plan that addresses their depression. What are the residents' thyroid levels? Review the side effects of medications they are taking.

MEDICATION CONCERNS

The process of pharmacokinetics (drug metabolism) is slower and less complete in older people. Circulatory, hepatic, and renal functions start to decrease normally with age, so it is easier for medication levels in elderly patients to become toxic. In addition, adverse effects of many medications are more likely to develop in older adults. Nurses who work in facilities that care for older adults must be very alert to the effects of the medications they give their patients as well as to the possible signs of side effects and toxicity. The American Geriatrics Society (AGS) Beer's Criteria help identify potentially inappropriate medications, and the Screening Tool of Older Persons Prescriptions (STOPP) and Screening Tool to Alert to Right Treatment (START) are screening tools that can be used to assess medication appropriateness in the older population. Report any medication concerns to the RN immediately and document observations accurately. Also, know the guidelines in your state or facility about directly contacting the physician or taking verbal orders.

Patients who live at home may lose track of their medication routine. They may forget to take medications altogether or forget they have taken them and take another dose. Another concern is that many pills look alike. When visual acuity is lessened and lighting is inadequate, patients may mistake one pill for another. For example, they may take two digoxin (Lanoxin) tablets instead of one digoxin and one furosemide (Lasix), especially if they put all their medications in one container. These types of mistakes can be lethal.

To help with this situation, nurses should teach patients and families about medication safety. Containers are available for planning which medications are taken at what time, enabling the nurse and patient to set up the patient's medications for a week or longer and for different times of day. If the patient is reliable, such a container will serve as a reminder to take a particular dose. If the patient still needs some reassurance, the nurse can instruct the patient to immediately mark on a calendar the date and time a dose is taken. In this way, the patient can double-check that

medications are taken correctly and will be less anxious about it. Also, smartphones, tablets, and other devices can be used to set reminder alarms.

Nurses working with older patients also must be aware of the resident/patient's weight, nutrition, and activity levels. It is very easy for older people to develop drug toxicity from their medications, regardless of whether they are at home or in a facility. Patients with drug toxicity or overdose can present with symptoms similar to those of a mental illness or other physical illness. In some cases, the proper dose of a medication for an older adult can be as little as 25% of the "usual" recommended adult dose. Be sure to ask specific questions of the healthcare provider regarding medication doses.

Similarly, side effects to medications can look like other symptoms. Teach patients and families about this possibility. Table 21.1 shows some of the

Table 21.1
Common Drug Side Effects and Nursing Actions for Older Adult Patients*

Side Effect	Other Possibilities	Nursing Actions
Dry mouth	• Stress response; electrolyte imbalance • Vitamin B deficiency	1. Offer sips of water or ice chips. 2. Offer hard, sugar-free candy (such as lemon drops) if patient is able to suck on them without choking. 3. Provide oral care with light application of lubricant such as saliva substitute. 4. Review laboratory work or call physician.
Constipation	• Fluid and nutritional deficiency, hemorrhoids, or rectal pain • Hypothyroidism	1. Assess diet for fiber and fluid intake. 2. Assess area for signs of hemorrhoids or other inflammation. 3. Assess need for laxatives as ordered by health-care provider. 4. Discuss need for physical activity as condition warrants.
Orthostatic hypotension	• Heart disorders • Dehydration	1. Assess vital signs. 2. Teach patient how to get out of bed or chair slowly. 3. Tell patient to stay sitting for a few minutes until dizziness goes away.
Urinary complications	• Prostate problems • Bladder problems • Uterus problems • Urinary tract infections (UTI) • Cancers	1. Keep track of frequency, amount, color, and odor of urine, and abdominal girth. 2. Educate the patient and family on the signs of a UTI and what to report to health-care provider.

Table 21.1

Common Drug Side Effects and Nursing Actions for Older Adult Patients*—cont'd

Side Effect	Other Possibilities	Nursing Actions
Confusion/ disorientation/ mental sluggishness	• Hypoglycemia • Head injury (e.g., fall) • Infection/fever • Depression • Vitamin deficiency • Transient ischemic attack (TIA) • Brain tumor • Dehydration • Alcohol and/or tranquilizer use	1. Give sweetened drink. If patient is still confused after 10 minutes, call health-care provider. 2. Check vital signs and for signs of infection. 3. Attempt to validate whether patient has had recent head trauma.
Fatigue	• Infectious process • Anemia • Hypothyroidism • Stress • Narrowing of coronary arteries	1. Assess vital signs. 2. Assess stress level. 3. Encourage activity if appropriate. 4. Assess sleep pattern.
Mood swings/ irritability	• Psychological disorders • Electrolyte imbalances	1. Use verbal and nonverbal communication skills to assess cause. 2. Request laboratory work.

*Always report these side effects to the charge nurse, document carefully, and notify the physician if that is allowed for LPN/LVN practice in your state.

common side effects of drugs on older individuals, disorders that may have similar symptoms, and nursing actions that can be taken and/or taught to the patient.

 ## PARANOID THINKING

Paranoid thinking in an older adult may be a result of fear about their social environment, and these thoughts can be facilitated and even amplified by what they see on television. Sometimes people with **paranoia** feel like others are stealing their belongings or coming into their rooms at night. As indicated earlier, criminals and con artists see elderly persons as "easy prey." What was once a situation that was not threatening (such as a walk around the block) can become very frightening for the person whose reaction time has slowed or who has diminished physical capacity for self-protection. Paranoid, fearful thinking can be a defense mechanism against these kinds of physical disabilities, making fear the reason to avoid leaving the house or even to demonstrate mistrust in their health-care provider.

This self-imposed isolation can lead to feelings of loneliness, which can then lead to illness that is more serious. Validate what the person is expressing, even when it sounds paranoid, but also investigate the person's fearful thinking. Age-related hearing loss (presbycusis) and vision loss as well as early onset of dementia can all contribute to paranoid thinking. Paranoid thinking can also occur when a resident is entering an LTC facility and is exposed to new caregivers and a roommate.

 ## INSOMNIA

Insomnia, or inability to sleep, is seen frequently in older adults. It can be caused by many things, including depression, fear, pain, urinary incontinence, or napping during the day. Sometimes, nighttime behavior changes such as increased confusion and agitation, especially at dusk, may be sundowner syndrome (also known as nocturnal delirium). This syndrome is sometimes seen in patients who have delirium and dementia. Lack of rapid eye movement (REM) sleep from insomnia can have negative effects on *anyone*, regardless of age or health status, even contributing to psychotic behavior. To someone with Alzheimer's disease or other cognitive problems, the effects of insomnia can intensify the symptoms of their cognitive disorder. In Maslow's hierarchy of needs, sleep is important for survival. Insomnia-related transient awakenings related to pain can come from movement while asleep (Schwab, 2020).

Concentrate on keeping communication open with these patients. Be sure that you and the patient mean the same thing when you say the same words. For instance, if the patient says, "I do not sleep at night because I am worried," the word *worried* should be explored. What is the patient worried about? What can be done to eliminate the worry? How severe is the worry? Using a one to five rating scale, you can more objectively document the effect of the "worry" on the patient. In addition, ask the patient what they mean by "not sleeping at night"; perhaps the patient takes naps throughout the day.

Evidence-Based Practice

Clinical Question: Is a detailed patient history and physical examination the best method to evaluate insomnia in the older adult?

Evidence: A study of 6,800 patients 65 years of age and older found older adults to have a higher incidence of insomnia than younger adults. In addition, the patients in the study were also found to have higher incidence of depression, especially those with persistent insomnia. The study showed that through a detailed evaluation of the patient, both nonpharmacological and pharmacological methods can be effective in treating insomnia in the older adult.

Implications for Nursing Practice:

- During the admission interview, identify the patient's/resident's sleep pattern.
- Identify if the patient/resident is having difficulty maintaining sleep.
- Identify if the insomnia is related to pain.
- Maintain a sleep journal for or by the patient/resident.
- Monitor which nonpharmacological and pharmacological interventions are effective.

Patel, D., Steinberg, J., & Patel, P. (2018). Insomnia in the elderly: A review. *Journal of Clinical Sleep Medicine, 14*(6), 1017–1024. https://doi.org/ 10.5664/jcsm.7172

END-OF-LIFE ISSUES

Life can end at any age; however, death is more common among the older population. Nurses who work in areas such as LTC, home health care, or hospice have a great opportunity to learn about and assist people with end-of-life issues. These opportunities also exist when working in acute care hospitals and clinics. It may not be feasible for professional counselors to meet the needs of older adults dealing with these profound issues. In fact, many people in this population will prefer the services of their own spiritual leader, but because the duties of many such leaders are overwhelming, the appropriate clergy may not be available at the moment of immediate need. However, nurses are there, and they have all the tools needed to be the helpers.

> **GOOD TO KNOW**
> Nurses need to assess their own beliefs surrounding the subjects of death and dying.

It is very important to discuss and understand your patients' religious and cultural beliefs about what the end of life means to them. It is your responsibility and privilege to help someone through this stage of life according to that individual's needs and wants.

Older patients are more likely than younger ones to experience widowhood. The surviving spouse must learn to live independently or face an alternative form of housing. Finances and household chores may have been divided between the partners, and now the surviving person is forced to assume responsibilities that formerly belonged to the deceased. Dating and returning to work may be sensitive issues for the survivor. Families may have strong opinions about what the newly widowed person "should" do. Nurses can and should be advocates for their widowed patients. Actively listening, validating the person's thoughts and feelings, and offering information about various services available to widowed persons are skills that can be very helpful.

Nurses can also be effective in helping people through the dying process. Death is inevitable, but people need to know it is okay to die. Elisabeth Kübler-Ross and others who teach about death and dying tell us that helping people to resolve life issues can help them die with peace and dignity. Again, nurses who choose to work in hospice, home health care, and LTC settings have a special opportunity to be there for people at this very important stage of life. Using humor and laughter appropriately, maintaining the hope patients may still have, and reassuring them that they will not be forgotten after death are some good techniques to help people prepare to die. Kübler-Ross's book *On Death and Dying,* published in 1969, remains a classic and described the five stages of grief (Chapter 4). It is important to remember that people do not experience the five stages in the same order.

Finally, nurses cannot ignore the incidence of suicide among the aging population. This chapter has alluded to many losses that people are likely to face as they age. Compound the sadness of losing jobs, friends, and other aspects of earlier life with physical illness and altered physical ability, and it may become clearer why some elders feel helpless or hopeless and opt for suicide. According to The National Institute of Mental Health (2021), the rate of suicide for persons age 65 and older is higher than the national average for all age groups. In 2018, persons ages 55 to 64 accounted for 8,540 deaths related to suicide. The highest suicide rate was found in white men age 85 and older. Follow the screening suggestions provided in Chapter 13 when considering the possibility that an older person may be at risk for suicide.

SOCIAL CONCERNS

Like younger adults, older adults today may find themselves in financial trouble. Many are facing financial challenges living on fixed incomes or existing only on Social Security benefits. Retirement age has increased over the years, and politicians are discussing raising it yet again. This could require people to continue working even longer before they become eligible to receive the Medicare and/or Social Security benefits they have earned. What is the effect of these financial challenges? Some predict that Social Security funds will be depleted by 2035, meaning older adults will have to survive on even less. Seniors may have inadequate personal and supplemental insurance, so they will not seek medical help when they need it. They may even find their heat and power cut off due to inability to pay utilities. Most municipalities are enacting laws and

setting aside emergency funds to help avoid these life-threatening situations. Nurses can help by providing information on utility- or rent-assistance programs to help elders who are opting to remain at home or in assisted living.

As baby boomers age, nurses are seeing a significant increase in this demographic. The average age of patients is getting older, and the issues nurses face will relate more frequently to people in the final stages of life.

The family unit of the older population looks different than it used to. People are opting to have children later in life or not at all. Nurses may see much younger family members than they might anticipate. In addition, the upcoming older generation is very diverse. Those of varied or mixed ethnic and cultural backgrounds will be seeking assistance in LTC facilities (FIG. 21.5). It is essential to learn about older patients' cultures and customs, to ask the proper questions upon intake, and to offer care that is respectful of cultural differences. Even people who are from the same culture as yours may have different practices and values.

Classroom Activity

With your classmates, create five small groups. Each group represents one decade from the past 50 years. With your group, list the songs, television shows, movies, and fads popular during your decade and then collect and share your information. Compare the commonalities and the differences of each group.

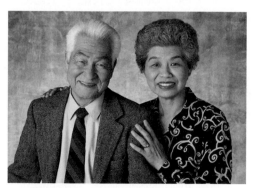

FIGURE 21.5 The demographic changes in the American population mean that a more ethnically and culturally diverse group will be seeking assistance in LTC facilities. Nurses must be ready to offer culturally sensitive care.

Clinical Activity

Using the information you gathered in the classroom activity, ask your patients to tell you more about popular songs, television shows, movies, and fads they recall from those decades.

One cultural demographic that has been almost ignored until recently by the gerontology community is elders who are LGBTQ+. Nowadays, nurses need to respect dress and grooming preferences and family structures of all types while also anticipating issues regarding choice of roommates and bathroom-sharing. Older individuals may be reluctant to share information about their sexuality or gender identity unless nurses communicate acceptance. Nurses need to be open in their communication and comfortable with the types of questions they must ask in order to provide the best care to all entrusted to their care.

NURSING SKILLS FOR WORKING WITH OLDER ADULTS

The following are some general skills needed to work with the older adult population effectively.

1. *Respect:* In the United States, a handshake is a sign of respect and cooperation. It is usually given at the beginning and ending of business meetings, and it is customary to shake hands at more formal social functions or when being introduced to someone new. Shaking the hand of an older patient will convey respect and cooperation and is an effective way to begin the nurse-patient partnership. Some citizens and residents of the United States do not participate in hand shaking, but this does not mean they lack respect for others. If you sense that shaking hands is not acceptable to that patient, then communicate to others that this action should not be used. Since the COVID-19 pandemic, many people fist bump instead of shaking hands.

Using the proper name of the patient also shows respect for that person. "Mr. Washington" or "Mrs. Jones" is the best way to address the patient. If the patient prefers, the nurse may call them by the first name or the name that the person is called socially. Do *not* do this until invited to do so,

however. Also, it is not acceptable to assign nicknames such as "granny" or "honey" arbitrarily to patients. In home health care and LTC, there is a danger of becoming too familiar. The facility becomes the residents' home, and residents become friendly with each other. This informal atmosphere sometimes spreads among the staff. But nurses must remember their professional role. Be pleasant and friendly while still being professional (Box 21.3).

> **GOOD TO KNOW**
> When addressing or referring to a patient, be sure to use both the name and the pronoun (he, she, they) the patient prefers.

> **CRITICAL THINKING QUESTION**
> You refer to an 87-year-old LTC resident as "Grandmom" because another resident likes the nickname. What you do not know is that the resident does not have any children as a result of several miscarriages. What emotional effect might this nickname have on this patient?

Under no circumstances should an older adult be treated as a child. As abilities diminish and a patient becomes incontinent or loses the ability to feed and dress themselves, some caregivers take on a parental role. It is easy to understand why: Changing "diapers" and feeding and dressing someone are activities we associate with children. However, older adults are *not* children; in fact, they have had careers and raised families. They are adults who now have special needs in order to help them maintain their adult dignity.

Box 21.3

Skills for Working With Older Adults

• Respect
• Goal setting
• Patience and understanding
• Humor
• Safety (providing a safe environment)
• Independence (allowing the patient to function at their optimal level)
• Acceptance

2. *Goal setting:* When preparing the plan of care with an older patient, remember to discuss goals that are measurable and attainable. Self-esteem and pride in one's accomplishments are as important when one is 80 years old as they were when one was 20. Success breeds success, and meeting small goals is an encouragement to the older person to attempt bigger goals. The patient will see that the nurse was there to help reach that goal, and the relationship between them will strengthen.

3. *Patience and understanding:* Older patients who have some challenge to their physical or cognitive functioning may be slower to respond to verbal cues and may not be able to walk down the halls at the pace that nurses generally travel. Be patient and recognize that care may take longer than expected. Plan for this and include the patient in this planning.. Convey the message that they have plenty of time (even though they may not). The patient who feels burdensome will be less likely to attempt activities or to collaborate in the plan of care. The patient/resident may be very sensitive to any nonverbal communication. It is especially important that your verbal and nonverbal responses are congruent and that your focus is entirely on that person at that time. Acknowledge any accomplishment, however small. The focus should be on the residents' strengths, not their weaknesses.

4. *Humor:* Humor that is appropriate to the age and condition of the patient will help smooth over some of the harder times for the nurse and the patient. Take your cues about humor from the patient. If the patient jokes about a situation, it is probably acceptable to go along with the humor. *Never* embarrass or make fun of the patient.

Taking a situation in stride at the patient's suggestion, however, can be a very healthy mechanism for dealing with some of the hardships associated with aging.

5. *Safety:* Ensuring safety in the care facility and teaching safety to the patient who remains at home are very important. With vision, hearing, and other senses losing acuity, the older person may misjudge space, temperature, and sound. This could lead to falls, burns, and inability to hear the doorbell or the telephone ringing.

6. *Independence:* Older adults should be allowed to perform without assistance as much as possible. Do not assume that an older person is unable to do things independently. Follow the guidelines on the patient's care plan. If the level of care required is complete, then provide complete care. If the care plan indicates the patient needs partial or complete care, then honor those directions. This is one of the fallacies of LTC: Too much focus is placed on the staff to provide care by a specific time and not on promoting independence. Offer assistance as necessary and let the patient know that you would like to help in whatever way you can. Because of the losses in hearing and visual acuity that often accompany aging, you may need to arrange for adaptive equipment that can help the patient to maintain as much independence as possible with daily activities.

7. *Acceptance:* In rapidly increasing numbers, people of diverse backgrounds and lifestyles are approaching the time of life that may require them to move to LTC centers or assisted-living communities. Those who will be caring for this diverse population must understand their own thoughts and feelings about working with different groups of people and must be prepared to meet a variety of needs with compassion and respect.

Remember that basic human needs as defined by Maslow and others are common to all groups of people. Table 21.2 summarizes some of the concerns of aging adults and techniques nurses can use to more effectively help this population.

 RESTORATIVE NURSING

Restorative nursing is part of rehabilitation and focuses on maintaining dignity and achieving optimal function for patients and residents (FIG. 21.6).

Table 21.2

Concerns of Aging Adults and Helping Techniques

Concern	Factors Associated With This Concern	Helping Techniques
Alzheimer's disease and other cognitive impairments	• Debilitating effects are observable. • Patients may need to leave their homes and live apart from a spouse. • Socializing will be curtailed.	Respect the individual. Set realistic goals. Maintain patience and understanding. Communicate effectively; allow time for the patient to respond. Use appropriate humor. Teach and promote safety. Promote independence.
CVA (stroke, brain attack)	• Physical and cognitive functions may be temporarily or permanently affected. • Depression is evident. • Aphasia may be present.	See "Alzheimer's disease." Allow venting of emotions. Assist with communication techniques. Allow patient to verbalize; do not automatically answer for patient.
Depression	• Symptoms may be different from those in other age groups. • Constipation, headaches, other pains, and fatigue may be indicators. • Difficulty breathing for which there is no diagnosis may occur.	See "Alzheimer's disease." Allow venting of thoughts and feelings. Teach about patient's medications. Encourage involvement in group activities as able. Focus on positives. Review patient's serum thyroid levels.
Medication concerns	• Pharmacokinetics is slower and less complete. • Circulatory and renal function is decreased. • It becomes easier for older adults to experience side effects or develop drug toxicity. • Patients who live at home may forget to take medications or forget they have taken them and take another dose. • Visual acuity is lessened; patients may mistake one pill for another. • Nurse should advise patient to maintain weight, nutrition, and activity levels.	Provide patient with information about medication. Instruct patient to notify health-care provider immediately if signs of side effects occur.
Paranoid thinking	• Fear about the environment • Slowed reaction time and diminished physical capacity • Feelings of loneliness and isolation	Allow venting of feelings. Do not reinforce paranoid thoughts. Speak in terms of the "here and now." Provide aids for hearing and vision loss.
Insomnia	• Depression, fear, pain, urinary incontinence, and napping during the day are common. • Decreased REM sleep can contribute to psychotic behavior; insomnia can intensify the symptoms of cognitive disorders.	Discuss underlying feelings. Teach relaxation methods. Encourage patient to seek medical evaluation. Discourage daytime napping. Keep sleep diary, if able. Monitor hours of sleep and sleep patterns.

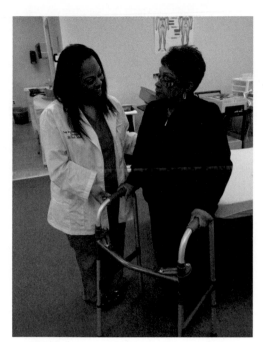

FIGURE 21.6 Restorative nursing is concerned with providing individualized restorative exercise to help patients achieve maximum function and maintain their dignity *(courtesy of Robynn Anwar).*

Some articles refer to restorative nursing as "good, old-fashioned nursing care"—arguably a subjective statement and more than likely related to the chronological age of the writer. Goals of restorative nursing include independence, promoting self-esteem for the patient, and allowing the patient to maintain as much control over their life and daily living activities as possible.

Most skilled nursing facilities are required to provide at least one designated nursing assistant and nurse who are specially trained and part of the "restorative" team. They work in conjunction with physical therapy and rehabilitation departments to provide individualized restorative exercise and training to assist residents to achieve their maximum ability.

Restorative nursing is also part of an LTC facility's documentation and reimbursement requirements. State and federal surveys grade the facility on its restorative program. OBRA long-term care laws require that residents either maintain their condition at the time of admission or improve on it. Declines in residents' conditions that cannot be proven to be medically unavoidable are not allowed. Including restorative nursing care in a patient's care

plan can prevent declines in condition that occur gradually over time, such as loss of mobility, contractures, and loss of self-care ability. Restorative nursing is to be provided to any resident, regardless of their cognitive ability: The resident with dementia and the transitional care resident recuperating from knee surgery are equally in need of restorative nursing services.

 ## PALLIATIVE CARE

Palliative care is specialized care for people with serious illness that focuses on addressing management of uncomfortable symptoms and the stress of advanced illness. It is about keeping patients and families comfortable and promoting the best quality of life that one can provide to someone facing an advanced illness. Palliative care is often associated with the last phase of life, but it can begin earlier in the course of serious illness. Hospice is one aspect of palliative care. Hospice care is specialized services for a patient with a terminal illness with less than 6 months to live. In addition to working through grief and bereavement with the patient and significant persons in that patient's life, nurses choosing to work in a palliative setting need to be comfortable with issues such as pain, symptom management, sedation and opioid medication, artificial nutrition and hydration, and coordinating or providing complementary therapies. In addition, palliative care nurses need to sharpen their communication skills and be very cognizant of religious, cultural, ethical, and legal issues, especially surrounding an individual's wishes and advance care planning as the end of life approaches.

It is widely documented that patients prefer to die in their own homes. However, sometimes that is not possible, so many LTC facilities are designing special units dedicated to palliative care. Organizations such as The Center to Advance Palliative Care (CAPC) are attempting to show the need for hospital-based and outpatient palliative care, as well. Palliative care can be provided in the acute hospital, the LTC facility, and in the home.

Nurses can receive training in this new specialty area. The good news is that LPNs/LVNs are more than welcome. To encourage LPNs/LVNs to participate in palliative nursing, the Hospice and Palliative Nurses Association (HPNA) developed a set of competencies.

Tool Box

HPNA competencies for LPNs/LVNs:
    https://advancingexpertcare.org/ItemDetail?iProductCode = HP301&Category = BOOKS&WebsiteKey = b1bae5a7-e24a-4d4c-a697-2303ec0b2a8d

Safe and Effective Nursing Care (SENC)

Advocate for patients' rights.
Have appropriate patient identification for medications and treatments.
Provide information to the patient and family about advance directives.
Educate patient and family about the aging process.
Verify patient's code status.
Provide privacy.
Refer patient and family to outside support services.
Document any communication barriers.
Verify and validate reason for refusing medication or a treatment.
Correlate the plan of care with the patient's cultural beliefs.
Monitor patient's ambulation.
Conduct neurological assessments.
Monitor for adverse effect of medicines.
Monitor for favorable outcomes.
Inquire about equipment needed after discharge.

Key Points

- The concept of "old" age is changing. More people are living longer and better after age 65. Older patients are being cared for in facilities and in their homes. Diversity among aging persons is on the rise. Nurses must be prepared to provide the best care possible to many different groups of elders. Nurses have an active role in helping the patient maintain a good quality of life.
- Normal conditions of aging include diminished hearing, vision, and other sensory acuity. Alzheimer's disease and other cognitive disorders are not considered a part of normal aging.

- Afflictions affecting the older adult can be mental, physical, or a combination of these. Medication side effects and drug toxicity can share the same symptoms as disorders that affect the older population. Accuracy of observation and documentation and prompt reporting are crucial to a nurse's responsibility in caring for older adults. Excellent communication skills are necessary.
- Palliative care and hospice provide specialized care for people facing advanced and terminal illnesses.

CASE STUDY

Ms. Finn is admitted as a new resident in your nursing home. She is 76 years old and has a diagnosis of congestive heart failure (CHF). She has fallen at home several times recently, and her adult children are concerned that she will become seriously injured. They have told her she needs to "go to the nursing home for a while until you get stronger." They tell the staff, confidentially, that

CASE STUDY—cont'd

they plan this to be a permanent placement and will be selling Ms. Finn's home to pay for her care. Ms. Finn will be started on digoxin, furosemide, and potassium for the CHF and has an order for acetaminophen with hydrocodone for pain.

Five days later, Ms. Finn has had a change in mental status. Her family comes to visit and finds that she is combative and forgetful. One of her children is crying. She looks at you and says, "What have you done to her? She's never been like this before."

1. What thoughts cross your mind?
2. How do you respond to the personal attack?
3. How will you attempt to resolve this situation?
4. How would you like to be treated if you were the family member?

Review Questions

1. One effective communication technique for assisting a patient with aphasia is:
   a. Try to guess the word or finish the sentence.
   b. Associate the word with the object.
   c. Tell the patient to think about it while you make the bed.
   d. None of the above.

2. According to OBRA, who is responsible for completing the assessment of an older adult?
   a. All health staff
   b. Nursing assistants
   c. LPN/LVN
   d. RN

3. Mrs. Brown, who is usually alert and oriented, is showing signs of confusion. Her vital signs are all within normal limits. She has recently been started on furosemide for CHF. The nurse suspects:
   a. Just normal aging
   b. Stroke
   c. Medication side effect
   d. Depression

4. A 73-year-old patient in your LTC facility has become withdrawn and cranky. You try to find a method to initiate communication and activity with the patient. Which of the following statements is the best choice to try communicating with your patient?
   a. "Why are you staying over here by yourself?"
   b. "Your daughter wants you to make friends here."
   c. "I need a partner for the card game; I'd like to have you be my partner."
   d. "The doctor said the more you do, the better off you'll be."

5. Losses associated with the process of aging frequently cause:
   a. Presbycusis
   b. Depression
   c. Dementia
   d. CHF

6. When an older patient begins to show signs of dementia, physicians and nurses should assess all of the following *except:*
   a. Medication routines
   b. Nutritional intake
   c. Circulatory function
   d. Behaviors assumed to be part of "normal aging"

7. The speech impairment that affects many people who have had a stroke is called:
   a. Apraxia
   b. Aphasia
   c. Autism
   d. Dystonia

8. Nurses understand that one of the reasons older people develop drug toxicity from their prescription medications is:
   a. Drugs are metabolized faster in older people.
   b. Drugs are metabolized slower in older people.
   c. Drugs are ineffective in older people.
   d. Drugs need to be ordered in stronger doses for older people.

9. Your patient is admitted with bruises on his head and upper arms. His son is with him and jokes about the bruises, stating, "Dad is getting so clumsy. He falls out of his wheelchair a lot." You glance at the patient, who says nothing, is looking down, and is avoiding eye contact. You become alert for the possibility of:
    a. Blood dyscrasias
    b. Vitamin deficiency
    c. Elder abuse
    d. Self-inflicted wounds

10. The federal law that mandates special care and assessment for the older population is called:
    a. OBE
    b. OBIE
    c. COBRA
    d. OBRA

11. When orienting new nursing assistants and other staff to your LTC facility, you remind them:
    a. Memory loss is a normal part of aging.
    b. Memory loss is not a normal part of aging.
    c. Stress decreases as people age.
    d. All of the above

12. In the orientation class, you notice one of the housekeepers crying. She shares with the group that her grandmother has "old timer's or something and she doesn't remember me anymore." You respond to her:
    a. "It must be difficult for you to see your grandmother with Alzheimer's disease."
    b. "It's called Alzheimer's disease. Many of our residents have that illness."
    c. "How old is your grandmother?"
    d. "Who else has a relative with Alzheimer's?"

Review Questions Answer Key 1.b, 2.d, 3.c, 4.c, 5.b, 6.d, 7.b, 8.b, 9.c, 10.d, 11.b, 12.a

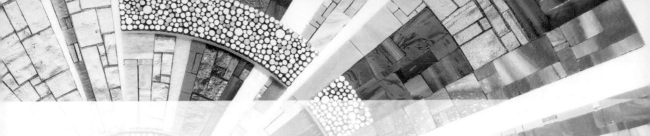

CHAPTER 22
Abuse and Violence

LEARNING OUTCOMES

1. Define abuse.
2. Define victim.
3. Differentiate among different kinds of abuse.
4. Identify characteristics of an abuser.
5. Identify nursing care to help survivors of abuse.

Abuse and violence are, unfortunately, commonplace in today's society. The news, television dramas, and movies expose people to more violence than they did in the past. Violence occurs in the workplace, on the road, in places of worship, and in schools. Terrorism is now a threat around the world. Active shooter drills have become routine as part of safety training in many parts of the United States. Violence in the home in the form of child abuse, sexual abuse, domestic violence, and elder abuse takes a terrible toll on society. This chapter will address physical, emotional, sexual, and economic abuse, as well as neglect.

Physical abuse includes any action that causes physical harm to another person. Hitting; burning; withholding food, water, and other basic needs; and other activities that go beyond accidental contact are all considered physical abuse. A rule of thumb for defining the line between an accident and physical abuse is the perpetrator's reaction when the recipient says, "Stop! You're hurting me!" or something similar. If the person causing the hurt stops and does not repeat the behavior, that behavior may well have been just an accident. If the behavior persists, if the request to stop is ignored or mocked by the perpetrator, or if the activity is repeated in future situations, there is a strong chance that the perpetrator is guilty of abuse. **Neglect** can include failure to provide for the basic needs of someone who is dependent on another, for example, a child, an adult with a disability, or an older relative. **Emotional abuse** can include **verbal abuse**, humiliation, excessive criticism, and lack of emotional support. **Sexual**

abuse can include rape as well as any inappropriate sexual contact without consent.

Victims are often too fearful or ashamed to report abuse. They can become adept at hiding the signs and/or convincing themselves that the abuse is not that bad. Lack of reporting contributes to the abuse cycle, which can go unnoticed by outsiders. Health-care professionals must be vigilant to recognize both the overt and the covert signs of abuse. Every state mandates that suspected child abuse be reported, and many states have enacted similar laws for domestic violence and elder abuse. The Joint Commission, the major accreditation body for hospitals and many other health-care institutions, expects accredited institutions to provide assessment of potential victims of abuse. Nurses are in a key position to identify and offer help to a suspected victim.

THE ABUSER

The **abuser** is usually in a position of dominance or power over their victim. The following reasons may cause a person to abuse another:

- History of being a victim. Children who grow up witnessing violence in the home and perhaps their community are sensitized to believe that this is the right behavior, and they may continue such actions into adulthood. Abusers retreat to these childhood memories and resort to abuse when they are stressed. They may never have developed skills to solve problems or deal with conflict in nonviolent ways. Rather, they learned that violence is the way to achieve a goal.

Cultural Considerations

Abuse crosses all cultural, ethnic, and socioeconomic groups. At times, some behaviors may appear abusive to outsiders but could be culturally acceptable. For example, in some cultures, wives are expected to be subservient to their husbands. This cultural norm needs to be taken into consideration before assuming the wife is being abused.

- Low self-esteem/need for power. Abusers often have a poor self-image. They feel frustrated and minimized as persons. They have poor interpersonal relationships and may not have had their ideas and accomplishments validated by people important to them. Close relationships are difficult because others become afraid of the abuser. Therefore, abusers resort to physical, verbal, or emotional abuse of others in an attempt to bring a personal sense of power and importance to themselves. Sexual abuse is almost never about sex; it is about conquering and winning. It is about demeaning another human being in order to feel a sense of strength. It is a short-term "fix" for the abuser and a lifelong scar for the abused.

- Impairment from alcohol/substance use. Being under the influence of a substance is a major contributor to violence. When a person's judgment is impaired and their ability to control impulses is altered, a person who is prone to these acts may abuse others. Easy access to weapons while impaired adds to the risk associated with substance abuse.

- Biological mechanisms. Brain disorders, alteration in brain function, biochemical influences, and genetic influences may also be factors in individuals with a greater tendency toward violence (Rosell & Siever, 2015). Brain disorders such as some brain tumors and some forms of encephalitis have been associated with violent behavior.

- Other factors. The abuser may be under stress (e.g., financial pressures, job loss) and have limited access to support resources to deal with problems, limited coping mechanisms to deal with conflict, and difficulty trusting others.

Another way to look at potential abusers is to examine the form that the aggression takes. Reactive aggression is associated with impulsivity and is more common in people who have a history of being abused. Proactive aggression is initiated rather than provoked and is more common in psychiatric illness (Rosell & Siever, 2015).

Can abusers be identified? Abusers may present with some of the following traits:

- inconsistent explanation of injuries of the victim
- failure to show empathy for the victim
- demanding to take victim home and refusal of hospitalization for the injured victim
- speaking for the victim
- criticizing the victim
- abusing family pets

> **GOOD TO KNOW**
> Because abuse in a family is often hidden, recognize that it can be difficult to identify an abuser.

THE VICTIM

Although victims of abuse have a broad range of traits, the two most common include:

1. *Low self-esteem:* People who have not learned to be assertive and to say what they think and feel or to speak out for what they need and want may not be able to call up the strength they need to ward off an attack. They may be easily manipulated by the abuser into believing either that they deserved the attack or that the abuser is truly repentant and will not abuse them again. They will begin to make up reasons to excuse the abuser's behavior and may accept the responsibility for the abuser's actions.

2. *Reliance on the abuser:* People who are reliant on the abuser for financial support as well as emotional and physical support are vulnerable to attacks from the abuser. This holds true for all age groups of people who are abused.

No one deserves to be abused. Having traits that may contribute to being abused does not mean the victim caused their abuse.

See Table 22.1 for characteristics of victims of child abuse, domestic violence, and elder abuse. Health-care professionals often see victims of abuse without realizing it. Patients who are abused may be fearful of sharing this information directly but may leave clues. Box 22.1 lists common warning signs of abuse.

Table 22.1
Characteristics of Victims of Abuse

Type of Victim	*Characteristics*
Child; all ages, with greatest risk under age 3 (including infants)	• Blamed for family conflict • Low self-esteem • Fear of parent or caretaker • Cheating, lying, low achievement in school • Signs of depression, helplessness • One child sometimes singled out in family due to being labeled as "difficult"; child may be the product of unwanted pregnancy, remind the parents of someone they dislike or even themselves, may have been born premature (inhibited parent-child bonding), or may have a chronic illness or learning disability
Domestic/spouse/ intimate partner	• Low self-esteem • Self-blame for partner's actions • Sense of helplessness to escape abuse • Isolation from family and friends • Views self as subservient to partner • Economic dependence on abuser
Elder	• Older than 75 years of age • Mentally or physically impaired • Isolated from others • Female • Increased risk for exacerbation of pre-existing conditions and premature death

Adapted sources: Linnard-Palmer & Coats, 2017; Morgan & Townsend, 2021; Centers for Disease Control and Prevention, 2021; National Institute on Aging, 2020.

Box 22.1

Common Warning Signs of Abuse

- Delay in seeking treatment for injuries, minimizing injuries
- History of being "accident prone"
- Pattern of injuries not accidental looking; for example, identical burns on bottom of feet, identical injuries on both sides of head
- Multiple injuries in varying stages of healing
- Conflicting stories from victim and abuser about cause of injury
- Inconsistency between history and injury
- Unusual, even bizarre, explanation for injuries
- Repeated visits to EDs or clinics
- Previous report of abuse
- Patient reporting abuse
- Patient fearful of caregiver or partner
- Visits to a variety of doctors, emergency rooms for treatment to avoid a record of treatment

Source: From Townsend & Morgan, 2017.

Clinical Activity

If your patient has been the victim of abuse, obtain information from the care team on the abuser and how to handle this person if they are present.

Classroom Activity

Identify local abuse hotlines and local domestic violence shelters.

CATEGORIES OF ABUSE

The most common categories of abuse include child abuse, sexual abuse, intimate partner violence, and elder abuse.

Child Abuse

Child abuse includes physical, emotional, and sexual abuse, as well as neglect. The term child maltreatment is now used to include both abuse and neglect. Child maltreatment occurs at all socioeconomic levels, although poverty remains a powerful risk factor. Maltreatment has a major effect on health and well-being throughout the child's life. Exposure to violence in childhood increases the risks of long-term injury, future violence victimization and perpetration, substance abuse, sexually transmitted infections, sexual promiscuity, delayed brain development, lower educational attainment, and limited employment opportunities (Fortson, Klevens, Merrick, Gilbert, & Alexander, 2016). Health-care professionals are mandated to report any suspicion of child abuse.

The Centers for Disease Control and Prevention (CDC) reports one in seven children has been a victim of abuse or neglect in the United States in the last year (CDC, 2021). The vast majority of cases reported involve neglect, followed by physical abuse and then sexual abuse. Accurate numbers have been difficult to attain because it is believed that many cases go unreported. The youngest children (birth to age 3) have the highest rates of maltreatment and death. In 2019, 1,860 children died from maltreatment in the United States (CDC, 2021). Children are a vulnerable segment of the population because they depend on others for all their needs. Parents are the most common abusers of children, although childcare providers, other family members, and teachers can also be the source of the abuse. See Box 22.2 for signs of child abuse.

Parents who abuse a child may have unrealistic expectations. For example, they may expect an infant

Box 22.2

Signs of Child Abuse

Child exhibits some of the following:
- Fear of returning home
- Antisocial behavior, such as lying or stealing
- Fear and anxiety when asked about injuries, fear response around adults
- Going to lengths to hide injuries
- Absences from school
- Lack of reaction to frightening event
- Unexplained, unusual injuries such as bites, burns, black eyes
- Abusing animals
- Overly compliant and passive behavior OR demanding, aggressive behavior
- Changes in behavior, school performance
- Signs of neglect—malnutrition, lack of medical care, frequent school absences, stealing money for food

Source: Adapted from Morgan & Townsend, 2021.

to control their crying or a young child to follow instructions perfectly (FIG. 22.1). Sometimes a child with special needs or emotional problems is singled out for abuse as the parents' patience is more severely tested with these children.

Shaken baby syndrome (also called abusive head trauma), a form of child abuse that occurs when a caregiver shakes a baby in an effort to stop its crying, contributes to many infant deaths each year (CDC, 2021). Klevens and Leed (2010) report that abusive head trauma is a leading cause of physical child abuse deaths in children under 5 in the United States. In addition, long-term effects include vision and hearing problems as well as developmental delays.

Each year, newborns are abandoned or even killed when new mothers panic. These are often infants that are delivered outside of a hospital setting and the new mother is alone and overwhelmed. Many states have passed laws for safe surrender sites of newborns if a mother is unable or unwilling to keep her child. These are also called safe haven laws. Rather than abandoning or discarding an infant, mothers can safely leave the infant at community locations that often include hospitals and fire stations. Many at-risk teenagers who are pregnant are unaware of this law, so community education that reaches teens must be provided to prevent the neglect, abandonment, and even death of these infants.

> **GOOD TO KNOW**
> It is important to know the law in your state regarding safe surrender sites. This information must be disseminated to pregnant teens and other women.

An early sign of abuse in the older child can be changes in behavior and school performance. Another sign can be abuse of family pets by the child. Children may try to deal with their own abuse by controlling another being or seeking an outlet for their anger through a more vulnerable victim, such as a pet.

Victims of child abuse are at an increased risk of becoming abusers as adults. Even though the child may hate the abusive situation, they never get an opportunity to observe healthy parenting or to learn adaptive coping mechanisms to deal with frustration without violence. Other long-term effects of being a victim of child abuse include low self-esteem, high risk for substance abuse, tendency toward depression, difficulty trusting in close relationships, and a violent lifestyle, including crime. Incarcerated youths frequently have a history of being abused and neglected.

> **CRITICAL THINKING QUESTION**
> A 4-year-old child with autism spectrum disorder is admitted to your unit from the emergency department (ED) with burns on both hands and bruises on one arm. The child's parents are at the bedside and very concerned. They have told the doctors that the child reached up and put her hands in a pot of hot water on the stove. How would you react to these parents? Describe factors that might give clues as to whether this could be child abuse or an accident.

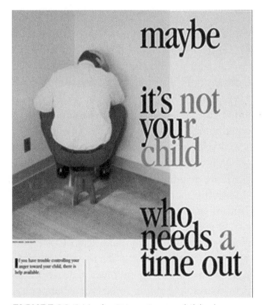

FIGURE 22.1 Maybe it is not your child who needs a time out.

> **Tool Box**
> National Child Abuse Hotline: 800-4-A-Child. This 24-hour hotline provides crisis intervention, education, and referrals.

Classroom Activity
Determine who is a mandatory reporter of suspected child abuse in the agency where you are assigned. Discuss the responsibility to be a mandatory reporter of child abuse as a licensed practical nurse/licensed vocational nurse.

Sexual Abuse

Sexual abuse is violent or nonviolent sexual contact or sexual activity that is not wanted by the receiver. It is generally inflicted on someone the abuser considers less powerful physically or emotionally. The abuser is usually a close, significant figure in the abused person's life and knows how to manipulate the potential victim into submission. Sexual abuse can involve a variety of behaviors. These can range from unwanted advances and inappropriate sexual contact to rape. **Sexual harassment,** which includes sending sexually explicit photos to the victim or posting sexual photos of the victim to social media without their permission, is also considered sexual abuse. Statutory rape refers to unlawful intercourse between a person who is over the age of consent with a person who is under the age of consent (usually defined as 16–18 years of age, depending on the state).

Girls are the most frequent victims of childhood sexual abuse, but boys are also abused. Children with disabilities are at higher risk. Sexual abuse of a child can also include sexual exploitation, as in taking explicit photos of the child or photos of other activities where the child is being used for the sexual pleasure of an adult. Long-term effects of sexual abuse include fear of intimacy, sexual problems, eating disorders, and an overwhelming sense of powerlessness. Children may feel threatened, be confused about their feelings, and question if the activity is right. The abuser

is usually a trusted person, which adds to the child's confusion. Children do not always have the words to express what is happening to them. They may also be so fearful that they say nothing. They may fear other family members will be hurt if they speak up. Victims may block out the memory of these incidents until later in life, when a major event or trauma triggers memory recall. Signs of sexual abuse in children include frequent urinary tract infections; torn, bloody underclothing; nightmares; bedwetting; and sudden onset of sexually related behavior, in addition to the other signs of child abuse as listed previously.

Incest is defined as sexual activity between persons so closely related that they are forbidden by law to marry. Girls are the most frequent victims of incest.

Rape is forcible, degrading, nonconsensual sexual intercourse accompanied by violence and intimidation. It often goes unreported. When a victim does seek medical care, most hospital EDs and urgent care centers have rape kits to assist in the proper collection of evidence, such as semen, hair, and fibers that may be compared with others to identify a suspect. In addition, a forensic nurse, who specializes in rape cases, may examine the patient. It is important that the person who was raped not clean up before going to the ED in order to keep forensic evidence intact. One of the victim's first instincts is to "wash away" the incident both physically and psychologically by showering. Discourage bathing or showering until evidence can be collected. **Date rape** (also known as acquaintance rape) most frequently occurs among teens and young adults. Rape happens to older people as well. That population is often assaulted in their private residences and in long-term care and assisted living facilities.

Human trafficking, which can include sex trafficking, is another form of abuse that often involves children and teens forcibly held against their will. It can also involve adults who are in vulnerable situations. Human trafficking involves the use of force, fraud, or coercion to obtain some type of labor or commercial sex act (U.S. Department Homeland Security, N.D.). This has been a growing problem in the United

States, especially involving forcibly bringing girls and women from other countries for illegal purposes.

Clinical Activity

If the hospital where you have a clinical rotation has a sexual assault nurse examiner (SANE) on staff, contact them to discuss their role.

Clinical Activity

Ensure that appropriate tests are completed as part of the work-up for a victim of sexual abuse (e.g., screening for sexually transmitted infections [STIs], pregnancy test, HIV test).

CRITICAL THINKING QUESTION

The nurse from the local grammar school calls your clinic asking for help. She tells you a parent of a 6-year-old has accused the teacher of sexually molesting her child. The school nurse does not know what to do. What would be your first action?

Intimate Partner Violence

Intimate partner violence (IPV) (also called domestic violence or spousal abuse) takes many forms, including physical, emotional, sexual, and **economic abuse**. One in five women and one in seven men will experience IPV in their lifetime (CDC, 2021). Men may be less likely to report it out of embarrassment. IPV can involve physical injury, use of intimidation, denigration, control, and sexual violence. Marital rape, which has been recognized only in recent years as a legal category in many states, occurs when a spouse is held liable for sexual abuse directed at a marital partner against that person's will. IPV can also take the form of controlling the partner's access to family finances.

Cultural Considerations

Intimate partner violence crosses all socioeconomic, geographic, racial, and ethnic lines and occurs in all types of intimate relationships.

This type of abuse often includes the children in the home. For example, an abusive domestic partner might say, "If you go out with your friends tonight, I'll see to it that your kids are taken away; you're unfit to be their mother (father) if you go out at night and leave them. You do not deserve them!" Or "Leave! And when you get back, the kids and I will be gone, and you won't see them again!" The children are used as a way to control and intimidate the partner. This type of button-pushing is very effective at negatively controlling someone's behavior out of fear of the consequences. Abusers also use the family pet as a means to control the partner; for example, the abuser may threaten to kill the family dog if the partner leaves. Pediatricians and veterinarians are trained to identify signs of domestic violence because they may observe clues of a troubled family when examining the children and pets.

The abuse cycle in domestic violence has been shown to follow a pattern that was originally identified by Walker in 1979.

1. *Tension-building:* The recipient of the abuse is compliant, believing that in some way they are at fault and deserve the abuse. The abuser's tolerance for frustration begins declining, leading to lashing out, and the victim takes the blame. The victim is probably using denial as a defense mechanism and feels pressure to appease the perpetrator to keep the peace. The perpetrator uses verbal abuse and minor beating, and also is aware that their behavior is not appropriate.

2. *Acute battering incident:* The victim senses that the beating is coming and may even provoke it to get it over with. Some triggering event occurs, which may be something minor like a miscommunication or dropping a dish. The victim may try to hide and will probably not seek help until the next day, if at all. The police may be called, but by the time they arrive, the victim may have already forgiven the perpetrator. This kind of physical abuse usually happens in private.

3. *Honeymoon:* The perpetrator is contrite, loving, and very sad about the incident of abuse that has occurred. The perpetrator may ask for forgiveness. They may try to make amends with gifts. The abuser promises to get help but only after discussing how the abuse has taught the victim a lesson, such as "Don't make me mad!" The victim, who wants desperately to believe the perpetrator, will forgive them and will begin to think that the relationship is returning to "normal."

The victim is still very much in love with the perpetrator, believing that love will conquer all and that, this time, the abuse will stop.

This cycle of IPV leads to the often-asked question: Why does a victim of IPV stay in the relationship? Some of the most common reasons for staying include:

- fear of retaliation against self, children, or pet
- fear of loss of custody of children or pet
- financial dependence on the abuser
- lack of support; do not know where to go if they leave abuser
- religious beliefs; will not consider divorce
- denial; thinks of the good times and hopes that things can improve so that there can be good times again

GOOD TO KNOW

Because it is common that a victim of abuse may return to a violent partner, health-care staff need to understand they cannot push a patient to leave the abuser. The decision to leave has to come from the victim. It may take multiple episodes before the patient is able to leave.

In assessing for domestic violence, look for the following signs: injuries while pregnant when there is resentment of a pregnancy, wearing clothes that cover the arms and legs and/or makeup to camouflage injuries, lack of care for own chronic illnesses, social isolation (including being restricted, monitored, or prevented from use of a computer or smartphone), abuse of alcohol or drugs, acting guilty for seeking medical treatment, and history of rape. Sutherland, Fantasia, Fontenot, and Harris (2012) recommend the following questions be incorporated in screening for IPV:

1. Have you ever been abused or threatened by your partner?
2. In the past year, have you been physically hurt by someone?
3. Have you ever been forced to have sex?

Tool Box

National Domestic Violence hotline: 1-800-799-SAFE (7233). This hotline provides confidential support, education, and referrals.

CRITICAL THINKING QUESTION

Your pregnant patient has been admitted with a broken ankle from a fall. When you walk into the room, the woman is crying on the phone, telling someone she is sorry and that it will not happen again. What would be your first action in response to hearing this?

Elder Abuse

Elder abuse includes neglect as well as physical, sexual, and emotional abuse. Exploitation of the person's financial reserves by family, hired help, or strangers is economic abuse (sometimes called fiduciary abuse). Abandonment is another type of elder abuse. This occurs when seniors who are unable to care for themselves are left alone (National Institute on Aging, 2020). Elder abuse can occur in the home or in residential facilities. It is estimated that elder abuse affects 10% of the geriatric population (CDC, 2021; Lachs & Pillemer, 2015). This problem is greatly underreported and will continue to increase as the population grows older.

Obtaining accurate statistics is hampered by the inconsistency of laws regarding elder abuse in the individual states and by the lack of a universally accepted definition of what elder abuse is. The CDC (2021) defines elder abuse as "an intentional act or failure to act by a caregiver or another person in a relationship involving an expectation of trust that causes or creates a serious risk of harm to an older adult." Some states do not include neglect or psychological abuse in their definition, so it is essential for nurses to be aware of how elder abuse is defined in the state in which they are working. Because the abuser is often the victim's caregiver, possibly even the victim's spouse or child, victims rarely report the abuse. They fear reprisals or abandonment because they are dependent on the caregiver. Society's lack of interest in older people may add to the underreporting (FIG. 22.2).

Caregivers who are inadequately prepared for the demands of providing care to an older person are a factor in elder abuse. The presence of cognitive impairment in the patient adds another level of stress in caring for them. Caregivers with no history of being an abuser can reach a point of frustration and fatigue that leads to behaviors they would normally find unacceptable, such as slapping or degrading their loved one. Elder abuse can also be

Caregivers of patients with dementia should be counseled about dealing with the stress of this role. Caregivers need to be given resources for support and respite care. Local programs available through the Alzheimer's Association or local senior centers may offer elder "day care" as well as support groups and caregiver resources to help prevent elder abuse.

Specific examples of elder abuse can include:

- hitting
- shoving
- social isolation
- leaving the victim in soiled linens
- withholding food and/or water
- using inappropriate restraints
- making threats
- forcing the victim to sign over financial affairs or change a will
- sexually molesting the victim
- insulting the victim

See Box 22.3 for the characteristics of victims and abusers in elder abuse.

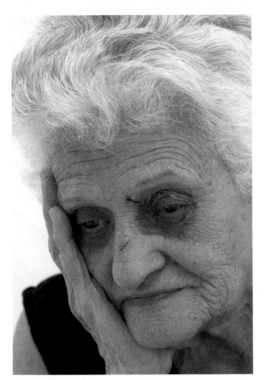

FIGURE 22.2 Could she be a victim of elder abuse?

difficult to detect by professionals because common signs such as bruising and skin tears may be common in older populations. The patient with dementia is particularly vulnerable because they are unable to speak up or will not be believed because of their intermittent confusion.

GOOD TO KNOW

Economic, or fiduciary, abuse can be evidenced when a patient gives hired caregivers passwords for bank accounts or creates a new will with a caregiver as beneficiary. It is important to determine that the patient is doing this voluntarily and is competent to make reasonable decisions.

Tool Box

Department of Justice: Elder Justice Initiative provides information to identify and address elder abuse. https://www.justice.gov/elderjustice

CRITICAL THINKING QUESTION

You are working in home health care. You visit your 90-year-old patient in her home. The daughter, who is the caregiver, is not home. The door to the house is unlocked, and the patient is tied in bed with a restraint. You call your supervisor, and the daughter walks in as you are on the phone. The daughter is frantic and tells you that she had to leave for a while to buy groceries. She had no one to watch her mother. What actions should you take? Should this be reported as elder abuse?

Classroom Activity

- Research the elder-abuse laws in your state and find out who mandatory reporters are.
- Identify resources for caregivers of patients with dementia in your community.
- Talk to staff at local nursing homes and assisted living centers to find out how they address suspected elder abuse.

Box 22.3

Common Characteristics of Victims and Abusers in Elder Abuse

Victim

- Evidence of malnutrition, dehydration, poor hygiene, pressure injuries, not receiving needed medical care
- Unusual injuries such as twisting fractures, cigarette burns on face or back, perforated eardrums from being slapped
- Evidence of sexually transmitted infections, unusual genital injuries
- Deterioration in mental status including confusion and depression
- Sudden lack of funds in person who previously had resources
- Frail, dependent, possible mental impairment requiring care from family member or hired help
- Extreme dependency, attachment to new caregiver
- Evidence of inappropriate use of restraints
- Abandonment of elder in emergency room, nursing home

Abuser

- Often living with victim, lacks resources to live elsewhere
- Refuses to allow diagnostic tests, hospitalization
- Often much younger than patient
- Cashes victim's Social Security or pension checks
- Sudden, intense involvement with patient with little input from other family members
- Discourages patient from contacting others
- Evidence of drug or alcohol abuse or mental illness
- Expects dependent elder to meet caregiver's needs
- Caregiver overwhelmed with patient's care needs, demonstrates frustration and resentment, isolated with limited assistance
- Elderly spouse with dementia who has challenges in managing stress
- Coerces senior to change will to caregiver's benefit
- Shows no guilt or rationalizes actions

Source: Morgan & Townsend, 2021; National Center for Elder Abuse, 2017; National Institute on Aging, 2020.

TREATMENT OF ABUSE

Victims of abuse often require immediate medical treatment, crisis intervention, and then long-term psychological help. The immediate crisis intervention may include getting them out of the abusive situation.

Some strategies for crisis intervention include arranging lodging at a domestic violence shelter, arranging **respite care** for an overwhelmed caregiver of a child or older relative, making an immediate social work referral for options if the patient cannot return home, and contacting law enforcement. Domestic violence shelters, or **safe houses**, are available in major cities. Victims of domestic violence as well as their children and sometimes even their pets are protected from the abuser at the shelter. The locations of these shelters are confidential so that victims can feel safe. Victims may need advice on how to seek help without arousing the suspicion of their abuser. For example, victims may have their computer search histories and cell phone call logs tracked by a suspicious abuser. Anyone who has been sexually abused needs testing for sexually transmitted infections including HIV, and women and girls may need pregnancy tests. Children and teens also need evaluation for substance abuse if they were exposed to drugs as part of the abuse. Children exposed to sexual abuse need access to specialists in the field. Repression of trauma can lead to a lifetime of emotional problems, so therapy is very important. Play and art therapy can be important tools for children to communicate their feelings.

Abusers and victims need specialized counseling programs as well as access to support resources such as local and national hotlines. Ongoing individual and group psychotherapy is often part of the treatment plan for both as well. Mandated therapy for abusers who are convicted of crimes may be part of their rehabilitation. Treatment for abusers can include resources for parenting skills and anger management.

Tool Box

Parents Anonymous is a national organization for parents with issues around child abuse. It is based on the Alcoholics Anonymous model: http://Parentsanonymous.org

Classroom Activity

Identify local parenting-education programs.

Pharmacology Corner

Victims of abuse may need medications for anxiety and depression. Victims may need substance abuse treatment if they were exposed to drugs as part of the abuse. Abusers may need medications to manage substance abuse, control angry impulses, and manage anxiety.

GOOD TO KNOW

Victims of abuse may seek out drugs or alcohol to self-medicate feelings of fear, anxiety, and shame. Substance use may be the initial symptom that brings the victim to a health-care provider.

NURSING CARE OF VICTIMS OF ABUSE

Common nursing diagnoses for the victims of abuse include the following:

- anxiety
- caregiver role strain
- family coping, disabling
- parenting, impaired
- post-trauma response
- powerlessness
- violence, risk for

General Nursing Interventions

1. *Ensure safety:* The **survivor** of abuse will be confused and fearful. Reassure the patient that everything possible is being done to ensure their safety. Social work involvement is essential. Obtain a list of people who are considered "safe" by the patient and ask if the patient would like those people to be called. If the patient wishes to press charges against the abuser, offer assistance with making the appropriate phone calls. Alert security staff members according to agency protocol to prevent the alleged abuser from causing more harm. Maintain a calm milieu. If the abuse victim is a young child or frail elder who cannot speak for themselves, immediately involve the interdisciplinary team to determine the next steps. Providing a safe, calm, secure environment will reassure the patient.

2. *Know your own thoughts and feelings about abuse:* A nurse who has been abused or who has been an abuser may find it difficult to be therapeutic for the patient. Remember that you may be treating the survivor as well as the abuser. You are responsible to help all patients. Abusers need help as much as the person who was abused. Be aware of your own safety and avoid putting yourself in a risky situation if an alleged abuser threatens violence to someone reporting the abuse.

GOOD TO KNOW

Suspecting someone of abuse can lead to stress for the health-care team. It is important to have a team plan of care when working with a suspected abuser. One nurse should not carry all the burden of this difficult situation. Seek out support from coworkers.

3. *Remain nonjudgmental/show empathy:* This is a crisis situation in many ways. Recalling communication skills and helping all involved to verbalize any concerns, thoughts, and feelings are crucial. Remaining technically correct in performing any procedures or sample collections is imperative to avoid contamination. Maintaining professionalism and confidentiality for both the survivor and the abuser is mandatory. Calling for help from counselors, advocates, or people chosen by the patient will help maintain a calm milieu. You are not expected to condone or accept the patient's actions but to respect and help the person, regardless of the situation. If a patient who may be a victim wishes to return home with a suspected abuser, you can offer support, education, and resources, but you cannot force the patient into different actions.

4. *Know your agency policy and use your resources:* Every health-care agency has its own policies and procedures for dealing with victims of abuse and violence. Familiarity with these policies and procedures will help save time and convey confidence. The patient may be confused and embarrassed about the situation. It may well have taken every bit of courage the person had just to get to the facility. Your smooth handling of the situation may provide the extra bit of confidence the victim needs to actually

go through with the examination. Collecting physical evidence, making observations, and asking screening questions may be part of your role in suspected abuse cases. In most jurisdictions, notification of the police, taking pictures for evidence, and other actions may be done only with the patient's consent. In the case of young children, developmentally disabled individuals, and frail older persons, where capacity to be interviewed is uncertain, involvement of the physician and social worker is essential to make decisions on how to proceed.

Many hospitals and trauma centers have some sort of abuse-advocacy program. A representative of this program should be contacted immediately to visit the victim. The abuse program representative will be able to offer support and provide information on safe houses and other services that may be available to the victim and their children.

Nurses who are caring for a survivor of abuse need to be aware of their state's laws regarding children who may have witnessed the abuse. In some states, a child who sees or hears abuse is also considered to have been abused. Nurses and other health-care providers are mandated reporters and, as such, find themselves in an ethical bind: They want to help and support the patient/survivor; however, they must tell that individual that if a child saw or heard the abuse, the nurse must, as a mandated reporter, report this fact to the child protection agency. The patient/survivor may feel pressure, in a sense, to not divulge the whole situation to the nurse if it requires mandatory reporting.

GOOD TO KNOW
Whenever you suspect abuse, get other staff members involved, including your supervisor, a social worker, and a health-care provider. Know the laws in your state and agency policies about who is a mandatory reporter.

See Table 22.2 for a nursing care plan for a child who may be the victim of abuse. See Figure 22.2 for the Concept map for the Patient with Physical Abuse.

GOOD TO KNOW
Movies and television programs with abuse themes: *The Burning Bed* (intimate partner violence), *Sleeping With the Enemy* (intimate partner violence), *Radio Flyer* (child abuse), *Allen v. Farrow* (child sexual abuse), *Big Little Lies* (intimate partner abuse), *I Care a Lot* (elder abuse), *The Guardians* (elder abuse), *The Accused* (sexual assault), *Flowers in the Attic* (child abuse).

Table 22.2
Nursing Care Plan for a Child With Injuries Consistent With Child Abuse

Assessment/Data Collection	Nursing Diagnosis	Goal	Interventions	Evaluation
Child admitted with broken bones, burns of unclear etiology. Child abuse by parent is suspected by health-care team.	Family coping, disabling	Keep child safe and provide intervention for parent.	• Ensure the child's safety per agency policy as first priority. • Establish a trusting relationship with child and parent. • Monitor parent interactions with child. • Demonstrate acceptance. • Explain all procedures thoroughly to child and parent. • Encourage parent to talk about stresses. • Ensure that appropriate people are contacted regarding reporting possible abuse.	• Child remains safe. • Parent acknowledges stressors and agrees to get help. • Safe, appropriate discharge plan is in place.

Clinical Vignette: Annette and Charles, both 21, have been dating for two years. Charles has always been jealous and gets very angry when Annette even talks to another man. He has hit her several times, hard enough to produce bruises, but never on her face, and she is able to hide the abuse from others. Tonight at a party, Annette danced with another man, and Charles became violent. He punched the man in the face and dragged Annette out to the parking lot. She yelled at him, "This is it! We are through! I don't ever want to see you again!" He started beating her around the face and upper body, and yelled, "You can't break up with me! I won't allow it! You belong to me, and no one else!" He left her lying in the parking lot. She felt powerless, and, in her despondency, opened her purse and swallowed half a bottle of acetaminophen. When she told her girlfriend, Dana, what had happened, Dana called 911, and Annette was taken to the hospital. She was treated for the overdose, and her wounds were cleaned and dressed. Following physical stability, she was transferred to the psychiatric unit. She tells the nurse, "I can't live like this. He won't let me go! I don't know what to do!" The nurse develops the following concept map care plan for Annette.

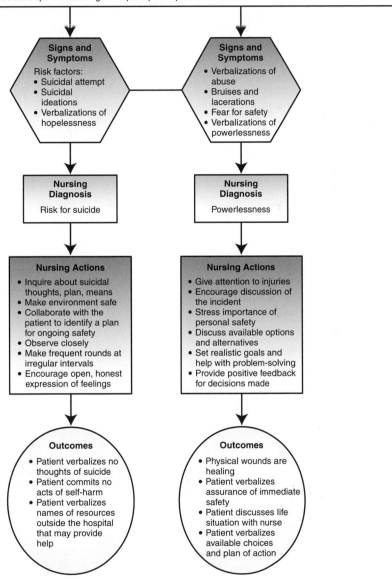

FIGURE 22.3 Concept Map for a Patient With Physical Abuse. (Source Morgan and Townsend [2021]. Essentials of Psychiatric Mental Health Nursing. FA Davis.)

Clinical Activity

Be aware of your emotional reaction when dealing with patients who are victims of abuse or abusers.

See Table 22.3 for a review of nursing interventions for victims of various types of abuse.

GOOD TO KNOW

The coronavirus disease 2019 (COVID-19) pandemic, which isolated people in their homes, presented new challenges for those at risk for abuse. Concerns have been raised about the incidence of child abuse, as children were not being seen by teachers or doctors, who are mandatory reporters. Support systems for children and parents such as churches, counselors, and play groups were suspended. The pressures of remaining in close quarters with a partner who is abusive led to increased incidence of domestic violence with fewer resources available during the pandemic to escape the situation. Older adults, too, were isolated at home, perhaps with a caregiver. They were not in physical contact with other family members who live elsewhere and were seldom seen by some mandatory reporters (varies by state) such as doctors, nurses, lawyers, and even bank tellers who might be likely to spot signs of neglect or abuse.

Evidence-Based Practice

Clinical Question: How does addiction in the home affect children?

Evidence: This study looked at the effect of parental addiction on children in the home.

Growing up in homes with addictions contributes to abuse and neglect that creates an environment for traumatic events and encounters. This study used an exploratory study design to explore the experiences of individuals whose upbringing was influenced by substance use at home or who had parents with addiction problems. Participants in this study were asked to identify coping mechanisms they adopted. Results showed diverse strategies to cope with these experiences, including leaving home, using substances early in life, and dropping out of school.

Implications for Nursing Practice: Screening and intervention for childhood trauma should be encouraged both in schools and community health settings. Such interventions have been found to reduce substance use among school children to deal with ensuing trauma and to address negative outcomes from this trauma. Recognizing the influence of parental addiction on the incidence of child abuse is something nurses need to keep in mind when working with families.

Ogenchuk, M.G. & Gaudet, M. (2021). Living with parents with problematic substance use: Impacts and turning points. *Public Health Nurs.* Mar 14. doi: 10.1111/phn.12888

Table 22.3

Nursing Interventions for Victims of Abuse

Type of Abuse	Indicators of Abuse	Nursing Interventions
Sexual	• Violent or nonviolent sexual contact or activity that is not wanted by the receiver that could include foreplay, touching, kissing, and mutual masturbation, as well as oral sex and vaginal or anal intercourse • Frequent bladder or vaginal infections • Bloody underwear • Evidence of incest—sexual intercourse between persons so closely related that marriage is illegal	• Carefully use rape kit and preserve evidence. • Provide safety and privacy. • Be nonjudgmental. • Show empathy. • Be advocate for patient. • Maintain calm milieu. • Know own thoughts and feelings regarding abuse and abuser. • Know agency policies.

Table 22.3
Nursing Interventions for Victims of Abuse—cont'd

Type of Abuse	Indicators of Abuse	Nursing Interventions
	• Evidence of rape—forcible, degrading, non-consensual sexual intercourse accompanied by violence and intimidation • "Date rape"—seen frequently in high school and college students (belief surrounding date rape is that the person who pays for the date is entitled to sex from the other person)	• Assist with contacting outside agencies (e.g., law enforcement, clergy), as requested by patient.

Physical	• Any actions that cause physical harm to another, such as:
	  • Hitting
	  • Burning
	  • Withholding food, water, and other basic needs
	  • Other activities that go beyond accidental contact
	• Request to stop ignored or mocked by the perpetrator
	• Activity repeating itself in future situations
	• Frequent visits to emergency department (for all forms of abuse)
	• Excessive bruising or bruising on unusual areas of body
	• Withdrawal from friends and social groups
		• Provide safety.
		• Be nonjudgmental.
		• Show empathy and reassurance.
		• Take the time to develop trusting relationship.
		• Be advocate for patient.
		• Maintain calm milieu.
		• Reinforce self-esteem.
		• Reinforce that victims should not blame themselves for the abuse.
		• Know own thoughts and feelings regarding abuse and abuser.
		• Know agency policies.
		• Assist with contacting outside agencies (e.g., law enforcement, clergy), as requested by patient.
		• Involve agency social worker.

Emotional	• Willful use of words or actions that undermine self-esteem—includes the "silent treatment" (causes the other person to guess at the problem) and other types of game playing, name calling, frequent degrading and harsh and/or cruel criticism	• Same as for physical abuse • Counter patient's self-depreciating comments. • Reinforce positive traits.
Child abuse/ neglect	• Sexual, physical, and/or emotional abuse—act of commission (doing) or omission (not doing) • Victim may believe that abuse is child's own fault • Child confused about what is happening and why • Abuser often larger, more powerful than the child, which is intimidating • Excessive absences from school • Child may display inappropriate behaviors, e.g., sexual	• Same as for physical abuse • Encourage use of play and art for child to express feelings. • Provide touch and support if the child will accept. • If child uncomfortable being touched, respect that and provide support in other ways. • Accept that child may be mistrustful.

Continued

Table 22.3

Nursing Interventions for Victims of Abuse—cont'd

Type of Abuse	Indicators of Abuse	Nursing Interventions
Domestic violence/ intimate partner violence	• Physical, emotional, sexual, and "button-pushing" kinds of abuse • Most typically reported by women • Kept isolated from friends and family • Withdrawal from friends and social groups • Use of substance abuse to cover distress	• Same as for physical abuse • Recognize that victim may return to abuser initially. • Help identify possible threats that victim is facing, e.g., child custody, loss of financial security.
Elder	• Victim is usually dependent on abuser in some way. • May be slapped, burned, tripped, neglected, humiliated • Can include economic abuse where victim's funds are misused or stolen	• Same as for physical abuse • Listen to patient's concerns and report them even if patient is confused. • Provide follow-up in the home.

Safe and Effective Nursing Care (SENC)

Provide a safe environment so that the patient can feel secure.

Communicate concerns to team members.

Implement security precautions as needed to ensure patient and staff safety.

Provide appropriate care that is sensitive to the victim's needs but also includes any support that is needed in collection of evidence.

Key Points

- Abuse takes many forms and is being reported in higher numbers annually.
- Victims of abuse are often in a vulnerable position to their abusers. The abuser often has a need to exert power and control.
- Abuse happens to people of all ages, races, ethnicities, sexual orientations, and socioeconomic groups. Men can also be victims, and the number of male victims is believed to be underreported. The youngest children are the most vulnerable to abuse.

- Nurses must be sensitive to the needs of the abused person as well as those of the abuser. Careful attention to physical assessment, communication, and emotional support are components of nursing care for people who are suffering the effects of abuse.
- The nurse has a responsibility to know state laws regarding the nurse's obligation to report evidence of child abuse, domestic violence, and elder abuse.

CASE STUDY

Mrs. Jones leaves your long-term care facility for a weekend with her daughter and son-in-law. She seems apprehensive but tells you, "I just worry that I'm a bother to them." You bathed her and helped her pack, and now you document that she is gone until Sunday afternoon and that you are concerned about her apprehension. You note no other physical or mental abnormalities. Sunday afternoon, she returns with skin tears on both arms and bruises over her right eye and on her right cheek. She is

CASE STUDY—cont'd

crying. Her daughter says, "Doesn't that look awful? Mom took a tumble from the toilet." Mrs. Jones says nothing until her daughter leaves, then says to you, "I worry about her. Her husband is a nice man, but he gets so mad at us sometimes. I really can't blame him; he

has a lot on his mind, and I can't give them any more money."

1. What are your responsibilities according to your facility? According to the state? According to your personal belief system?
2. How would you proceed?

Review Questions

1. When caring for someone who has been abused, the nurse can be therapeutic by:
   a. Showing empathy
   b. Ensuring safety
   c. Contacting counselors and advocates
   d. All of the above

2. Which of the following is the best approach when caring for a rape victim?
   a. Ask why it happened.
   b. Document the information in the patient's own words.
   c. Offer to take the patient home after your shift.
   d. Ask what the victim was wearing.

3. When a survivor of abuse and the abuser both present at your facility, your responsibility is to care for:
   a. The survivor only
   b. The abuser only
   c. Both people
   d. Neither one; call the health-care provider

4. Mrs. X has been caring for her mother at home. Mrs. X's mother has stage three Alzheimer's disease and is requiring more of Mrs. X's time. Mrs. X says to you, "I just don't know what to do. I can't stand it anymore. I love my mother, but I don't have any time for myself, and I can't afford a nursing home." You say:
   a. "Mrs. X, hang in there. Things have a way of working out."
   b. "Why don't your sisters and brothers help out a little?"
   c. "There are agencies that provide respite care for people in your situation. If you like, I could tell the social worker that you would like some information on this service."
   d. "It's got to be hard to put up with this all day when you aren't trained for it."

5. A 38-year-old female presents to urgent care. She has a 3-year-old and a 4-year-old child with her. She is frightened and badly bruised. "He'll kill us all if he knows we came here," she screams. You:
   a. Ask her to please not scream—she is alarming the other patients.
   b. Ask, "Who will kill you?"
   c. Bring her and her children to a room immediately.
   d. Ask her to sit for a moment while you contact someone who can provide safety for her.

6. Mrs. Smith arrives for her appointment. She has had a positive home pregnancy test and suspects she is pregnant. She has a black eye and a lacerated upper lip, and she admits her husband hit her because "I did something stupid. I fell asleep, and supper burned. It's my fault. He works hard. He deserves a decent meal. I'm OK." You tell her:
   a. "Nobody deserves to be hit. Here is the name of an organization that can help."
   b. "You need to leave him right away before he hurts your baby too."
   c. "Why do you stay and let him do that?"
   d. "Has he done this before?"

7. Your 20-year-old female patient in the ED has multiple cuts, bruises, and burns. When you ask how she got these, she is vague and says she is just clumsy. She tells you she is anxious to get home to her boyfriend so that he will not get angry that she left home, but she hopes that she can get a prescription for a tranquilizer. What does this response indicate to you?
   a. She has an anxiety disorder.
   b. She is accident prone.
   c. She may be caught up in the cycle of abuse.
   d. She has a substance abuse problem.

8. A young woman is brought into the ED after a sexual assault. Your primary nursing intervention should be:
   a. Help her bathe and clean up to make her feel more relaxed.
   b. Discuss the importance of follow-up treatment for possible sexually transmitted disease.
   c. Provide her with physical and emotional support during evidence collection.
   d. Give her a list of community resources.

9. A woman who was sexually assaulted 6 months ago has been attending a support group for rape victims. She has learned that the most likely reason the man raped her is:
   a. He was high and did not know what he was doing.
   b. He had a need to control her and dominate her.
   c. She met him in a bar and was impaired when they went to her apartment.
   d. He had a strong need for sex.

10. Which of the following is not an example of economic abuse in the elderly?
    a. A caregiver is using the patient's ATM card for personal use.
    b. The patient's son is asking to see the patient's will.
    c. A caregiver is encouraging the patient to no longer see her son and daughter.
    d. A hired caregiver is named power of attorney for finances for his elderly patient.

REVIEW QUESTIONS ANSWER KEY 1.d, 2.b, 3.c, 4.c, 5.c, 6.a, 7.c, 8.c, 9.b, 10.b

APPENDIX A
Answers and Rationales

CHAPTER 1

History of Mental Health Nursing

1. **b.** The main goal of deinstitutionalization was to allow as many people as possible to return to the community and lead as normal a life as they could. Not all mentally ill people would be able to do that because of the severity of their illnesses. On the other hand, not all mentally ill people had to be kept in locked units, nor do they today. Community hospitals were to be kept open, but many state hospitals closed because of the decline in census.

2. **c.** The development of psychotropic (psychoactive) medications in the 1950s was a keystone to allowing people to return to their homes. The Community Mental Health Centers Act came about 10 years later. The Nurse Practice Act dictates the scope of practice for nurses; and electroshock therapy, now called electroconvulsant therapy, took place in hospitals.

3. **d.** The Nurse Practice Act, which is written specifically for each state, is the set of regulations that dictates the scope of nursing practice. The National League for Nursing (NLN) and the American Nurses Association (ANA) are national nursing associations that set recommendations for the practice, education, and well-being of nurses. The Patient Bill of Rights is a document to protect the patient. Nurses must know the parameters of this document for ethical practice, but it does not dictate the scope of nursing practice.

4. **d.** Deinstitutionalization and changes in the health-care delivery system encourage people with mental health issues to be treated in a variety of health-care settings. Nurses will care for patients with mental illnesses in all of the settings listed.

5. **d.** Dorothea Dix is the only one on this list who was not a nurse.

6. **b, d, e.** AAPINA represents Asian American and Pacific Islander nurses; PNAA represents Philippine nurses; NANAINA represents Alaska Native American Indian nurses.

7. **b.** Asylums were originally described as places of refuge. The meaning is much different today.

8. **d.** The National Institute of Mental Health (NIMH) was established in 1946.

9. **c.** Florence Nightingale recognized the relationship between sanitary conditions and healing.

10. **a.** Phenothiazines were the first psychotropic drugs introduced in the 1950s.

CHAPTER 2

Basics of Communication

1. **b.** This option offers assistance in a way that encourages the patient to say what he or she needs. **a** used the word "why," which has negative connotations. **c** is closed-ended and allows a "yes" or "no" answer. **d** is also closed-ended. Adding the "please" does not make it a correctly formatted question.

2. **c.** Nurse–patient communication is purposeful and helpful. **a** would change the focus of the nurse-patient relationship and lower the chances for a successful therapeutic relationship. Sometimes nurses and patients do become friends, but this cannot get in the way of the professional relationship of the nurse and the patient. **b** suggests that the nurse is somehow "the boss." Patients sometimes have that perception, but the nurse is really a "partner" in collaboration with the patient. **d** suggests a distance that would place the nurse too far from the patient emotionally. It would be difficult to discuss some of the intimate details the patient needs to discuss if the relationship is too distant and formal.

3. **c.** This option combines an observation with a closed-ended question. In this instance, it can be effective. Even with the closed-ended question, it is the best of the four choices. **a** implies playing into a hallucination and assumes that the patient intended to

talk to someone else. **b** is intended to quiet the patient by using guilt. Asking the patient to be quiet will discourage the patient from wanting to confide in you. **d** uses the word "why" without prefacing it with an observation, thus opening up the possibility of the patient's feeling defensive.

4. **d.** This option honestly tells the patient that you cannot give that information. The physician must explain the results first. **a** oversteps the boundaries of the nurse. **b** uses the "why" word. **c** gives advice, by using the word "should."

5. **c.** This puts the conversation back to the patient and allows venting of concerns. **a** and **b** give advice; **d** gives false reassurance and also belittles the patient's concerns.

6. **a.** This is correct because it tells the patient the nurse is concerned yet leaves the patient responsible for stating what he or she needs at the moment. **b** uses the word "why," and **c** has a very authoritarian tone. **d** is a command that is very authoritarian and even threatening.

7. **a.** Here, the nurse tells the patient that he or she understands the special concerns of the religion and culture of Judaism but does not make a promise that the dietitian will come, which would build false hope. **b** is incorrect because it does make that promise. **c** does not give any indication that compromise is possible or that the nurse is "hearing" the true concern. **d** is agreeing and is a block to therapeutic communication.

8. **d.** This is stating an implied thought or feeling. The nurse is confirming the fact that the patient is feeling ignored. **a** makes light of the patient's concern to see the physician. **b** is not helpful for the patient and shows no sensitivity for the patient's desire to see the physician. **c** is a block because it shows disapproval for the patient's concern and sides with the physician rather than the patient.

9. **a.** This option is more correct than **b** because it offers an observation before using a closed-ended question. **b** and **c** are simply closed-ended questions. **d** is an observation, but it uses "why," which tends to leave people feeling defensive.

10. **b.** "I feel like" is not a "feeling" statement at all, but rather a thought statement. There

is no emotion identified. **b** encourages the nurse and patient to explore what emotional response is being experienced by the patient in a safe environment. **a** and **c** are nontherapeutic techniques. **d** is nontherapeutic in many ways: changes the subject, does not reflect what the patient has said, and implies the nurse is not interested in pursuing the patient's feelings.

CHAPTER 3

Ethics, Evidence-Based Practice, and Regulations

1. **b.** Ethics is a code of professional expectations that does not have legal force behind it. The issues border on legal implications, but ethics comes more out of expectations that patients have of nurses than out of actual legal bounds.

2. **c.** Each state has a Nurse Practice Act that defines the scope of practice for registered nurses (RNs), licensed practical nurses (LPNs), and licensed vocational nurses (LVNs) in that state.

3. **d.** The Patient Bill of Rights is designed to define the rights of all patients in health-care facilities. These will change somewhat from state to state. People who are institutionalized for some reason may be termed "vulnerable" because they may be unable to speak for themselves or provide for their own safety. All who care for people in these facilities must treat them in accordance with the Patient Bill of Rights.

4. **b.** This is an honest, assertive technique that shows one nurse voicing a concern to another nurse. **a**, **c**, and **d** are all forms of blocks to therapeutic communication.

5. **d.** Most Nurse Practice Acts require that LPNs follow the chain of command. In this situation, speaking with the nurse in charge is the best choice. **a** is a block to therapeutic communication because it is argumentative and voices disagreement with the patient. **b** is not safe: Even though it is always important to listen to patients, a nurse must never assume the patient is right. **c** is inappropriate at this time; it must first be determined that an error has occurred. Once this is established, the RN or the LPN, if allowed

by state and/or agency policy, should inform the physician.

6. **c.** The Health Insurance Portability and Accountability Act allows patients to have a greater say in how their records are shared and with whom. It also has regulation relating to other areas of confidentiality and how files are shared among providers. It does not force anyone to be treated in a particular facility, but it would raise questions about transporting records in personal vehicles, etc.

7. **b.** Offer another pain relief technique. Mr. Richards does have the right to refuse medication. He also has the right to privacy, but the option provided borders on punitive and may be a threat to patient safety. It is also appropriate to discuss acceptable behavior and the effect he is having on the other residents—just not now. Wait for a time when he is reasonably comfortable and willing to negotiate treatment. Bringing in more staff and performing an invasive technique is not only threatening, but it violates many of the Patient Bill of Rights.

8. **c.** The LPN/LVN works under the direction of the registered nurse or physician and cannot order medication independently. It is not acceptable practice for the LPN/LVN by the Nurse Practice Act.

9. **c.** It is the LPN/LVN's responsibility to contact his/her supervisor.

10. **c.** Mr. B should have received a copy of the Patient Bill of Rights. The nurse can discuss with the patient why he feels his rights have been violated.

 CHAPTER 4

Developmental Psychology Throughout the Life Span

1. **d.** This patient is demonstrating the Electra complex, which is part of the phallic stage of Freud's developmental stages.

2. **c.** Unsuccessful completion of the anal stage would lead to these behaviors and to more serious disorders, according to psychoanalytic theory. These people would be termed "anal retentive" in some social and professional circles today.

3. **d.** This option states that Y's behavior is not appropriate and lets Y tell you that the consequences have been discussed. Y is able to make a choice. **a** and **b** sound harsh and threatening and are not helpful forms of communicating. **c** is very close to letting the nurse "care-take" for Y. In behavior modification, Y would most likely be responsible for his or her own actions and choices.

4. **a.** Cell differentiation, the process whereby cells "specialize" into their particular type, is generally complete by the end of the first trimester (third lunar month).

5. **d.** Women are successfully having children at young ages; however, it is generally believed that a woman's body is not completely mature until the age of 18 years. Because the young woman's body is not completely mature, it is difficult to sustain her health and the life of the fetus. Therefore, infant mortality as well as danger to the mother's health is greatest before this age. Older women are next in line as a risk group for infant mortality because of changing hormones that can jeopardize the woman's ability to support a fetus and carry it to term. Certainly, there are exceptions in both of these age groups regarding pregnancy and successful delivery. These are broad, general beliefs that are held among many in the medical and nursing community.

6. **b.** Anima is Carl Jung's term for female tendencies in men. Animus is male characteristics in women.

7. **d.** According to Erikson, the stage or task for children in the 3- to 6-year-old group is the stage or task of "initiative." The stage or task of "industry" (the stage at which integration of life experiences or the confusion of those experiences develops) covers ages 16 to 20 years. "Intimacy" (the stage at which the main concern is developing intimate relationships with others) begins at approximately age 18 and continues through approximately age 25.

8. **c.** It is believed that infants develop at a very similar rate and pattern (physically, behaviorally, and cognitively) until the age of 10 months. Again, this is based on generalizations; there are always exceptions (e.g., a child who is longer than most of his or her particular age group because of the gene

pool from parents who are taller than the average).

9. **b.** Assimilation is the process of taking in and processing information. It is generally learned by experiencing through the senses. "Accommodation" is the process of working with the information that has been assimilated and making that information a working part of the toddler's daily life. "Autonomy" is the stage or task Erikson believed a toddler should be achieving. "Adjustment" is a general term related to change. It is not always a healthy response to change.

10. **d.** According to Jean Piaget, the 2-year-old child is in the preoperational stage, where the child is demonstrating interest in something other than parents.

 CHAPTER 5

Sociocultural Influences on Mental Health

1. **b.** Proxemics, or spatial distances, vary among cultures. What is comfortable and appropriate for some is not appropriate for others.
2. **c.** Prejudice means to "pre-judge." It is making a decision about a person, situation, etc., before having all necessary information.
3. **b.** Homelessness is not a mental illness but may be a condition of mental illness. It is difficult for this population of people to access the health care and community services available.
4. **b.** Approximately one-third of the homeless in the United States are mentally ill.
5. **d.** Enlist the assistance of a religious representative to negotiate removal of the item(s) in question. Other safety actions may also be required, but right now, relating to this individual at his or her spiritual level is necessary not only for the patient's religious freedom of expression, but also to get him or her to cooperate with additional nursing actions.
6. **d.** Actually, all of the responses are correct. Nurses are mandatory reporters for suspected abuse/neglect/endangerment of children. Certainly, the child could ultimately die from uncontrolled diabetes. It is appropriate to call the RN and Doctor of Medicine (MD) to the examination room, but a stat call would not

be necessary since you are there. The best choice is to sit with the family for a time, gain their trust, and collect more information that could be used to modify the care plan or assist the MD with appropriate referrals for the best care of this child and family.

7. **b, c, d.** Many homeless fall into the "working poor" category and are actually working full-time jobs. Approximately one-third of the homeless also have a mental illness, quite often schizophrenia.
8. **a, c, e.** Though mental illness is a common cause of homelessness, the economy and loss of assets from health-care expenses are contributing factors for some.
9. **d.** Ethnicity is defined by personal traits or common characteristics such as language or skin color relating to a specific group of people.
10. **d.** Authoritative parenting focuses on the setting of rules and limits setting for the child.

 CHAPTER 6

Nursing Process in Mental Health

1. **a.** The nursing process is a systematic way of collecting data for consistency in patient care. **b** and **c** are incorrect, even though nurses do document patient needs and RN and LPN/LVN roles are different in the nursing process. Patient needs are not usually documented as part of the nursing process per se. **d** is incorrect because the nurse needs to know the difference between medical and nursing care before writing the nursing process. Only nursing care is incorporated into the nursing process.
2. **c.** This is the best choice of those listed. It asks what you need to know, but it asks from the patient's perspective. It is less judgmental than the other choices.
3. **b.** Return demonstration (re-demonstration) is the best method for evaluating the patient's learning. **a** is a method of teaching. **c** and **d** are steps in the nursing process and steps in developing a teaching plan.
4. **a.** Mental status examinations are made as part of the assessment or data collection part of the nursing process.
5. **a, b.** Planning is the third component in the nursing process. In the planning process the

nurse plans measurable and realistic goals, both for long and short term.

6. **a.** The RN initiates the nursing diagnosis from the patient's data collection or assessment. The LPN/LVN can assist in this step.

7. **a, b, d.** The principle of teaching enhances the patient's understanding of the nurses' rationale for the specific interventions in their care.

8. **a, b, d, e.** Tone is not part of the mental status examination.

9. **d.** The North American Nursing Diagnosis Association (NANDA-I) is a universal and systematic approach to define a person's needs according to his or her assessment using nursing diagnosis.

10. **d.** Formal teaching occurs when the patient is ready. The nurse can then prepare a teaching plan. The nurse will also schedule a specific time for teaching and feedback of the learned information.

CHAPTER 7

Stress, Coping, and Defense Mechanisms

1. **c.** Rationalization is the defense mechanism that sounds like "excuses."

2. **a.** Denial is the refusal to accept situations for what they really are. This is a classic example of denial.

3. **d.** This child is using compensation, which is finding some other strength that will make up for a real or imagined inadequacy.

4. **d.** He is "blaming" his wife for his actions rather than taking responsibility for his thoughts, feelings, and actions. By blaming, he is "projecting" his frustration and anger onto his wife to justify hitting her.

5. **a.** Rationalization. Certainly, eating a meal of burgers and fries does not depict mental illness. Even though the person may be joking, and there is an element of truth, this statement depicts an "excuse" for one's behavior and choice of menu selection.

6. **b.** Undoing. This is a tricky one. Many may have chosen **c**, Symbolization. The reason this would be more likely an example of "undoing" is because Tara is trying to make up for a negative behavior that affected her daughter. Although words have not been spoken, there is not really an "emotion" that

is being represented, as would be the case in symbolization. Rather, Tara seems to be offering the tickets to "undo" the embarrassment she caused her daughter by her drunk and inappropriate public behavior.

7. **a, c, d.** Shirley is returning to a time when her stress level was minimal. Posing as an adolescent reminded her of being young and innocent. Shirley knew when she pouted at an earlier age that she got her way and was considered cute.

8. **c.** John blamed the search committee, who are all right handed, for denying him the job instead considering the possibility that he was not qualified.

9. **a.** For healthy outcomes, a person has to have effective coping to engage in selecting appropriate choices.

10. **b.** The personality is made up of these three components according to Freud's theory. Defense mechanisms are derived from the ego development of Freud's theory of personality.

CHAPTER 8

Medications and Other Therapies

1. **b.** Options **a**, **c**, and **d** are commonly seen in the crisis (or third) phase of crisis; feeling of well-being is observed in the pre-crisis phase of crisis, when the patient thinks and states that everything is "fine."

2. **d.** The patient needs to know that he or she is away from the stress, even if it is only temporary. The person may not be able to think rationally, and to hear that safety and help are being offered can be the start of stress reduction and intervention. The following explain why the other options are not correct. **a**: "Why" needs to be avoided when possible to decrease the chance of the statement sounding judgmental and making the patient feel defensive. **b**: Besides the fact that this is a closed-ended question, the person may not know the answer to this. It may, in fact, be one of the major causes of the stress that led to the crisis. **c**: This is an open-ended statement and will be valid to ask—later. As one of the first questions a person in crisis hears, it can lead to increased confusion and guilt. He or she might not have a clue as to what led to the

attack or may be blaming himself or herself needlessly. Because nobody deserves to be abused, asking the question of the person experiencing crisis can sound as though the nurse thinks the perpetrator had just cause to abuse.

3. **c.** Milieu is the therapeutic environment. It should be stress-free, or at least minimally stress-producing, and should make the patients feel comfortable to practice new, healthy behaviors. It might be locked, depending on the patients, but it is not required to be. The patients will not usually be hospitalized "for life" (however, some might be); a 72-hour hold situation should have a milieu that corresponds to the needs of the patient being held.

4. **b.** Electroconvulsive therapy (ECT) is not used to treat convulsive disorders. That is a mistake people make because of the name "electroconvulsive therapy." The treatment causes a light seizure but does not treat seizure disorders. **a**, **c**, and **d** are all true about ECT.

5. **d.** The use of psychoactive medications can change the person's ability to think and process information and help him or her to feel different about the situation, which may allow other therapies to work in adjunct to the medication, to help the person toward wellness. These medications do not cure mental illness. They are used for more than just violent behavior, and although they may have an effect on pain receptors, that is a side effect rather than a primary use for this group of medications.

6. **c.** Patients treated with the monoamine oxidase inhibitors (MAOI) group of medications should avoid certain foods and beverages that contain tyramine to avoid hypertensive crisis.

7. **b.** One of the goals of crisis intervention is to decrease anxiety. The person may feel a temporary increase in anxiety (e.g., at the time of being arrested or taken to the "detox" center), but that should resolve fairly quickly with effective intervention.

8. **a.** Repression is a defense mechanism and is therefore counterproductive in therapy. All other choices are correct.

9. **b.** The antianxiety drugs are potentially addictive. Patients with addictive tendencies may become addicted to these medications more easily than they would to drugs from other categories.

10. **c.** Antidepressants all carry a Food and Drug Administration (FDA) black box warning that these medications may increase suicide risk in children and adolescents.

 CHAPTER 9

Complementary and Alternative Treatment Modalities

1. **c.** The definition of an alternative therapy is one that is used in place of conventional medicine. **a** suggests that such therapy has no value, which is very dependent upon the patient's beliefs. **b** is the definition of complementary therapies. **d** is incorrect; many cultures and people use alternative modalities as first-line treatment for all types of illness.

2. **d.** Complementary therapies are used with conventional medicine. **a** is vague; medical treatment is not defined simply by Western standards. **b** is incorrect because a model refers to a picture of an idea. **c** infers that conventional medicine is holistic, when in fact it is disease-oriented.

3. **a.** Integrative refers to the use of conventional and less traditional methods in harmony. **b** is incorrect because such combinations are not exclusive to any one belief system. **c** would leave the decision making to a physician without patient input, which is not holistic. **d**: Biofeedback is a complementary therapy.

4. **d.** The mind-body connection correctly describes why belief and expectation have an effect on health and disease. **a** is an incorrect definition; complementary therapies are used with conventional medicine. **b** is an opinion based on the notion that the mind and body operate independently of one another. **c** describes a treatment modality rather than a mechanism.

5. **b.** Regardless of the nurse's own feelings, remaining open and supportive encourages communication and rapport. **a** would have the effect of destroying rapport by making Mrs. Lucas wrong for her beliefs. **c** might be better reported to the physician for his decision. **d** would have the LPN/LVN

performing well outside of his or her scope of practice in most states.

6. **d, e, f.** Aromatherapy, Reiki, and massage are either alternative or complementary. In **a**, **b**, and **c**, ECT, hypnotherapy, and psychotherapy are considered conventional.

7. **a.** Reiki is a therapy involving energy manipulation and unblocking energy flow. **b**, **c**, and **d** are all forms of massage therapy.

8. **a.** Trance *is* an altered state of consciousness, but it is assuredly *not* sleep. Much of the therapeutic value of the work done in trance is lost if the client falls asleep. **b**, **c**, and **d** are all correct statements about trance.

9. **c.** This statement uses "see" and "clearly" to communicate that the speaker prefers a visual channel. Through the predicates "feels good" and "gut feeling" in **a**, the speaker reveals a kinesthetic channel preference. In **b**, the speaker demonstrates an auditory preference through the predicates "sounds good" and "paying attention to." **d** reflects the rarely used olfactory preference; many practitioners treat these predicates as kinesthetic for therapeutic purposes.

10. **b.** Presupposing, or assuming, that the patient will not improve will directly and indirectly negatively affect the thoughts, feelings, and actions of the nurse as well as the patient. Often, mentally ill patients are more sensitive to unspoken assumption, especially when it is communicated nonverbally. **a**, **c**, and **d** will positively effect unspoken communication and improve chances for better rapport.

CHAPTER 10

Anxiety, Somatic Symptom Disorders, and Post-Traumatic Stress Disorder

1. **b.** The vividness of the description suggests that the person is having a flashback. Auditory hallucinations would most likely involve "voices" or "hearing" the guns. Delusions of grandeur might cause the person to go after the people with guns, while being unarmed himself or herself. Free-floating anxiety would be less descriptive. The person would not know the cause of the anxiety.

2. **d.** SSD (somatic symptom disorder) is the most likely of those listed. Somatic symptom disorder (SSD) is characterized by bodily symptoms that are either very distressing or that result in significant disruption of functioning and are accompanied by excessive and disproportionate thoughts, feelings, and behaviors regarding those symptoms. To be diagnosed with SSD, an individual must be persistently symptomatic (typically for at least 6 months). Physical symptoms are not the hallmark symptoms of the other diagnoses listed.

3. **d.** This is the best of the four choices because you are simply stating for the patient to relax. You are helping him reoxygenate and refocus and you are calming him by offering to stay with him. It also buys you some time to make a visual assessment. **a** would be appropriate nursing actions, but not as the first priority. Your first actions need to be to calm the patient and continue to assess. **b** and **c** are nontherapeutic responses.

4. **b, c, d.** Multiple personality disorder (also known as dissociative identity disorder) is considered to be a dissociative disorder rather than an anxiety disorder. Some theorists believe that the dissociative disorders are also anxiety disorders, but most are now differentiating the two types of disorders. Depressive disorders are a separate diagnosis.

5. **d.** Individuals with PTSD usually go to lengths to avoid stimuli associated with a traumatic event, although **a** and **c** could be seen in these individuals but not the most common symptoms. **b** would be unlikely given the diagnosis.

6. **d.** Phobia is an irrational fear that cannot be changed by reason or logic. The patient usually understands it is irrational, but the fear remains.

7. **b.** Agoraphobia is fear of open spaces, so a shopping mall can be a trigger.

8. **a, b, c, e.** Venlafaxine (Effexor) is an antidepressant.

9. **c.** Acrophobia is a form of specific phobia because it is fear of a specific situation (heights).

10. **a, e, f.** are *not* appropriate nursing interventions. Stimuli should be diminished to

decrease the stressors present. All changes in behavior and responses to treatment should be documented. Activities should be encouraged, but only those that are enjoyable and do not produce additional stress. People need to acknowledge the stressors and deal with them. Avoiding or creating "diversion" is not the best nursing care. Creating an environment where individuals feel comfortable and want to participate in activities is more therapeutic.

CHAPTER 11

Depressive Disorders

1. **a.** This is selective reflecting. You have repeated the patient's exact words in a way that encourages her to either explain herself or rephrase her response in some way. **b**, **c**, and **d** are all blocks to therapeutic communication. **b** is challenging her, **c** uses the word "why," and **d** is giving advice.
2. **b.** Selective serotonin reuptake inhibitors like Zoloft typically take anywhere from 2 to 6 weeks to affect target symptoms like sadness, low energy, loss of appetite, and negative thoughts.
3. **c.** Communicating in a judgmental manner is always a block to therapeutic, helping relationships.
4. **c.** Major depression usually manifests itself with symptoms of extreme sadness, which is the prevalent mood for a period of at least 2 weeks. Euphoria would be more indicative of bipolar depression.
5. **d.** This is false reassurance, which is never appropriate in therapeutic relationships. The other choices are all appropriate nursing interventions for a person who is depressed.
6. **b.** Patients taking MAOIs must avoid processed foods to avoid a hypertensive crisis.
7. **d.** Rather than pressure the patient to socialize, sitting with the patient shows acceptance and readiness to listen when the patient talks.
8. **c.** Though symptoms of depression are quite normal, using an open-ended sentence demonstrates concern about the changes in behavior.
9. **b.** You want to know more about the patient's changes in behavior before jumping into a plan of action.

10. **a.** Though men frequently suffer from depression, it is more common in women.

CHAPTER 12

Bipolar Disorders

1. **b.** Dehydration can precipitate serious side effects from lithium, including tremors, seizures, and coma.
2. **d.** One of the main side effects of lithium is dehydration and fluid and electrolyte imbalance. Her dry lips, staggering gait, and feeling confused could all be symptoms of dehydration and sodium depletion. We do not have enough information about this situation to know if other factors are involved, such as taking incorrect dose.
3. **a.** Delusions of grandeur are evidenced by the patient believing that the mayor is seeking out her opinion. This is unlikely and demonstrates an unrealistic sense of self-importance.
4. **a.** 1.0 to 1.5 mEq/L is the therapeutic serum concentration for acute mania. For maintenance the level is usually lower.
5. **b.** Olanzapine is an antipsychotic. It may be used in the treatment of psychotic behavior in bipolar disorder but may be used in combination with a mood stabilizer.
6. **b.** By encouraging the patient to reflect on past disappointments, you are encouraging focus on what the person has been through. At the same time you are not negating the positive feeling he/she has now. Neither are you reinforcing unrealistic thinking.
7. **d.** The manic patient needs foods that are easy to eat while pacing or moving around. The other foods require the patient to sit down for a meal, and the patient may not be able to do that.
8. **c.** Given these choices, this patient would benefit from medication to help prevent injury from hyperactivity.
9. **d.** To be given the diagnosis of bipolar II the individual must have recurrent depression with bouts of hypomania. The other choices contain incorrect information.
10. **a.** Stimulants could easily precipitate a manic episode or intensify a current one. All the others may be utilized effectively.

11. **a.** Cyclothymic disorder is a chronic mood disturbance of at least a 2-year duration involving numerous episodes of hypomania and depressed mood but of less intensity.

 CHAPTER 13

Suicide

1. **d.** Teaching skills to help the patient deal with the problems of day-to-day life will be helpful in the long run. **b** is a mistake made by people who believe the myth that some suicide attempts are not serious. **c** is a block to therapeutic communication (disagreeing) and may give false hope. The patient does not see that there is much to live for, or the suicide would probably not have been attempted. **a** is also incorrect because reporting the patient to the police is not required in most communities and could be a threat to the patient.

2. **b.** People are more likely to carry out the suicide when they appear to feel better. This is when they have the energy to create a plan and carry it out. When they are deeply depressed or confused, they often are not able to think clearly enough to do these things. When people feel loved and appreciated, they are less likely to think about suicide. This may be a temporary feeling on their part, however.

3. **c.** If a person is talking about suicide, the possibility for carrying it out is very real and must be taken seriously. In very few situations is suicidal ideation a manipulative or attention-seeking behavior. Suicide may be an impulsive act but the person has usually been thinking about it for some time.

4. **d.** This man has definite potential for self-harm. He is not attempting to manipulate his wife's feelings, although she may feel that he is.

5. **b.** Your first action is to place the patient on one-on-one observation. Some facilities accomplish this by having staff perform rounds at a minimum of every 15 minutes; most facilities assign a staff person to stay with the patient. There is no need to place the patient in a locked unit at this time, nor is it appropriate to publicize the precautions to the whole facility. It would not be appropriate to give him his razor, as this could be an implement he could use to perform the suicide.

6. **c.** Document the discussion but explain that the precautions will remain in effect. It is for his safety and the safety of others that the precautions are policy, generally. You may thank him for sharing his beliefs, and depending on where he is in his treatment, it may become appropriate for him to share his belief system with others.

7. **b.** Older men who live alone with a history of alcohol abuse are at one of the highest risks for suicide. Though any of the other examples could be suicidal, they do not represent the most frequent statistically.

8. **d.** This response is supportive and empathetic. **a** and **b** reflect insensitivity to the patient's distress. Asking the question of response **c** has nothing to do with the depth of distress this patient must have felt, so it is inappropriate.

9. **b.** By asking the patient directly what she plans to do you are gaining important information and communicating your concern to the patient. Because she told you her plan, you know she is reaching out for help.

10. **a.** By reaching out to you, she is communicating her mixed feelings about suicide and is indirectly asking for help.

 CHAPTER 14

Personality Disorders

1. **d.** Consequences should always be stated at the time the limits are set, to increase consistency. The problems with **a** through **c** are as follows. **a**: When the behavior occurs, the patient may be testing, but if the consequences are not known, the patient has not been given enough information to make an appropriate choice. **b**: Anticipating a behavior is presuming, and you may be presuming incorrectly. This sets up negative expectations from the patient. **c**: The limits should not be set for the convenience of the staff or family or anyone but the patient. Family should be involved in the care plan if the patient is agreeable.

2. **c.** David is most likely displaying signs of antisocial personality disorder evidenced by information that he tends to lie and has

committed a crime, and his patterns with job and personal relationships. He is not exhibiting signs of suspiciousness or paranoia, nor is he behaving in a dependent manner.

3. **a.** Manipulation is used frequently by patients with personality disorders. This mechanism can be used with other disorders but it is a primary mechanism in personality disorders.

4. **b.** Compliance with established norms is particularly difficult for someone with antisocial personality disorder. Interpersonal relationships can be challenging, but these patients can participate in group activities because they can excel and bring attention and gratification to themselves.

5. **c.** Antisocial (sociopathic) personality disorder is usually the type of disorder in which a person would be in trouble with the law.

6. **b.** Schizotypal personality disorder is characterized by bizarre and unusual behaviors—some of which may be also seen in schizophrenia.

7. **c.** The nurse needs to understand how he or she reacts to the challenging behaviors exhibited by people with personality disorders. Medications, long-term therapy, and in-patient hospitalization are rarely effective.

8. **c.** Characteristics of narcissistic personality disorder include exaggerated sense of self-importance and lack of concern for the nurse's time.

9. **d.** Vague communication is not acceptable. Honesty and clarity in communication are always necessary. The patient may feel inferior, which may be part of the manipulation. The nurse needs to confront the feelings of inferiority or any others that the patient might state.

10. **b.** Borderline personality. This group tends to engage in self-mutilating behaviors.

 CHAPTER 15

Schizophrenia Spectrum and Other Psychotic Disorders

1. **d.** Inviting the patient to the party brings him into the present and allows him to make the choice for himself. This will help increase self-esteem and diminish other symptoms. **a** reinforces the hallucinations, which is

never appropriate for nurses. **b** and **c** are forms of demands, which may cause the patient to revert to negative and possibly aggressive behaviors.

2. **a.** Shawna's symptoms are consistent with patients who have catatonic schizophrenia. **d**, schizotypal, is a type of personality disorder but not actually a form of schizophrenia.

3. **a.** This is an example of a hallucination. The patient is seeing something that is not there. There is nothing actually visible that could be misinterpreted as a snake; if there were, this would be an illusion.

4. **c.** This is the honest response, and it focuses on returning the patient to reality. The other responses play into the hallucination or border on belittling the patient.

5. **c.** Patients with schizophrenia do not function well in society without treatment. Even with treatment, some patients have a difficult time. The "reality" of schizophrenic people is their *own* reality and not the reality of the rest of society.

6. **b.** It is important always to deal with reality and the present when dealing with people with schizophrenia. Never reinforcing hallucinations and directing people away from situations that are stressful or competitive are also important.

7. **b.** This time you are dealing with an illusion. There is something on the ceiling, and the patient is misinterpreting what is there.

8. **c.** Once again, maintaining honesty and reality is the best response.

9. **a.** Echolalia is the behavior or symptom of catatonic schizophrenia involving the patient repeating a word or part of a word or phrase over and over. Echopraxia is repetitive movement or actions.

10. **a.** Delusions of grandeur include believing one is not subject to the laws of nature.

11. **a.** Muscle rigidity and protruding tongue are classic symptoms of extrapyramidal symptoms (EPS) in addition to restlessness and tremors.

12. **c.** Decreasing anxiety and promoting trust are both realistic goals. Both of these are a process that can be helped over time.

13. **a.** We now know that schizophrenia is a brain abnormality.

CHAPTER 16

Neurocognitive Disorders: Delirium and Dementia

1. **b.** Delirium is probably the best choice, because the patient presented as alert and oriented before surgery. Nothing indicates dementia at this point. She is not delusional; she is having a hallucination. The dilemma may be in what the nurse chooses to do next.

2. **a.** Your best action is to call your charge nurse and/or the physician immediately. Your state Nurse Practice Act will dictate whom you should call first. Turning on the light may be helpful, but asking about the spiders plays into the hallucination, which is not therapeutic. Stopping the patient's pain medications is not an independent nursing function; you need to make that call to the physician first. Checking her medical record should have been done earlier, and it will not be helpful to her right now.

3. **c.** By reflecting back to Mrs. H your observation, you are promoting good communication and emotional support. The other choices are all blocks to therapeutic or helping communication.

4. **b.** Aricept can cause insomnia. It can also cause bradycardia, not tachycardia.

5. **d.** Although Alzheimer's type dementia is not a result of aging or arteriosclerosis, these conditions may be present in addition to the dementia.

6. **c.** You would expect to see memory and other cognitive processes impaired in someone with an organic mental disorder. The person will probably not be oriented to at least one of the three spheres of person, place, or time.

7. **b.** Donepezil, galantamine, and rivastigmine are cholinesterase inhibitors. Memantine is not a cholinesterase inhibitor. Haloperidol and chlorpromazine are antipsychotics.

8. **c** This is the best option. You are showing concern for the patient, the family, and their situation. You have stated the implied message and offered to get the physician, who must be the one to give the initial information. You have maintained dignity for all, while behaving professionally.

9. **d.** Vascular or multi-infarct dementia is usually the result of several smaller strokes. The patient has usually had conditions such as high blood pressure for quite some time. The condition displays many of the same behaviors as other types of dementia but is also usually irreversible.

10. **d.** The patient with delirium receives the greatest benefit from reorientation techniques. In advanced dementia, repeated attempts at orientation can contribute to anxiety.

CHAPTER 17

Substance Use and Addictive Disorders

1. **c.** Denial is the most common defense mechanism used by people who are chemically dependent. Rationalization is also used by some patients.

2. **a.** Alcohol is a central nervous system (CNS) depressant that can lead to impaired judgment, confusion, lethargy, and coma in large amounts, The "high" that people feel is temporary and very misleading.

3. **d.** Tremors, confusion, and hallucinations are the classic symptoms of delirium tremens (DT).

4. **d.** Sally may very well be codependent in her sister's alcohol abuse. Sally is taking responsibility for Susie's behavior instead of having Susie take care of herself.

5. **b.** This response addresses both sisters and tells them they both need help. It is honest and caring, and puts the responsibility on them to help themselves through this situation.

6. **a.** Susie should be encouraged to attend weekly Alcoholics Anonymous (AA) meetings and Sally to attend weekly Al-Anon meetings. We do not know from the information if they are adult children of alcoholics. There is no need to check into the unit weekly, but they can be told that it is acceptable to call or check in if they choose to do so. The psychologist will tell them the meeting schedule; this would not be a nursing function for discharge planning.

7. **c.** These behaviors are the classic ones that indicate an addiction.

8. **a.** Honest communication is necessary for the person and family to heal.

9. **b.** Codependent. In an effort to be caring, you are inadvertently making excuses and encouraging the drinking behavior.

10. **b.** Chlordiazepoxide is often used to safely detoxify a person from heavy alcohol use. It is relatively safe and reduces the risk for complications from alcohol such as seizures.

11. **d.** AA is a lifelong commitment as one admits powerlessness over alcohol and remains in need of this support.

12. **a.** Methamphetamine abuse often includes appetite suppression and weight loss.

 ## CHAPTER 18

Eating Disorders

1. **c.** Anorexia nervosa is the fear of food. Bulimia nervosa is termed "binge eating." Pica is an eating disorder seen in young children.

2. **b.** This response is therapeutic—demonstrating your efforts to help the patient identify the feelings she experiences when trying to eat. **a** and **d** are threats, and appetite stimulants are not useful because the disorder is unrelated to appetite.

3. **b.** Patients who have anorexia have an intense fear of being fat. They have an inaccurate sense of their size and body image and will not develop normal eating patterns without much help and behavior modification.

4. **a.** A nutritional deficit, and probably a fluid imbalance, exists in patients who are anorectic. The fluid imbalance is caused by the lack of intake and perhaps vomiting. There is also a body image disturbance, but it is a negative self-perception rather than a positive one.

5. **d.** Unlocking the feelings surrounding an eating disorder can be very helpful to the patient and treatment team. Focusing on the food and the destructive behaviors associated with the food puts the emphasis on the wrong area.

6. **c.** Patients with bulimia nervosa cannot control their eating. They binge and purge, and they are overly concerned and preoccupied with body shape and size.

7. **d.** This statement conveys your desire to help with ANY concern this patient may have postoperatively. The other options do show a concern and interest in this patient, but focusing on food and weight may limit the

patient's willingness to offer other needs. The patient may also not be ready to talk about weight yet. This is a hopeful yet traumatic step for many.

8. **b.** This response is a combination of the therapeutic techniques of parroting and open-ended question. It uses the patient's words and leaves the question open for Donald to elaborate. The other choices are nontherapeutic and do not allow for patient expression.

9. **c.** These are the classic symptoms of bulimia.

10. **c.** After binging, the person seeks a release of tension related to shame and guilt by purging.

 ## CHAPTER 19

Childhood and Adolescent Mental Health Issues

1. **b.** Safety for children with conduct disorder is primary in importance. Chances are that the child will not settle quickly, and asking the parent to leave with the child is not a supportive action for either the parent or child.

2. **c.** Exposing the child to one new person rather than several will help the child develop a relationship. More than one person and touching the child may increase anxiety. Isolating the child will reinforce fears.

3. **d.** Children often act out or draw pictures about what is troubling them. Offering toys or drawing materials and observing the child discreetly can tell you much about what he or she has experienced. It may also serve as a diversion, but offering toys or drawing materials is meant to encourage self-expression rather than serve as a diversion from the situation.

4. **d.** Physical activity is a good outlet for the attention deficit-hyperactivity disorder (ADHD) child. Checkers and video games are too sedentary, and pool requires concentration that may be difficult for the child.

5. **b.** CNS stimulants are effective with ADHD to increase levels of neurotransmitters to elicit a calming effect.

6. **d.** All of these choices apply to ADHD.

7. **b.** The most common symptom of autism is impaired social functioning. The patient does not make strong friendships. Emotions

may be completely opposite of what would be appropriate, and the patient may achieve an appropriate developmental task and then regress, or may not achieve appropriate developmental tasks at all.

8. **c.** This is the best choice of the options listed, because it implies the nurse heard the parents' concerns and recognized the need to get them appropriate help right away. The other options are either nontherapeutic or provide false hope to the parents. They may sound polite but are not helpful for the parents, who are concerned they did something wrong and want to know how they can help their child.

9. **c.** Chaotic home life is a common thread in children with conduct disorder.

10. **c.** The FDA has issued a black box warning on all antidepressants to monitor children and teens for suicide when taking these medications.

CHAPTER 20

Postpartum Issues in Mental Health

1. **b.** Projecting evilness onto the infant is a sign of postpartum psychosis. The other responses are all normal reflections of anxiety about the baby or the mother.

2. **d.** Highly labile emotions related to the baby are a common sign of postpartum blues. **b** and **c** are signs of more serious disorders that could affect the infant's care. **a** is a normal concern of a new mother.

3. **b.** Postpartum blues usually start a few days after birth. These blues are common and not a psychiatric diagnosis, nor do they reflect problems in bonding.

4. **a.** Postpartum depression is closely related to depression in a previous pregnancy. The other choices may be factors that could contribute to depression but are not the most important cause. The other responses are not appropriate.

5. **b.** Giving the new mother information on this being a normal response is an important intervention.

6. **b.** The major concern with a history of bipolar disorder in a pregnant woman is the high risk for recurrence, and it is also a major contributor to postpartum psychosis.

7. **b.** This statement is concerning that this new mother may be progressing to depression or some other disorder. More follow-up and support are needed. **c** could be an indicator of a postpartum psychosis. **a** and **d** are more likely to be associated with postpartum blues.

8. **b.** Mood stabilizers have been linked to malformations in neonates.

9. **c.** Antidepressants are effective for treatment of postpartum depression. The other responses are inaccurate. Diet and exercise may be helpful in depression but would not be the major treatment for this psychiatric disorder.

10. **d.** All of these choices must be addressed in postpartum psychosis. This is an emergency for safety of the newborn.

CHAPTER 21

Aging Population

1. **b.** Reinforce the word by showing or handling the object. Trying to guess the word or finishing the patient's sentence can be frustrating and insulting and can discourage the patient from attempting to communicate. Asking the patient to think about the word while you do something else is distracting.

2. **d.** Federal regulations require that the assessment be conducted by an RN for purposes of consistency. All other people on the healthcare team supply input and documentation to assist with the assessment.

3. **c.** Medication side effect would be the most obvious possibility, as the medication is a recent change in routine, and normal vital signs should help rule out the possibility of a recent stroke. Depression is a more distant possibility.

4. **c.** You have been assertive and told the patient what you wanted in a way that encouraged the patient to participate in a specific activity. This also supports the person's self-esteem.

5. **b.** The losses experienced as people age are frequent causes of depression.

6. **d.** Dementia is not a part of normal aging. Other possibilities for unusual behavior should be ruled out before diagnosing a person with dementia.

7. **b.** Aphasia is the speech complication that often results from stroke. Affect can also change after a stroke, but that is not a speech difficulty.

8. **b.** Drugs are metabolized more slowly in older people, which results in a cumulative effect that leads to toxicity.

9. **c.** These could be symptoms of elder abuse. The location of the bruises is consistent with shaking or beating. The lack of eye contact or verbal response indicates that the patient may be in fear. More investigation is needed or the beatings might get worse.

10. **d.** OBRA stands for Omnibus Budget Reconciliation Act. It establishes standards for the care of the older adult.

11. **b.** Progressive memory loss is not a normal part of aging. When memory loss is apparent, evaluation of the causes and nursing interventions to deal with it are important.

12. **a.** Providing support to a coworker is most important. The other choices are more clinical questions.

 ## CHAPTER 22

Abuse and Violence

1. **d.** Showing empathy for the patient, offering to provide further assistance, and reassuring safety will help the patient to trust you and probably to be more comfortable and compliant with examinations.

2. **b.** Getting a statement in the patient's own words and documenting it in the medical record are required. **a** is information that the patient may not know. The word "why" is counterproductive in therapeutic communication. **c** is not recommended for reasons of liability for both the nurse and the patient. It is most likely a violation of your agency policy as well as a violation of professional ethics. **d** is inappropriate as it has nothing to do with the rape.

3. **c.** You need to be helpful to both people. You will need to take care of the physical and emotional health of both patients, and you will do it according to the degree of immediacy called for. A physician must be called if one is not in the area, but until he or she arrives, your nursing care, observation, and documentation will help ensure the best possible care for the patients.

4. **c.** You let Mrs. X know that you hear her concern and need for help. You are offering the best help you can at the moment, while allowing her to make the decision about speaking to the social worker.

5. **c.** Although some patients may express displeasure at someone going ahead, most will realize something is terribly wrong. Apologize for their inconvenience and have someone assist them as soon as possible. Attending to this woman, her immediate needs, and those of her children is the best nursing choice. You may also let her know that someone will be in who can help her with safety issues, but it is important to get her in a quiet, safe room. After all, the perpetrator may be right behind her. She knows that.

6. **a.** You are showing empathy, being nonjudgmental, and offering the patient assistance. Offering to her that she needs to leave sounds helpful and may be true, but she has to make that decision on her own. The organization you offered her in option **a** may assist with that as well. "Why" is a nontherapeutic response. Asking if he has done that before does make an attempt at gathering information and showing concern, but the more immediate need now is to support her and offer her some options for assistance.

7. **c.** There is evidence to indicate the possibility of the abuse cycle. All the other responses may be accurate, but there is not enough information to determine this. This woman may believe she must return to the home where abuse is probably occurring.

8. **c.** Physical and emotional support is the most important initial intervention. The other interventions may be needed later in the visit. Bathing should not happen until samples have been taken.

9. **b.** Rape is an act of violence and not related to sexual desire.

10. **b.** The son may need to see the will to obtain information for financial planning of patient's resources. **a** and **c** indicate the caregiver is overstepping his/her boundaries. The nurse would need more information to determine whether **d** is appropriate.

APPENDIX B
Agencies That Help People Who Have Threats to Their Mental Health

1. **National Institute of Mental Health (NIMH)**
   6001 Executive Blvd
   Bethesda, MD 20892-9663
   (301) 443-4513; 1-866-615-6464;
       301-443-8431 (TTY)
   Fax: (301) 443-4279
   www.nimh.nih.gov

2. **Depression and Bipolar Support Alliance**
   55 E. Jackson Blvd, Suite 490
   Chicago, IL 60604
   (800) 826-3632; Fax: (312) 642-7243
   www.dbsalliance.org

3. **National Alliance on Mental Illness**[*]
   4301 Wilson Blvd
   Suite 300
   Arlington, VA 22203
   Main: (703) 524-7600;
   Helpline: (800) 950-6264
   www.nami.org

4. **Child Welfare Information Gateway**
   Children's Bureau/ACYF
   330 C St SW
   Washington, DC 20201
   www.childwelfare.gov/

5. **Mental Health America (MHA)**
   500 Montgomery St, Suite 820
   Alexandria, VA 22314
   Phone: (800) 969-6642; Fax: (703) 684-5968
   www.mentalhealthamerica.net

6. **American Association of Retired Persons (AARP)**
   601 E. St NW
   Washington, DC 20049
   (888) 687-2277
   www.aarp.org/retirement

7. **National Hospice & Palliative Care Organization (NHPCO)**
   1731 King St
   Alexandria, VA 22314
   Phone: (703) 837-1500; Fax: (703) 837-1233
   www.nhpco.org

8. **National Eating Disorders Association**
   200 W. 42nd St
   New York, NY 10036
   (800) 931-2237
   nationaleatingdisorders.org

9. **Child Abuse Prevention Association**
   503 E. 23rd St
   Independence, MO 64055
   (816) 252-8388; Fax (816) 252-1337
   www.childabuseprevention.org

10. **Alcoholics Anonymous**
    AA World Services, Inc
    PO Box 459, Grand Central Station
    New York, NY 10163
    (212) 870-3400
    http://aa.org

11. **Active Minds (college based)**
    2001 S. St NW, Suite 630
    Washington, DC 20009
    (202) 332-9595
    http://www.activeminds.org/
    This organization supports student activism in mental health

12. **International OCD Foundation**
    PO Box 961029
    Boston, MA 02196
    (617) 973-5801
    https://iocdf.org/

---

[*] Most states have a chapter of National Alliance on Mental Illness (NAMI) as well.

13. **Trevor Project (LGBTQ)**
    PO Box 69232
    West Hollywood, CA 90069
    (212) 695-8650
    http://www.thetrevorproject.org
    Support programs for LGBTQ youth
14. **Pacer's National Bullying Prevention Center**
    8161 Normandale Blvd
    Bloomington, MN 55437
    (800) 537-2237
    http://www.pacer.org/bullying/
15. **American Academy of Child & Adolescent Psychiatry**
    3615 Wisconsin Ave NW
    Washington, DC 20016-3007
    https://www.aacap.org//
    Phone: (202) 966-7300

16. **The Jed Foundation**
    530 7th Ave, Suite 801
    New York, NY 10018
    https://jedfoundation.org/
    Phone: (212) 647-7544
    Network with teens, young adults, and college students with mental health and emotional issues

APPENDIX C
Organizations That Support the Licensed Practical/Vocational Nurse

The following is a partial list of organizations that support and foster the role of the licensed practical nurse (LPN)/licensed vocational nurse (LVN) in the United States.

1. National Association for Practical Nurse Education and Service (NAPNES)
   2071 N Bechtle Ave, #307
   Springfield, OH 45504-1583
   Phone: 703-933-1003
   Fax: 703-940-4089
   www.napnes.org

   NAPNES is the oldest association that advocates for the practice, education, and regulation of practical and vocational nurses, practical nursing schools, practical nursing educators, and students. NAPNES has consistent state members throughout the United States. Publications: *Journal of Practical Nursing.*

2. National Association of Licensed Practical Nurses (NALPN)
   P.O. Box 1895
   Manitowoc, WI 54221
   (920) 663-8450
   nalpn.org

   The mission of the NALPN is to foster high standards of nursing care and to promote continued competence through education/certification and lifelong learning, with a focus on public protection.

   NALPN is committed to quality and professionalism in the delivery of nursing care, working with other organizations and groups in a cooperative progressive spirit to build strong professional and public relationships.

3. American Psychiatric Nurses Association (APNA)
   3141 Fairview Park Dr, Suite 625
   Falls Church, VA 22042
   (855) 863-APNA (2762); Fax: (855) 883-APNA (2762)
   www.apna.org

   APNA is a resource for psychiatric mental health nursing. It offers affiliate memberships for LPN/LVNs.

4. American Association for Men in Nursing (AAMN)
   2511 8th St S
   Wisconsin Rapids, WI 54494
   (929) 515-4945
   www.aamn.org

   Founded in 1973, the purpose of AAMN is to provide a framework for nurses, as a group, to meet and to discuss and influence factors that affect men as nurses. Check the Web site for local chapter information.

5. National Coalition of Ethnic Minority Nurse Associations Inc. (NCEMNA)
   6101 West Centinela Ave, Suite 378
   Culver City, CA 90230
   (310) 258-9515; Fax: (310) 258-9513
   https://ncemna.org

   NCEMNA is a national collaboration of ethnic minority nurse associations. NCEMNA, Inc. is made up of five national ethnic nurse associations: Asian American/Pacific Islander Nurses Association, Inc. (AAPINA); National Alaska Native American Indian Nurses Association, Inc. (NANAINA); National Association of Hispanic Nurses, Inc. (NAHN); National Black Nurses Association, Inc. (NBNA); and the Philippine Nurses Association of America, Inc. (PNAA).
   a. AAPINA
      (contact through NCEMNA Web site https:// ncemna.org)

      An organization for Asian American Pacific Islanders, organized in 1992. AAPINA's goal is to network with AAPI nurses and students worldwide, to identify their health-care needs, and to provide essential health-care education.

b. NANAINA
2004 Randolph Ave
St. Paul, MN 55105
(612) 227-4709
https://nanaina.org/
    NANAINA was organized in 1993 in North Dakota. NANAINA's goal is to improve health care for American Indians and Alaskan Natives

c. NAHN
201 E. Main St, Suite 1405
Lexington, Kentucky 40507
(859) 469-5800
www.nahnnet.org
    NAHN is an active and vocal advocate for licensed Hispanic nurses, advocating for policy changes and offering unique perspectives related to Hispanic health-care needs.

d. NBNA
8630 Fenton St, Suite 910
Silver Spring, MD 20910-3803
(301) 589-3200; Fax: (301) 589-3223
www.nbna.org
    The NBNA's mission is to "represent and provide a forum for black nurses to advocate and implement strategies to ensure access to the highest quality of healthcare for persons of color." Local chapters are available in many regions.

e. PNAA
1346 How Lane, Suite 109-110
North Brunswick, NJ 08902
https://mypnaa.wildapricot.org/
    PNAA upholds the positive image and welfare of its constituent members, promotes professional excellence, and contributes to significant outcomes to health care and society as well as unifying Filipino-American nurses in the United States and its territories.

f. Hospice and Palliative Nurses Association
400 Lydia Street, Suite 103
Carnegie, PA 15106
(412) 787-9301
advancingexpertcare.org
    Advancing nursing expertise in hospice and palliative care through education, advocacy, leadership, and research. LVN/LPN membership level as well as certification. Check the Web site for local chapter information.

APPENDIX D
Standards of Nursing Practice for LPNs/LVNs

NATIONAL ASSOCIATION OF LICENSED PRACTICAL NURSES (NALPN) CODE FOR LICENSED PRACTICAL/VOCATIONAL NURSES

- Know the scope of maximum utilization of the licensed practical nurse (LPN)/licensed vocational nurse (LVN) as specified by the nursing practice act and function within its scope.
- Safeguard the confidential information acquired from any source about the patient.
- Provide health care to all patients regardless of race, creed, cultural background, disease, or lifestyle.
- Uphold the highest standards in personal appearance, language, dress, and demeanor.
- Stay informed about issues affecting the practice of nursing and delivery of health care and, where appropriate, participate in government and policy decisions.
- Accept the responsibility for safe nursing practice by keeping oneself mentally and physically fit and educationally prepared to practice.
- Accept the responsibility for membership in NALPN and participate in its efforts to maintain the established standards of nursing practice and employment policies that lead to quality patient care.

NALPN NURSING PRACTICE STANDARDS

Introductory Statement
Definition: Practical/vocational nursing means the performance for compensation of authorized acts of nursing that utilize specialized knowledge and skills and that meet the health needs of people in a variety of settings under the direction of qualified health professionals.

Scope: Practical/vocational nursing comprises the common case of nursing and, therefore, is a valid entry into the nursing profession.

Opportunities exist for practicing in a milieu where different professions unite their particular skills in a team effort for one common objective—to preserve or improve an individual patient's functioning.

Opportunities also exist for upward mobility within the profession through academic education and for lateral expansion of knowledge and expertise through both academic and continuing education.

Standards
Education
The licensed practical/vocational nurse:

1. Shall complete a formal education program in practical nursing approved by the appropriate nursing authority in a state.
2. Shall successfully pass the National Council Licensure Examination for Practical Nurses.
3. Shall participate in initial orientation within the employing institution.

Legal/Ethical Status
The licensed practical/vocational nurse:

1. Shall hold a current license to practice nursing as an LPN/LVN in accordance with the law of the state wherein employed.
2. Shall know the scope of nursing practice authorized by the Nurse Practice Act in the state wherein employed.
3. Shall have a personal commitment to fulfill the legal responsibilities inherent in good nursing practice.
4. Shall take responsible actions in situations wherein there is unprofessional conduct by a peer or other health-care provider.
5. Shall recognize and have a commitment to meet the ethical and moral obligations of the practice of nursing.
6. Shall not accept or perform professional responsibilities that the individual knows (s)he is not competent to perform.

Practice

The licensed practical/vocational nurse:

1. Shall accept assigned responsibilities as an accountable member of the health-care team.
2. Shall function within the limits of educational preparation and experience as related to the assigned duties.
3. Shall function with other members of the health-care team in promoting and maintaining health, preventing disease and disability, caring for and rehabilitating individuals who are experiencing an altered health state, and contributing to the ultimate quality of life until death.
4. Shall know and utilize the nursing process in planning (assessing [data gathering]), implementing, and evaluating health services and nursing care for the individual patient or group.
   a. Planning (assessing [data gathering]): The planning of nursing includes:
      - Assessment of health status of the individual patient, the family, and community groups
      - An analysis of the information gained from assessment
      - The identification of health goals
   b. Implementation: The plan for nursing care is put into practice to achieve the stated goals and includes:
      - Observing, recording, and reporting significant changes that require intervention or different goals
      - Applying nursing knowledge and skills to promote and maintain health, to prevent disease and disability, and to optimize functional capabilities of an individual patient
      - Assisting the patient and family with activities of daily living and encouraging self-care as appropriate
      - Carrying out therapeutic regimens and protocols prescribed by a registered (RN), physician, or other persons authorized by state law
   c. Evaluations: The plan for nursing care and its implementations are evaluated to measure the progress toward the stated goals and will include appropriate persons and/or groups to determine:
      - The relevancy of current goals in relation to the progress of the individual patient
      - The involvement of the recipients of care in the evaluation process
      - The quality of the nursing action in the implementation of the plan

- A reordering of priorities or new goal setting in the care plan

5. Shall participate in peer review and other evaluation processes.
6. Shall participate in the development of policies concerning the health and nursing needs of society and in the roles and functions of the LPN/LVN.

CONTINUING EDUCATION

The LPN/LVN:

1. Shall be responsible for maintaining the highest possible level of professional competence at all times.
2. Shall periodically reassess career goals and select continuing education activities that will help to achieve these goals.
3. Shall take advantage of continuing education opportunities that will lead to personal growth and professional development.
4. Shall seek and participate in continuing education activities that are approved for credit by appropriate organizations, such as the NALPN.

SPECIALIZED NURSING PRACTICE

The LPN/LVN:

1. Shall have had at least 1 year's experience in nursing at the staff level.
2. Shall present personal qualifications that are indicative of potential abilities for practice in the chosen specialized nursing area.
3. Shall present evidence of completion of a program or course that is approved by an appropriate agency to provide the knowledge and skills necessary for effective nursing services in the specialized field.
4. Shall meet all of the standards of practice as set forth in this document.

Source: National Association of Licensed Practice Nurses at http://nalpn.org/wp-content/uploads/2016/02/NALPN-Practice-Standards.pdf. Address: 3801 Lake Boone Trail, Suite 190, Raleigh, North Carolina 27607. Nursing Practice Standards for the Licensed Practical/Vocational Nurse. (2015). In *The National Voice of LPN's*. Retrieved from http://wildcatresourcesinc.com/wp-content/uploads/sites/38/2016/03/NALPN-Practice-Standards.pdf.

APPENDIX E
Assigning Nursing Diagnoses to Client Behaviors

Common behaviors are matched with examples of corresponding nursing diagnoses.

Behavior	Nursing Diagnosis
Aggression, hostility	Risk for injury; risk for other directed violence
Anorexia or refusal to eat	Impaired nutrition: Less than body requirements
Anxious behavior	Anxiety (specify level)
Confusion, memory loss	Confusion, acute/chronic; impaired memory; disturbed thought processes
Delusions	Disturbed thought processes
Denial of problems	Ineffective denial
Depressed mood or anger turned inward	Complicated grieving
Detoxification, withdrawal from substances	Risk for injury
Difficulty accepting new diagnosis or recent change in health status	Risk-prone health behavior
Difficulty making important life decision	Decisional conflict
Difficulty sleeping	Insomnia; disturbed sleep pattern
Difficulty with interpersonal relationships	Impaired social interactions; ineffective relationships
Disruption in capability to perform usual responsibilities	Ineffective role performance
Dissociative behaviors (depersonalization)	Disturbed sensory perception
Expresses feelings of disgust about body or body part	Disturbed body image
Expresses anger at God	Spiritual distress
Expresses lack of control over personal situation	Powerlessness
Fails to follow prescribed therapy	Ineffective self-health management; noncompliance
Flashbacks, nightmares, obsession with traumatic experience	Post-trauma response
Hallucinations	Disturbed sensory perceptions; disturbed thought processes

Continued

Behavior	Nursing Diagnosis
Highly critical of self or others	Low self-esteem (chronic, situational)
Inability to meet basic needs	Self-care deficit
Loose associations or flight of ideas	Disturbed thought processes
Loss of valued entity, recently experienced	Risk for complicated grieving
Manic hyperactivity	Risk for injury, disturbed thought processes
Manipulative behavior	Ineffective coping; impaired social interactions
Multiple personalities; gender dysphoria	Disturbed personal identity
Overeating, compulsive	Risk for imbalanced nutrition: More than body requirements
Phobias	Anxiety; fear
Physical symptoms as coping behavior	Ineffective coping
Potential or anticipated loss of significant entity	Grieving
Projection of blame, rationalization of failures, denial of personal responsibility	Defensive coping
Ritualistic behaviors	Anxiety; ineffective coping
Inappropriate sexual behaviors	Impaired social interaction
Self-inflicted injuries (non–life-threatening)	Self-mutilation; risk for self-mutilation
Sexual behaviors (difficulties, limitations, or changes in; reported dissatisfaction)	Ineffective sexuality pattern
Stress from caring for chronically ill person	Caregiver role strain
Substance use as a coping behavior	Ineffective coping; ineffective denial
Suicidal gestures, threats, ideation	Risk for suicide; risk for self-directed violence; hopelessness
Suspiciousness	Disturbed thought process; ineffective coping
Violent behavior	Risk for violence; ineffective coping; risk for injury
Vomiting, excessive, self-induced	Risk for deficient fluid volume
Withdrawn behavior	Social isolation

Source: Adapted from Townsend (2015): *Psychiatric Mental Health Nursing,* 8th ed.
Philadelphia: F.A. Davis Company, with permission.

Glossary

Abuse: Physical, verbal, or emotional mistreatment of self or others; misuse of chemicals, food, or other substances.

Abuser: One who mistreats others.

Accommodation: Process of adjusting one's schema to fit changing situations (Piaget).

Accountability: When a health-care worker accepts responsibility for any actions performed while caring for a patient.

Adaptation: The effective coping with changes that are external and internal.

Addiction: A chronic brain disease characterized by compulsive and maladaptive use of a substance or behavior (e.g., gambling).

Affect: The outward display or expression of a feeling or mood.

Ageism: Form of discrimination against people on the basis of age.

Aggressive communication: Form of communication that hurts another and is not self-responsible ("you" statements).

Agnosia: Loss of ability to recognize objects.

Agoraphobia: Intense fear of open spaces. This can be experienced in such circumstances as on public transportation, when left alone, or when in the middle of a crowd.

Agraphia: Difficulty writing and drawing.

Akathisia: Restlessness; an urgent need for movement.

Alcohol abuse: Compulsive use of alcohol usually lasting 1 month or longer.

Alcohol dependence: Improper use of alcohol with impairment of social or occupational functioning, which leads to signs of tolerance or withdrawal.

Alcoholism: A complex, progressive disease characterized by significant physical, social, and/or mental impairment directly related to alcohol dependence and addiction.

Alcohol use disorder: Term used by *DSM-5* to identify alcohol use that is severe enough to meet criteria for this diagnosis including

withdrawal symptoms. Previously was known as alcohol abuse or alcohol dependence.

Alternative medicine: Modalities that replace those of conventional medicine.

Alzheimer's disease: A form of progressive dementia.

Ambivalence: Contradictory feelings experienced at the same time.

American Nurses Association (ANA): A national nursing organization established for registered nurses.

American Psychiatric Nurses Association (APNA): A national nursing association dedicated to psychiatric mental health nursing.

Amygdala: Area of the brain that plays a role in the anxiety response, is involved in the "fight or flight" responses, and plays a role in memory.

Anhedonia: Inability to experience pleasure.

Anorexia nervosa: Serious aversion to food, which can lead to malnutrition and death. Also called *anorexia*.

Antidepressants: Classification of psychoactive medications used to treat depression.

Antimanic agents: Classification of psychoactive medications used to treat manic behavior, such as in bipolar disorder.

Antiparkinson agents: Classification of medications used to treat the symptoms of both drug-induced and non–drug-induced parkinsonism.

Antipsychotics: Classification of psychoactive medications used to treat psychotic behavior found in disorders such as schizophrenia and organic brain disorders.

Antisocial personality disorder: A pattern of irresponsible, exploitive, and guiltless behavior with a tendency to fail to conform to the law and to exploit and manipulate others for personal gain. Popularly known as *sociopathic personality*.

Anxiety: Feelings of uneasiness or apprehension.

Aphasia: Inability to communicate through speech because of brain dysfunction.

Apraxia: Inability to carry out motor activities despite intact motor function.

Aromatherapy: Related to herbal therapy; provides treatment by both direct pharmacological effects of the aromatic plant substances and indirect effects of certain smells on mood and affect.

Assertive communication: Self-responsible statements that begin with the word "I" and deal with thoughts, feelings, and honesty.

Assessment: The first step in the nursing process, it is part of a systematic approach to providing care. The assessment data will be subjective and/or objective.

Assimilation: Taking in, processing, incorporating new information (Piaget).

Asylum: Old term for institution for the care of the needy, especially the mentally ill.

Attention deficit-hyperactivity disorder (ADHD): The display of a persistent pattern of inattention and/or hyperactivity-impulsivity that is more frequent and severe than is typically observed in individuals at a comparable level of development.

Atypical antipsychotic: Second generation drug that blocks both serotonin (another neurochemical) and dopamine.

Autism spectrum disorder (ASD): A group of disorders that are characterized by impairment in several areas of development, including social interaction, skills, and interpersonal communication.

Autonomy: Development of a sense of self and independence (Erikson).

Avoidant personality disorder: An extreme sensitivity to rejection leading to avoidance of social contacts.

Ayurveda: Based on the principle of healthy balance. Ayurvedic practitioners assess three energies: vata, pitta, and kapha.

Awareness: Having a realization, perception, or knowledge.

Behavior: Any action or activity that can be observed.

Behavioral theorist: A scientist who develops theories about human thought and behavior, including Watson, Pavlov, and Skinner.

Behavior modification: Form of treatment in which variables are manipulated to encourage and reinforce desired behavioral changes.

Beliefs: Concepts, opinions, and ideas that are accepted as true and are usually not exactly the same for each individual.

Beneficence: An ethical principle to act for the good and welfare of others.

Binge drinking: Episodic, excessive drinking. Four or more alcoholic drinks (for women) or five or more alcoholic drinks (for men) on the same occasion on at least 1 day.

Binge eating disorder: Recurrent episodes of binge eating that lead to feelings of distress. Not associated with purging.

Biofeedback: Method of teaching patients to recognize tension within the body and to respond with relaxation.

Bipolar disorder: A disorder characterized by mood swings from profound depression to extreme euphoria with intervening periods of normalcy.

Body image: Individual's perception of his or her body.

Body mass index (BMI): In adults, an approximation of body fat based on a calculation of weight divided by the square of one's height.

Borderline personality disorder: A disorder characterized by a pattern of intense and chaotic relationships with emotional instability and tendency toward self-destructive behavior.

Broca aphasia: Difficulty expressing in written or verbal forms of communication. Sentences are incomplete.

Bulimia nervosa: Eating disorder in which a person experiences eating binges along with purging.

Bullying: A form of aggressive behavior manifested by the use of force or coercion to affect others, particularly when the behavior is habitual and involves an imbalance of power.

Catatonia: Rigidity and inflexibility of muscles, resulting in immobility or extreme agitation.

Cerebrovascular accident: The sudden death of some brain cells due to lack of oxygen when the blood flow to the brain is impaired by blockage or rupture of an artery to the brain. Also known as *CVA* or *stroke*.

Chemical restraint: The use of medication as a restriction to manage behavior or restrict patient freedom of movement.

Child abuse: The physical, emotional, or sexual mistreatment of children.

Chronemics: Study of the role of time in communication.

Civil law: Body of laws dealing with rights of private citizens.

Codependency: Maladaptive coping behaviors that reinforce another person's addictive behavior by allowing that person to avoid consequences of his/her actions. Also called *enabling*.

Cognitive: Pertaining to the thought process and the ability to think.

Cognitive Behavior Therapy (CBT): Psychotherapeutic approach that combines behavior therapy with cognitive psychology; it is a problem-focused and action-oriented short-term therapy.

Collaborative: Form of care in which nurses work together and with other disciplines for the betterment of patient care.

Commitment: The act of forced hospitalization, frequently against the patient's will when the patient's safety is compromised.

Communication: Method of transmitting messages between a sender and a receiver. It can be verbal or nonverbal.

Communication block: Method of communication that impedes helpful interactions with patients.

Community Mental Health Centers Act of 1963: A result of President John F. Kennedy's concern for the treatment of the mentally ill.

Complementary medicine: A wide variety of alternative practices such as acupuncture and hypnosis that are recognized and accepted by mainstream medicine; done in conjunction with traditional medicine.

Conduct disorder: A repetitive and persistent pattern of behavior in which the basic rights of others or major age-appropriate societal norms or rules are violated.

Confidentiality: The act of maintaining privacy of patient information.

Conversion: Transference of anxiety into physical symptoms.

Co-occurring disorder: Existence of both a substance abuse disorder and a serious mental illness. Also called *dual diagnosis*.

Coping: The act of successfully adapting psychologically, physically, and behaviorally to problems or stressors.

Counseling: One of several forms of therapy techniques provided by a professional therapist.

Crisis: A state of psychological disequilibrium.

Culture: Nonphysical traits, rituals, values, and traditions that are handed down to others from generation to generation.

Culture of nurses: Professional values, rituals, and traditions passed down from one generation of nurses to the next.

Cyberbullying: The use of the internet and social media to harm other people in a deliberate, repeated, and hostile manner.

Cyclothymic: Characterized by chronic mood disturbance involving numerous episodes of hypomania and depressed mood.

Data collection: Gathering of information about a patient; part of nursing process.

Date rape: Unwanted sexual intercourse between people who are acquainted and in which the party who pays for the date expects sex in return.

Defense mechanisms: Group of behaviors used to reduce or eliminate anxiety. Unconsciously falling into habits that give the illusion of coping but produce ineffective results.

Deinstitutionalization: A policy in which people who had formerly required long hospital stays became able to leave the institution and return to their communities and homes.

Delirium: Acute brain syndrome; rapid onset of cognitive impairments such as loss of memory and disorientation.

Delirium tremens (DTs): Form of delirium from withdrawal from alcohol in which the person experiences, among other symptoms, tremors, hallucinations, delirium, and diaphoresis.

Delusions: Fixed, false beliefs relating usually to persecution or grandeur.

Dementia: Gradual progression and deterioration of cognitive functioning that interferes with memory, language, and/or executive functions, such as organizing and abstraction. Also referred to as *major neurocognitive disorder*.

Dependent: Relying on another person or substance.

Dependent personality disorder: Characterized by a pervasive and excessive need to be taken care of.

Depression: An alteration in mood that is expressed by feelings of sadness, despair, and pessimism.

Detoxification: The process of withdrawal of a substance through supervised medical interventions to prevent complications.

Dietary supplement: Products that are taken by mouth to supplement the diet. They contain one or more dietary ingredients such as vitamins, amino acids, or herbs and are labeled as being a dietary supplement.

Disruptive mood dysregulation disorder: Diagnosis characterized by severe temper outbursts in children with irritable or angry mood, but no clear manic episodes, in at least two settings up to age 12.

Dissociate: To separate a strong emotional response from the consciousness.

Dissociative disorders: Disruption and/or discontinuity in the normal integration of consciousness, memory, identity. This category includes dissociative identity disorder (multiple personality).

Doctrine of Privileged Information: A bond between patient and physician. Under this doctrine, the physician has the right to refuse to answer certain questions (e.g., in a court of law) and can cite "privileged physician-patient information."

Domestic violence: Intentionally inflicting or threatening physical injury or cruelty to one's partner. Also known as *intimate partner violence, spouse abuse.*

DSM-5: *Diagnostic and Statistical Manual of Mental Disorders,* 5th ed. Major psychiatric reference by the American Psychiatric Association. Published in 2013.

DSM-5-TR: *Diagnostic and Statistical Manual of Mental Disorders,* 5th ed. Text Revision. Revised version of the 5th edition in 2022.

Dysfunctional: Having abnormal or ineffective function in mental health pertaining to coping and relationships.

Dysmorphophobia: Preoccupation with an imagined defect in appearance.

Dysphasia: Difficulty in speaking.

Dysthymic disorder: See persistent depressive disorder

Dystonia: A disorder in which the symptoms manifest as bizarre distortions or involuntary movements of any muscle group.

Echolalia: Repetition of phrases, words, or part of a word; often part of catatonia.

Echopraxia: Repeating the movements of others.

Economic abuse: Using another's resources for one's own personal gain without permission or making the victim financially dependent on the abuser. Also called *fiduciary abuse.*

Effective coping: Skills that reduce tension and do not create more problems for an individual.

Ego: Second part of Freud's personality development theory, balancing the id; the ego meets and interacts with the outside world.

Elder abuse: Physical, emotional, or sexual abuse of older adults.

Elderly: Pertaining to older people, often described as people over 65 years old.

Electroconvulsive therapy (ECT): Reserved for types of depression or schizophrenia not responding to other forms of treatment. A current is passed through the patient, resulting in mild seizures and temporary amnesia.

Emotional abuse: Willful use of words or actions that undermine another person's self-esteem.

Empathy: Therapeutic communication technique of understanding another person's emotion without actually experiencing the emotion.

Ethics: The basic concepts and fundamental moral principles that govern conduct.

Ethnicity: The condition of identifying with an ethnic group.

Ethnocentrism: When individuals believe that their particular ethnic or religious group has rights and benefits over those of others.

Eustress: Type of stress that results from positive experiences (experiences such as raises, promotions).

Evaluation: Part of nursing process that summarizes nursing interventions and the outcomes.

Evidence-based practices (EBP): Refers to practices found through research that provide a positive outcome when applied to patient care.

Extrapyramidal symptoms (EPS): A variety of responses associated with drugs that antagonize the dopamine receptors outside the pyramidal tract, causing a variety of effects, including tremors and rigidity.

Feeling: Emotion.

Feeling statement: Statement that identifies an emotion that one is experiencing or trying to explore (e.g., "I feel proud" or "I feel frightened").

Fidelity: A promise to be a competent nurse when providing patient care.

Formal teaching: Teaching that is planned and scheduled.

Free-floating anxiety: Anxiety that has no identifiable cause; feeling of "impending doom."

Free-standing treatment centers: Treatment centers that provide care ranging from crisis care to traditional 21-day stays. They may be called *detoxification (detox) centers, crisis centers,* or other similar terms.

Generalized anxiety disorders: An anxiety disorder that has no identifiable cause and that is characterized by excessive worry or severe stress and a feeling of "impending doom"; it typically lasts 6 months or longer.

Geriatrician: A physician who specializes in treating older patients.

Geriatrics: Branch of medicine that deals with the illnesses and treatment of elderly people.

Gerontology: The study of aging and old age.

Global aphasia: Combination of receptive and expressive forms of aphasia

Good Samaritan Law: Law that offers immunity from prosecution for citizens who stop to assist someone in need of medical help.

Hallucinations: False sensory perception; can affect any of the five senses.

Health-illness continuum: Theory that physical and mental health and illness fluctuate somewhat on a daily basis, while staying within a social norm of behavior.

Health Insurance Portability and Accountability Act (HIPAA): Regulations developed by the Department of Health and Human Services to provide national standards pertaining to the transmission and communication of medical information among patients, providers, employers, and insurers.

Hearing impaired: A loss of hearing function that may be congenital or due to normal aging or other causes. It interferes with communication between the sender and the receiver.

Herbal supplement: A type of dietary supplement containing one or more herbs.

Hill-Burton Act: The first major act or law to address mental illness in the United States. It provided money to build psychiatric units in hospitals.

Histrionic personality disorder: Associated with extreme dramatic, excessive behaviors in someone who has a pattern of strong emotions.

Holistic: Viewing a person as a whole.

Homeless: The state of being without a permanent place of residency or home.

Human trafficking: The use of force, fraud, or coercion to obtain some type of labor or commercial sex act.

Hyperactivity: Excessive psychomotor activity that may be purposeful or aimless.

Hypnosis: Form of therapy that is meant to produce a state of increased relaxation and increases openness to suggestions for behavior modification.

Hypnotherapy: The means for entering an altered state of consciousness, and in this state, the use of visualization and suggestion to bring about desired changes in behavior and thinking.

Hypochondriasis: Condition of unrealistic or exaggerated concern over minor symptoms.

Hypomania: A mild form of mania that is associated with hyperactivity but is not severe enough to cause marked impairment in social or occupational functioning. Also known as a *hypomanic episode*.

Id: First part of Freud's personality theory, which is preoccupied with self-gratification.

Illusions: Misperceptions of a real external stimulus.

Implementation: Part of the nursing process that identifies specific actions a nurse will do to help a patient meet a goal; nursing intervention.

Impulsivity: The trait of acting without reflection and thought of the consequences.

Incest: Sexual activity between people who are so closely related that marriage is illegal.

Ineffective communication: A breakdown either in the sender's process of delivery of a message or how that message is received.

Ineffective coping: The use of coping skills that do not reduce tension and/or that are hazardous to an individual.

Informal teaching: Teaching that is provided at unplanned or unscheduled times.

Insidious: Referring to onset that is so gradual it is hardly noticed.

Insomnia: Difficulty sleeping.

Integrative medicine: The combination of conventional and less traditional treatment, including complementary treatment methods.

Intimate partner violence: A pattern of abusive behavior that is used by an intimate partner to maintain control over the partner.

Intoxication: A physical and mental state of exhilaration and emotional frenzy or lethargy and stupor.

Judgment: Subjective assessment of a patient's ability to make appropriate decisions.

Justice: Ethical principle that health-care providers should provide care fairly and justly.

"La belle indifférence": Inappropriate lack of concern for symptoms.

Laryngectomee: Person who has had a laryngectomy.

Laryngectomy: Partial or total removal of the larynx ("voice box").

Lethality: The level of risk of death in the suicide method.

Lewy body disease: Second-most common form of dementia. This has a similar presentation to Alzheimer's disease, with the addition of visual hallucinations and parkinsonian features.

Lunar month: Twenty-eight-day cycle in prenatal development.

Magical thinking: A primitive form of thinking in which an individual believes that thinking about a possible occurrence can make it happen.

Major depressive disorder: Psychiatric illness characterized by depressed mood or loss of interest or pleasure in usual activities that affects one's life for at least 2 weeks.

Major neurocognitive disorder: An acquired decline in mental ability severe enough to interfere with independence and daily life.

Malingering: Deliberate faking or exaggerating of symptoms.

Mania: Predominant mood that is elevated, expansive, or irritable with frenzied motor activity. Also known as *manic episodes*.

Maslow's Hierarchy of Needs: An orderly progression of development that takes in the physical components of personality development as well as the emotional components.

Memory: Mental function that enables a person to store and recall information.

Menarche: First menstrual period.

Mental health: State of being able to function with successful adaptation to stressors.

Mental illness: Disorders characterized by dysregulation of mood, thought, and/or behavior as recognized by the *Diagnostic and Statistical Manual of Mental Disorders.*

Message: Information that may be verbal or nonverbal and that is transmitted from the sender. It is part of the communication process.

Mild neurocognitive disorder: Less severe form of cognitive impairment than dementia.

Milieu: Environment for treating patients.

Mind–body connection: An interconnection of the mind and body in which the mind influences the body's responses.

Mindfulness: An awareness of what is going on at the present time and realizing the mind-body connection.

Models: Pictures or ideas that we form in our minds to explain how things work. They help us understand and interact with other people and our environment, and help us to formulate beliefs.

Monoamine oxidase inhibitors (MAOI): Group of antidepressant medications that work by blocking the enzyme monoamine oxidase.

Mood: An individual's sustained emotional tone, which influences behavior, personality, and perception.

Morbid obesity: Condition of being abnormally overweight; weight that is 100 pounds or more above established norms.

Narcissistic personality disorder: A disorder that displays exaggerated self-love and self-importance.

National League for Nursing (NLN): An organization that emphasizes nursing education, development, and leadership.

National Mental Health Act of 1946: Part of the result of the first Congress to be held after World War II, providing money for training and research in nursing care (and other patient care disciplines) to improve care for people with mental illnesses.

Negative reinforcement: Increasing the probability that a behavior will recur by removal of an undesirable reinforcing stimulus.

Neglect: Deliberate deprivation of necessary and available resources such as medical or dental care.

Neurolinguistic programming (NLP): The theory that language cues can be used to understand how an individual experiences his or her world, allowing a practitioner to help a patient change her or his experience and respond to problems in a different way; uses visual, auditory, and kinesthetic channels.

Nocturnal delirium: Increased confusion and agitation at dusk. Also called *sundowning.*

Nonmaleficence: To do no harm.

Nonverbal communication: Actions, the way we use our body, and facial expressions that are used in communications.

Nontherapeutic: A breakdown in communicating a message, the message is not therapeutic.

North American Nursing Diagnosis Association-Independence (NANDA-I): A nursing organization that establishes and oversees standardized language for nurses to improve communication and outcomes.

Nursing diagnosis: Nonmedical statement of an existing or potential problem.

Nursing Interventions Classification (NIC): A comprehensive standardized language of intervention labels and possible nursing actions.

Nursing Outcomes Classification (NOC): A standardized language that provides outcome statements and a set of indicators that describe the specific patient, caregiver, family, or community states related to outcome.

Nursing process: Established system of data collecting and care planning performed by nurses.

Obesity: A body mass index greater than 30.

Objective: Step one in the nursing process. It is data related to the patient that represents touch, sight, smell, and body language.

Obsessive Compulsive Disorder (OCD): The presence of obsessions and compulsions that the individual feels compelled to think about and perform that interfere with daily functioning.

Obsessive-compulsive personality disorder: Characterized by preoccupation with rules, orderliness, and control.

Ombudsman: Individual appointed to investigate complaints and concerns in an agency or governmental institution.

Omnibus Budget Reconciliation Act (OBRA): A federal act that provides standards of care for older adults.

Operant conditioning: A method of learning that occurs through rewards and punishments for desired or undesired behaviors.

Orientation: Measurement of knowledge of person, place, and time in the mental health assessment.

Palliative care: Specialized care that focuses on patients with advanced illness and their families by providing expert symptom management and the promotion of the best quality of life.

Panic disorder: Condition of having one or more panic attacks, followed by the fear of having others.

Paranoid personality disorder: Consistent pattern of suspiciousness and mistrust that interferes with functioning in society.

Paraphilic disorders: Intense and persistent sexual interest that goes outside the bounds of usual behavior. These include pedophilia, exhibitionism, voyeurism, and sadism.

Parenting: Raising children; referring to styles of raising children.

Parkinsonism: Group of symptoms that mimic Parkinson's disease, including tremors and rigidity.

Patient Bill of Rights: Federal and state guidelines to ensure the civil rights of people who are entrusted to the care of health-care providers in hospitals, nursing homes, and so on.

Patient interview: An interaction between the patient or client and the health-care provider in order to collect patient data.

Patient Self-Determination Act: Federal law giving each individual the right to make their own decisions about their health care.

Patient teaching: Any set of planned education activities designed to improve patients' health behaviors and health status.

Persistent depressive disorder: A chronic form of depression that is a milder form than major depressive disorder. Previously called dysthymic disorder.

Personality: Sum of the behaviors and character traits of a person.

Personality disorder: Nonpsychotic, maladaptive behavior that is used to satisfy the self.

Person-centered therapy: Humanistic theory of unconditional positive regard for the person, involving treatment of the whole person rather than just the illness.

Phobia: Irrational fear.

Physical abuse: Any actions by omission or commission that cause physical harm to another.

Physical restraint: Any physical method of restricting an individual's freedom of movement, activity, or normal access to his/her body that cannot be easily removed.

Placebo: A neutral, inactive agent given in place of medication that produces symptom relief or other desired effects based upon the patient's expectations and beliefs.

Plan of care: Nursing process and medical orders that dictate a patient's daily care.

Planning: Systematic way for the patient to achieve their goals. Planning is two parts: short-term goals and long-term goals. Both are measurable and realistic.

Positive reinforcement: Increasing the probability that a behavior will recur by addition of a reinforcing stimulus.

Postpartum blues: A transient, self-limiting period of sadness that occurs in a woman immediately after the birth of her baby.

Postpartum depression: A clinical depression that occurs in a woman shortly after the birth of her baby.

Postpartum psychosis: A sudden onset of psychotic symptoms that occurs in a woman after the birth of her baby.

Post-traumatic stress disorder: Reaction to witnessing or experiencing severe trauma that was not expected (e.g., rape, war).

Prejudice: Prejudging people or situations before knowing all the facts.

Presupposition: Assumptions we make when forming communication.

Primary gain: Relief of anxiety by use of defense mechanisms or the act of remaining physically or mentally unhealthy.

Professional: Referring to performing a skill for pay.

Proxemics: Study of spatial relationships including space, time, and waiting, which are all influenced by one's culture.

Pseudodementia: Depression in the elderly that mimics dementia.

Psychoactive (psychotropic) drugs: Any drug that alters mood, perception, mental functioning, and/or behavior.

Psychoanalytic: Method of psychotherapy based in Freudian theory; uses free association and dream interpretation as part of the treatment. Treatment in this style is usually long term.

Psychopharmacology: Medications as they are used and prescribed for mental illness.

Psychosexual: Referring to Freud's theory of personality and development in which behavior is related to the sexual gratification or lack of it received in early development.

Psychosis: A mental state in which there is a severe loss of contact with reality.

Psychotropic: Medication that affects mental activity, behavior, or perception.

Puberty: Stage of development at which sexual organs mature and one is capable of reproducing.

Purging: The act of attempting to rid the body of calories by self-induced vomiting or the excessive use of laxatives or diuretics.

Rape: Violent sexual act that is performed against one's will.

Rapport: The matching of speech patterns using auditory, kinesthetic, and visual references, which provide a starting point for meaningful communication.

Rational-emotive behavior therapy (REBT): Form of therapy involving a rational balance between thinking and feeling.

Receiver: The recipient of a message (information) sent by a sender.

Reflexology: Massage and manipulation of the feet that acts upon energy pathways in the body, unblocking and renewing the energy flow.

Reiki: A form of energy work incorporating touch that manipulates the client's energy along body meridians or pathways.

Religion: Set of beliefs about one's spirituality, rituals, and worship.

Respite care: Relief supplied to primary caregivers.

Responsibility: Accountability.

Restorative nursing: Pertaining to rehabilitation that focuses on maintaining dignity and achieving optimal function.

Safe house: Specified "secret" place for people who are being abused to go for shelter.

Scaffolding: A child becomes more independent after receiving guidance in their learning process. The child can then model the given guidance even though the parent or caregiver is still present to assist in advancing the child's positive behavior.

Schizoaffective disorder: A disorder manifested by schizophrenic behaviors with a strong element of mood disorders, including depression or mania.

Schizoid personality disorder: A pattern of extreme detachment from social relationships and a restricted range of emotional responses.

Schizophrenia: Serious mental health disorder characterized by impaired communication, alteration of reality, and deterioration of personal and vocational functioning.

Schizophrenia spectrum disorder: The gradient of psychopathology seen in schizophrenia from least to most severe.

Schizophreniform disorder: Schizophrenia symptoms without the level of impairment of functioning usually seen in schizophrenia, and lasting more than 1 month and fewer than 6 months.

Schizotypal personality disorder: A personality disorder characterized by odd and eccentric behaviors but not to the degree of schizophrenia.

Scope of practice: Terminology used by national and state/provincial licensing boards for various professions that defines the procedures, actions, and processes that are permitted for the licensee.

Secondary gain: Response to illness that results in attention, monetary benefits, and the like.

Self-mutilating behavior: Deliberate, self-injurious behavior such as cutting with the intent of causing nonfatal injury to relieve tension.

Sender: The party who transmits a message (information) to a receiver.

Sexual abuse: Unwanted sexual contact.

Sexual harassment: Unwanted sexual innuendo, often inflicted by a workplace superior on an employee or a subordinate.

Shaken baby syndrome: A condition that results from an infant's being shaken violently by the extremities or shoulders, usually out of frustration and rage over the child's crying. Sometimes referred to as *abusive head trauma*.

Signal anxiety: Stress response to a known stressor.

Situational, Background, Assessment, Recommendations (SBAR): A method for healthcare providers to communicate in a structured and uniform method, with a focus on the patient's problem, leading to a solution.

Social communication: The day-to-day interaction with personal acquaintances. Slang or "street language" may be used. Less literal and purposeful in social interactions.

Sociopathic: See *antisocial personality disorder*.

Somatic: Relating to or affecting the body.

Somatic symptom disorders: A persistent pattern of excessive and disproportionate thoughts, feelings, and/or behaviors related to somatic symptoms.

Somatization: Emotional turmoil that is expressed by physical symptoms, often in the loss of functioning of a body part.

Somatoform disorder: Physical discomfort that resembles a medical condition that has no logical explanation or medical basis.

Specific phobia: A fear that is persistent to a specific object or situation, e.g., fear of spiders.

Splitting: Defense mechanism often used in those with borderline personality disorders when there is difficulty assimilating both positive and negative aspects of a situation.

Stereotype: A general opinion or belief.

Stimulants: Classification of medication that directly stimulates the central nervous system.

Stress: Subjective emotional strain or anxiety. A state of unbalance when there is tension with a person's internal and external environment.

Stressor: Any person or situation that produces anxiety responses.

Subjective: Based on personal feelings or beliefs; often relates to patients reporting symptoms in their own words.

Substance abuse: The maladaptive and consistent use of a substance accompanied by recurrent and significant negative consequences such as interpersonal, social, occupational, and legal problems.

Substance dependence: A cluster of cognitive, behavioral, and physiological symptoms that indicate that the individual continues use of the substance despite significant substance-related problems.

Substance use disorder: *DSM-5* diagnostic term for substance abuse and substance dependence.

Suicidal ideation: Thoughts about harming oneself.

Suicide: The act of purposefully taking one's own life.

Suicide attempt: Any act with the intention of taking one's own life in which the individual survived.

Suicide pact: Agreement made among a group of people (often adolescents) to kill themselves together.

Superego: Third part of Freud's personality theory; the conscience, which deals with morality.

Survivor: One(s) remaining after the death of another.

Survivor guilt: Feeling of guilt at being a survivor; often seen in post-traumatic stress disorder.

Survivor of suicide: Family or friend of an individual who commits suicide.

Sympathy: Nontherapeutic technique of experiencing the emotion along with the patient.

Tardive dyskinesia (TD): Involuntary movements due to side effects of some antipsychotic drugs.

Therapeutic communication: Communication that attempts to determine a patient's needs. Also called *active* or *purposeful communication*.

Thinking/cognition: The mental action or process of acquiring knowledge and understanding through thought, experience, and the senses.

Thought: An opinion, idea, or plan that is formed in one's mind.

Tolerance: The need for increasingly larger or more frequent doses of a substance to obtain the desired effects.

Tort: An action that wrongly causes harm to another but is not a crime and is dealt with in civil court.

Traditional Chinese medicine (TCM): An ancient Chinese therapy used to balance life for optimal health.

Trance: A state of altered awareness of a client's surroundings that brings the individual's focus of attention to an internal experience, such as a memory or an imagined event.

Typical antipsychotics: The first generation of antipsychotic agents that acts on the central nervous system (CNS). Their main action is to block the dopamine receptors.

Unconscious: Referring to ideas and behaviors that are concealed from awareness.

Unintentional: An act that may result in injury or property damage and that is determined to be accidental.

Vascular dementia: Dementia caused by disruption of blood flow to the brain, as in a stroke.

Veracity: The quality of being true and honest.

Verbal abuse: Method of harming another by using degrading, harsh, or foul language.

Verbal communication: Process of exchanging information by the spoken or written word; the objective part of the process of communication.

Victim: A person who is harmed by another.

Visually impaired: A person with loss of complete or partial visual functioning.

Wernicke aphasia: Difficulty interpreting or understanding written or verbal forms of communication, occasionally a word incorrectly.

Withdrawal: Negative physiological and psychological reactions that occur when a substance is reduced or no longer taken.

Yoga: A mind-body method of healing that uses body positions to facilitate balance and flexibility.

Zone of proximal development: A time when a child's actions are at first dependent on others until the child becomes independent and performs without assistance, demonstrating cognitive growth.

Index